CW01543387

Health *for* Life
15–16

Nick Boddington

Adrian King

Alan van Loen

Jenny McWhirter

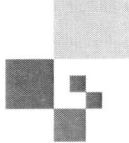 Nelson Thornes

Published in 2009 by:
Nelson Thornes Ltd
Delta Place
27 Bath Road
CHELTENHAM
GL53 7TH
United Kingdom

09 10 11 12 13 / 10 9 8 7 6 5 4 3 2 1

A catalogue record for this book is available from the British Library

ISBN 978 1 4085 0190 0 (Set)
ISBN 978 1 4085 0191 7 (Book)
ISBN 978 1 4085 0192 4 (CD-ROM)

Cover photograph by iStockphoto.com
Illustrations by Angela Knowles
Page make-up by eMC Design Ltd. www.emcdesign.org.uk

Printed and bound in Great Britain by Antony Rowe

Acknowledgements
The authors and publishers wish to thank the following:
Thanks to Jenny McWhirter for writing the section 'A focus on risk'.
Thanks to Alan van Loen for writing the SRE sessions which drew on material he created when he was commissioned by CSN Consultancy to develop a new programme for Essex schools. Some aspects of his material for that programme were originally based partly upon ideas from an earlier version of the APAUSE programme. The way that he adapted this material with prior permission and combined it with other original materials is entirely his responsibility as author. Alan would also like to acknowlegde the influence of Jo Adams' 'Delay' ('Let's Leave It Till Later') programme on some of his work. In writing Year 11 Session 'A question of knowing your ABC' Alan van Loen has based this on the work of Albert Ellis, the founder of Rational Emotive Behavior Therapy (REBT).

Every effort has been made to contact copyright holders and we apologise if any have been overlooked. Should copyright have been unwittingly infringed in this book, the owners should contact the publishers, who will make the corrections at reprint.

Contents

Dedication

This book is dedicated to the memory and work of Noreen Wetton. *Health for Life 15–16* remains true to the principles she so forcefully championed and the subject she believed was at the heart of the curriculum.

A teacher once described Noreen as someone who had gone right through 'clever' and come out the other side. Among Noreen's many gifts was the skill to distil complex ideas into simple, practical classroom strategies for teachers. Unlike so many trainers, who spellbind with the richness of their vast knowledge and experience but leave people in awe of skills to which they can only aspire, teachers would leave Noreen saying, 'That is so obvious, that is so simple, why didn't I see it like that? I'll try that with my children tomorrow.' In the PSHE field, this was known as being 'Wettoned'. You can always tell a teacher who has been 'Wettoned'. As two young advisors fortunate enough to go through a long process of 'Wettoning', we are glad that she reminded us of some simple truths:

- Before teaching any aspect of PSHE, always ask yourself, 'How are students already making sense of this?' If you don't know the answer, find out.
- Always build in an emotional dimension because what we feel, and what we believe others feel, often drives our choices and behaviour more than what we know.
- Learning to be personally and socially well educated, and being able to manage our physical and emotional health and that of others, is like making filo pastry. You have to build it up layer by layer, and it takes time.
- A child's personal and social development is as much a product of modelling as of teaching. When you have a relationship with children, you are always teaching and they are always learning.
- You should leave every lesson having learned something new about your students and use this constantly to develop as a teacher. The classroom is a genuine community of enquiry, and the dialogue generated through PSHE can inform whole-school improvement.

We both recall the many times that Noreen, when she was almost 80 years old, would say, 'So show me what the lesson would look like on a wet Thursday afternoon with 30 mixed-ability children who haven't been out to break. You can't? Well, come back when you can.'

Noreen helped us understand what great teachers have always known:
'If you want children to learn, understand the human in front of you – you will then improve their self-esteem.
If you do this, you will improve their self-confidence.
And, if you do that, they will feel emotionally engaged with what you are doing.'
(Curran, 2008)

Noreen would have loved that. She also knew that:
'To know others is to be clever
To know yourself is enlightenment.'
(Lao Tzu, 600 BC)

Nick Boddington and Adrian King, September 2008

Foreword

The human brain is the most complex structure in the universe. It has over 150 billion cells, joined up with an almost limitless number of connections. Our brains have been evolving for over 400 million years, and some parts are designed to keep us alive as if we were still in that long-gone world. While some parts of our brain are unique to us as human beings, other parts are the same as those of reptiles or other mammals. Some functions of our brain are within our control, while others are reflexes that will completely take over if our brain thinks we are under threat.

While we all share the same brain structure, the development of an individual brain depends on the experiences of its owner. Experience literally grows our brains and each brain is therefore unique. Our brains process a huge amount of information every minute of our lives, but we are unaware of most of it unless our brains choose to draw it to our attention.

We live in two worlds. The first is a physical world of electro-chemical processes that make up our brain activity. The second is our own inner world in which the electro-chemical processes manifest themselves inside our minds as the voices, feelings and images that our brains present to us.

Everything we see, hear, smell, taste and feel is actually constructed inside our brains and then presented to our conscious minds. Since we interpret every experience we have (through the understanding gleaned from all our previously stored experiences), any experience we share with others is still unique to us. The image we 'see' when watching a sunset is actually a construct inside our heads. You make the sunset that you 'see'.

Because our brains are so flexible, we can learn how to think differently. As far as we know, we are the only creatures with 'meta-cognition': we can think about our own thinking. Because of this, and with practice, we can choose to 'change our minds'.

We understand a huge amount about our brains, but there is more that we don't understand. Since we are our brains, the same applies to us.

Considering all of the above, imagine what happens when two or more brains get together: the result might be productive or destructive, but it will always be amazing. Helping brains, the most complex structures in the universe, to work productively together has to be one of the most incredible things we can do. This is teaching PSHE.

How *Health for Life* contributes to PSHE teaching

Health for Life is based on the premise that we don't experience life as a series of ongoing 'issues' or 'topics' but as a series of 'experiences' or 'moments'. These may be events that we witness, where our response may stay inside us, or opportunities or challenges that demand a more active response from us. These moments usually happen within a social context, and may be very complex.

Sometimes we can see important moments coming and we can prepare ourselves for them. Sometimes they sneak up on us and catch us by surprise. Sometimes they give us time to stop and think. Sometimes they require us to react immediately. They will usually start by making us feel something.

The importance of feelings

Knowledge – what we know – may come along a little later, perhaps, as the voice in our head tries to explore or explain what we are initially feeling. Although what we know may come to influence our decisions, our final choices are often dictated by what we are feeling. Once we make a decision, we then need the skills and language to be able to execute a strategy to 'manage the moment'. But actually using those skills, speaking those words and putting our strategy into action depends on how we feel about ourselves and others in that context, and at that moment.

This is why the sessions in *Health for Life 15–16* always begin with a situation and always try to work within the experience of the learner. No factual information should be provided until the student has been offered an opportunity to consider how they feel about what is happening. After any factual input, it is strongly suggested that students be encouraged to reflect on how it has changed or reinforced their feelings and also on what they can now claim and do. Learning always flows between what we feel and what we know.

The importance of critical reflection

Critical reflection is at the heart of this resource, which is why so much emphasis has been placed on structured questioning. We build and refine our concepts and come to our own unique understanding through:

- the questions we ask of ourselves
- the questions we are asked by others
- the answers provided by our own critical reflection
- sharing that reflection with one another.

Health for Life 15–16 seeks to focus on moments: critical moments; forks-in-the-road-ahead moments; the analytical; the reflective and the 'crunch' moments; the spontaneous and the emergency moments. It is about understanding, skills, confidence, options and decisions. This teaching resource could truthfully be described as momentous, for it is all about moments.

Introduction

Welcome to *Health for Life 15–16*. With this publication the series now spans the 4–16 age range. This resource builds on and extends work from *Health for Life 11–14*, and it is recommended that you use it in conjunction with that publication.

Effective PSHE makes a significant contribution to 'Every Child Matters', by enabling students to take responsibility for:

- being healthy
- staying safe
- enjoying and achieving
- making a positive contribution
- achieving economic wellbeing.

The first four points above could be summarised by the term 'personal wellbeing'.

It is important to recognise that these strands are mutually supportive. If students are learning in emotionally safe and socially healthy environments, they are more likely to have the confidence to take risks with their thinking, make a positive contribution to the group's learning and enjoy their achievements in the classroom.

For the purposes of this book and the CD-ROM, the term personal, social and health education (PSHE) covers the variety of names given to this area of the curriculum. The terms 'teacher' and 'classroom' are also used, although educators such as youth workers have found *Health for Life* useful in other learning settings.

Health for Life 15–16 will help you to:

- involve students in consultation to ensure their programme is relevant to their lives
- plan a relevant, flexible PSHE programme
- gather data and opinions to inform school policy
- respond to government requirements
- develop your status as a 'healthy school'.

Much of this resource is duplicated on the CD-ROM. This will enable you to:

- develop your own session plans
- edit the material in this resource, customising it to support your students' needs or local context
- construct activities such as fact sheets or quizzes to support learning
- create presentations including case studies or scenarios, key questions and factual information for students using technology such as interactive whiteboards
- support a PSHE-focused school website.

Why is PSHE so important?

Students are growing up in the most rapidly changing period in our history. The only certainty about the future is that we know very little about what it will be like. For this reason, students will need to:

- be skilled and motivated learners
- have a strong sense of their own self-worth, believing themselves to be neither more nor less valuable than anyone else
- have a strong belief that they control their own destiny and are not 'victims of life'
- have high aspirations that challenge them but are not so out of reach as to be demotivating
- be able to form strong and stable relationships with others.

Many students will be living and working in a diverse global community that is increasingly interdependent. The pace of change means that those who can't successfully engage with learning are likely to be left behind.

Teenagers of 15 and 16 years will be growing in independence and becoming aware of the opportunities and choices that will affect their health. In *Health for Life* 'health' means an overall sense of wellbeing and not just the absence of disease or infirmity.

The themes of *Health for Life*

Five themes are offered:

1 **Physical health** – how I look after my body so that I can do everything I want to now and in the future.
2 **Emotional health** – how I protect my feelings and manage them so that they positively help me.
3 **Social health** – how I develop and look after my relationships so that I can support others and they can support me.
4 **Reputational health** – how I protect my life story.
5 **Aspirational health** – how my aspirations direct, motivate and challenge.

Students in this age group are increasingly encountering and needing to manage issues and situations that they explored in their earlier education. They are finding that they now need to apply in their daily life the knowledge, language, skills and strategies that they have acquired and rehearsed. Significant neurological changes are still taking place in the brains of people in this age group, which can affect their capacity to manage impulses, assess risk and empathise with others.

Health for Life emphasises social and health themes as the context for developing and rehearsing generic personal and social skills, language and strategies for managing living in an increasingly complex world. Students aged 15–16 need help to rehearse these skills. Their growing need for a rich body of factual and relevant information to inform the choices and decisions they are making now, or very soon, also needs to be recognised.

Factual information, however, can quickly go out of date, and society's values and beliefs can shift or evolve over time. These students will leave school all too soon, and they must be equipped with the skills they will need to be able to locate, access and evaluate sources of information for themselves so that they can make good decisions based on good information.

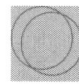

> 'We are currently preparing students for jobs that don't yet exist, using technologies that haven't yet been invented, in order to solve problems we don't even know are problems yet.'
> (Holden, R. (2006) Shift Happens, Jeffers Press)

> 'We can't solve problems by using the same kind of thinking we used when we created them.'
> (Albert Einstein)

The timing of the themes and topics has been based on research into how over 250,000 students make sense of their world of health. However, since society quickly moves on, it is essential that this resource is used flexibly. If you consider that the timing is inappropriate for your students, feel free to move material to an earlier or later period. It is important to base decisions on the needs of your students, perhaps using some of the action research methods included, and not what others with their own agenda may feel 'appropriate'.

Well-taught PSHE offers a social context for developing skills that go far beyond simple 'study skills', and helps students practise the skills of 'learning to learn', especially learning in a social context. Good PSHE therefore underpins the academic curriculum. Perhaps most importantly, it helps us get to know our students a little better and affirms to them that their views and opinions are of value to us. PSHE has a taught content but the teacher's practice and the school's culture must also model the values the programme is seeking to develop.

The principles of *Health for Life*

Good PSHE and this resource are underpinned by a set of principles that will help you plan a programme and, perhaps more importantly, refine it to reflect the needs of different classes and students' changing social context. As you progress through this book, you will be stimulated to think about many interesting concepts and ideas. These ideas and concepts will enrich your teaching and enhance students' learning about their present and future health and wellbeing.

Learning Futures: Next Practice in Learning and Teaching (Paul Hamlyn Foundation and Innovations Unit, 2008) argues that learning that is deep, authentic and motivational requires **engagement** and **integration**, through:

- **relevance:** enterprise and enquiry led, balancing knowledge and skills, and a thematic rather than 'one off' approach
- **co-construction:** negotiation with learners of the curriculum, content and styles of teaching
- **in and out of school contexts:** linking formal, informal and virtual learning and family, community and business partnerships
- **learner/teacher mix:** including the use of peer tutors, teachers as learners, parents, external experts, mentoring, coaching and learning communities.

PSHE should:

- **start from where students are.**
  In order to do this, both you and the students need to identify what you already know and think you know; what vocabulary and language you already have; what beliefs you hold; what strategies you believe are appropriate; what strategies you feel comfortable with using.

- **support classrooms and schools as 'communities of enquiry' and teachers as 'reflective practitioners'.**
  The sessions offer a structure to enable both you and the students to learn together how students are making sense of their world. In this way *Health for Life* can provide ongoing support for school communities developing or revising their curriculum and school policies. For example, reviewing school policies on sex and relationships, drug use and misuse, anti-bullying and anti-racism can all be informed by feedback from the PSHE programme. By engaging all learners, the PSHE programme becomes part of the process of continuous school improvement.

- **be taught through a flexible spiral programme, revisiting each theme as needed with more complex situations, language and strategies.**
  Students never stop trying to make sense of their world. If we don't provide opportunities to revisit issues as their experience, horizons and needs change, students won't simply wait until we get around to them in our programme.

- **include an emotional dimension.**
  'What we know' is often not as important as 'how we feel about what we know'. How we feel and how we think others may feel has a huge impact on our decision making. This can get pushed out by an emphasis on 'logical decision making' or 'information only programmes'. When students investigate any issue, we need to help them also explore how they feel about it, how they feel about what they see (or imagine) others are doing, and how these feelings influence any action they decide upon.

- **emphasise the positive.**
  Use gathered evidence to ensure students have correct beliefs about the proportion of their peers engaging in potentially risky health behaviours. This is sometimes known as challenging perceived social norms. Help students to explore why most students choose not to engage in dangerous behaviours. Focus on the benefits of the healthy choices students are making and celebrate these decisions, rather than dwelling on the possible risks of unhealthy or socially unacceptable choices.

- **recognise that all other areas of the curriculum contribute opportunities to support personal development.**
  The taught curriculum, pedagogy and classroom culture all offer opportunities to enrich PSHE, just as the skills, attitudes and values developed in PSHE can be applied to enrich other curriculum areas.

- **model the behaviours and values the programme is intended to develop or promote.**
  In *Health for Life* you, as the teacher, are a facilitator of learning and are not expected to be a health expert.

- **be taught within a 'Health-promoting School' setting.**
  Here, the broader curriculum, culture and ethos of the school consistently model the aims of the programme and the school's overall aims and mission.

Planning your PSHE programme

Well-taught PSHE provides one of the most powerful learning opportunities within the taught curriculum. This is what makes this subject so professionally challenging for teachers and, for some, the most fulfilling part of their week.

Because *Health for Life* offers a structure for discussion that starts from how students feel, and tries wherever possible to work 'inside their reality', activities need careful planning. No other area of the curriculum is so 'personal'. Students are asked not only to think about what they know and how they feel, but also to explore their anxieties, fears, hopes and aspirations, how they presently relate

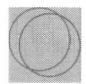

to others, how they might like to relate to others and how others relate to them. Since every student lives a unique life filled with both highs and lows, it is essential that teachers are sensitive to this in their planning and teaching.

It is important to provide a comprehensive PSHE programme in Year 10 that can be revisited and reinforced in Year 11, with plenty of time for topics that you have chosen to prioritise in Year 11. There is always far more potential PSHE than you can cover in the school curriculum, even if other subject areas are making a contribution. It is important to be pragmatic. It is better to prioritise and cover fewer topics in depth than to try to cover a larger range of topics with a superficial, information-only focus. In this way, students have more chance of developing deeper and transferable skills.

PSHE and active learning

PSHE needs to be taught through active rather than passive learning. One of the real strengths of a good PSHE session is that its progress and outcomes are often unpredictable as the students shape the direction of their learning. The learning outcomes may be a mixture of planned objectives and the students' emerging interests.

As with any area of the curriculum, PSHE should be subject to careful reflection and evaluation (see page 42). The trick is to reflect on when:

- the students will find their own way to your objective
- you need to reassert your agenda
- the balance is appropriate
- it is OK to just let go because the students are exploring an issue that you judge to be more relevant to them.

In any session it is equally important to consider what cognitive skills students are practising or extending, and to be sensitive to how their feelings might be influenced.

There is a more detailed focus on pedagogy on page 262.

The challenge of PSHE

PSHE has long been considered the place in the curriculum where schools are asked to address society's ills. The problem is these ills are not solved and the list just keeps growing. The expectations that government, the media and society in general have of the contribution and impact PSHE can make seem at odds with the status and resources allocated to the subject.

The result has been a plethora of topics and issues all being squeezed into a relatively small period in the taught curriculum. If we continue to accept this model, then we end up with a 'patchwork quilt' of a programme with lots of topics. Few, if any, are covered in worthwhile depth and little, if any, connection is made between them in the minds of students.

Overall PSHE planning

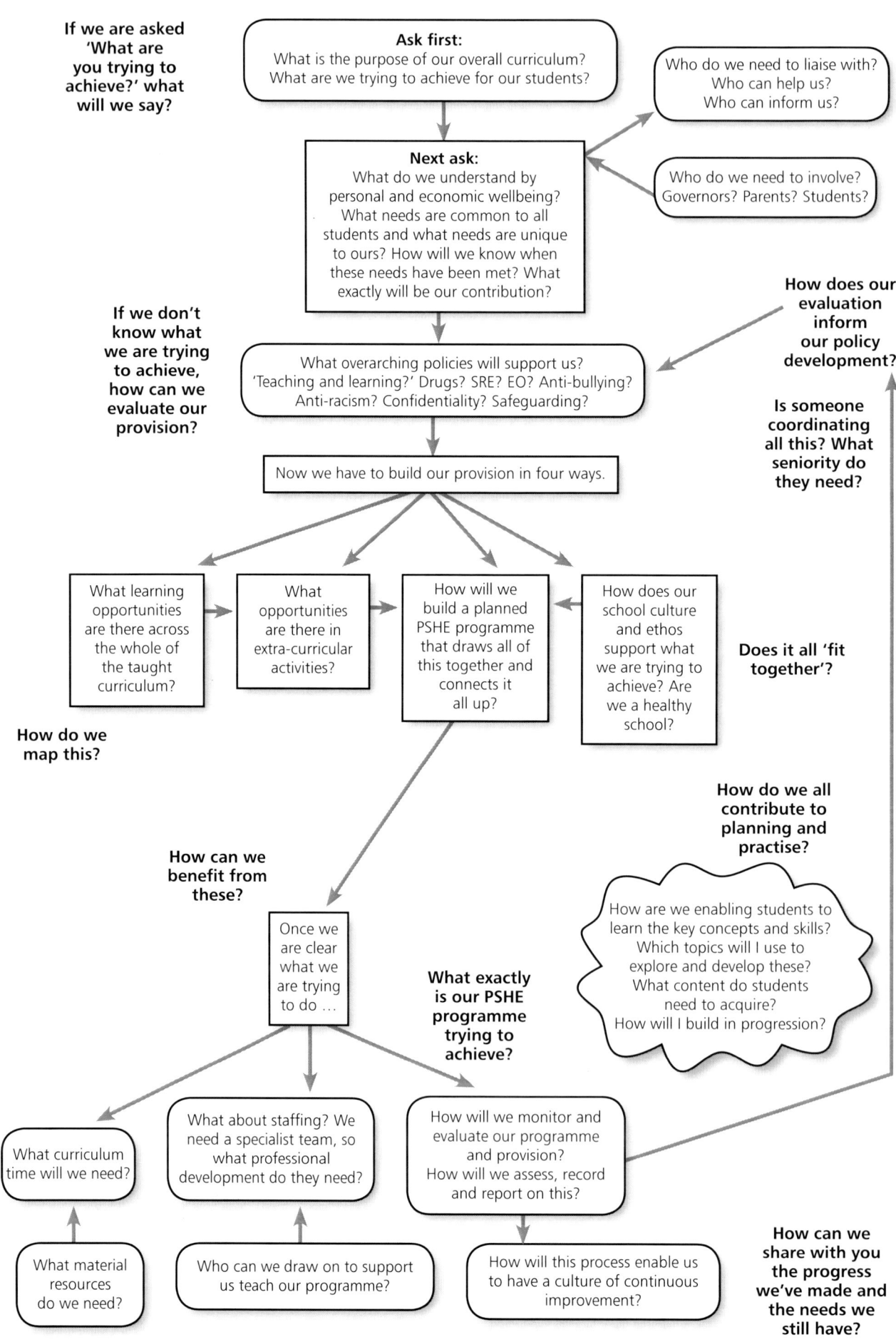

If we are asked 'What are you trying to achieve?' what will we say?

Ask first:
What is the purpose of our overall curriculum?
What are we trying to achieve for our students?

Who do we need to liaise with?
Who can help us?
Who can inform us?

Who do we need to involve?
Governors? Parents? Students?

Next ask:
What do we understand by personal and economic wellbeing? What needs are common to all students and what needs are unique to ours? How will we know when these needs have been met? What exactly will be our contribution?

If we don't know what we are trying to achieve, how can we evaluate our provision?

How does our evaluation inform our policy development?

What overarching policies will support us? 'Teaching and learning?' Drugs? SRE? EO? Anti-bullying? Anti-racism? Confidentiality? Safeguarding?

Is someone coordinating all this? What seniority do they need?

Now we have to build our provision in four ways.

What learning opportunities are there across the whole of the taught curriculum?

What opportunities are there in extra-curricular activities?

How will we build a planned PSHE programme that draws all of this together and connects it all up?

How does our school culture and ethos support what we are trying to achieve? Are we a healthy school?

Does it all 'fit together'?

How do we map this?

How do we all contribute to planning and practise?

How can we benefit from these?

Once we are clear what we are trying to do …

What exactly is our PSHE programme trying to achieve?

How are we enabling students to learn the key concepts and skills? Which topics will I use to explore and develop these? What content do students need to acquire? How will I build in progression?

What curriculum time will we need?

What about staffing? We need a specialist team, so what professional development do they need?

How will we monitor and evaluate our programme and provision? How will we assess, record and report on this?

What material resources do we need?

Who can we draw on to support us teach our programme?

How will this process enable us to have a culture of continuous improvement?

How can we share with you the progress we've made and the needs we still have?

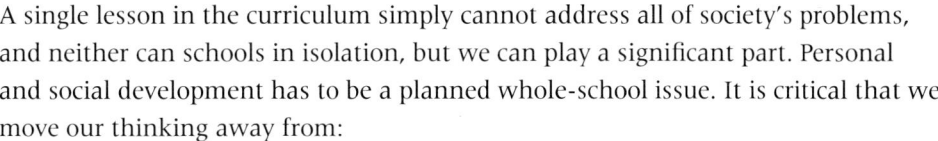

Considering outcomes

A single lesson in the curriculum simply cannot address all of society's problems, and neither can schools in isolation, but we can play a significant part. Personal and social development has to be a planned whole-school issue. It is critical that we move our thinking away from:

- what is our content or what do we need to cover?

towards:

- what outcomes do we want for our students and what learning experiences have to be in our programme in order to achieve this?

Unless we have great clarity and use it to help us create a set of criteria for determining suitable topics, we risk drowning under the weight of potential subject matter. It is very easy to create a PSHE programme that is a weekly exploration of inevitable 'temptation' with the risk of 'degradation, doom and gloom' if you make the wrong choice.

Possible key themes to consider are:

- Instead of exploring why a small number of students engage, perhaps for only a short period in their lives, in risky or unhealthy behaviours, we should ask and explore with students why the vast majority of students don't.

- Instead of attempting to protect students from all the possible risk factors they have or might encounter in their lives, we should focus on enhancing the generic protective factors that help students manage a variety of present and future choices and risks (see page 271). These can also be enriched by the pedagogy we choose to use throughout the programme and by the opportunities offered in a healthy school culture.

While some aspects of PSHE may be relevant to all students, it must be recognised that students will have some unique needs. Therefore, some learning experiences should be emphasised more than others so long as this is the result of a real consideration of students' needs and based on sound evidence.

Developing skills

Health for Life argues that we make our decisions in a social context and that one of the key skills we need to develop is managing ourselves and others in often sensitive or 'high-stake' situations. Of course, there is a body of knowledge within PSHE. Without this it is difficult to argue rationally either as a teacher or with a fellow peer in favour of making a healthy or safe(r) decision over an unhealthy or more dangerous one. What we know is important. How we feel about what we know (and how we guess others feel) is even more important. In addition, the choices we make, and the skills we have to act on those choices, are absolutely vital.

It is essential to emphasise these transferable management skills within a specific PSHE theme or context. (For example, we might develop and rehearse the skill of 'assertiveness' in the context of contraception.) It is advisable to build the same rigour of planning into skill development and opportunities for students to explore and clarify their values and beliefs as you do for content.

To illustrate the wisdom of this, consider formal 'management' training. Companies do not train managers by trying to expose them to every possible management challenge. Instead, key transferable skills are identified and thoroughly developed and rehearsed through a selection of relevant contexts or scenarios. A variety of transferable models are offered that can be overlaid on different situations and it is recognised that good management depends upon both values and interpersonal skills. Within management there is a body of current knowledge, such as employment law, but it is recognised that this may change and, if in doubt, it can be researched.

If you were asked, 'What is the purpose of our school's PSHE programme, what are we trying to achieve for our students, and how well do we think we are doing?' what would you say? Our own answer would be:

> We need to prepare students for the challenges of the present, and for those of the future that we can't foresee. We need positive, optimistic and enthusiastic students who are curious and motivated to learn and with a comprehensive, transferable 'skill set' that enables them to manage themselves and their relationships confidently, creatively and knowledgeably in a complex world, if not always entirely skilfully, then at least competently. We need students who can accurately assess and balance risk so that they can live a full, rich and long life.

Health for Life is designed to support you in realising your own unique solution.

Organising whole-school PSHE provision

Although there are opportunities to support students' personal, social, health and economic wellbeing throughout the curriculum and your school's overall ethos or culture will provide vital reinforcement, it is essential to retain a discrete PSHE programme. This should be of sufficient duration to allow a meaningful learning experience and be taught by PSHE specialists. Effective PSHE, in the true tradition of real learning, is 'dangerous'.

To expect other subject specialists, in their role as tutors, to manage one of the most interactive, student-led subjects, with highly sensitive content and an unpredictable learning process, is at best challenging and at worse unrealistic. Many subject specialists enjoy the challenge of PSHE but others dread it. There is little evidence that teaching PSHE increases the bond between tutors and their forms. This is more to do with the existing qualities of the teacher and not PSHE. The risk of tutor-led PSHE is that the programme reflects the diverse skill or comfort level of the tutors and not the real needs of the students. Both teachers and students consistently recognise this and it is unfair to both groups.

Although other models have been explored by schools, they are usually dictated by the organisation of the rest of the curriculum rather than for the benefit of PSHE. *Health for Life* argues that the most effective model is a core lesson supported and enriched by the wider curriculum, including long block events all set within a healthy school.

The temptation is to build a spiral programme using themes from the national PSHE curriculum to provide blocks of study recurring year on year. This can present a problem, however, since, for example, a block of work on drug use could address most of the concepts and processes under personal wellbeing and many under economic wellbeing. What is important is to identify the learning opportunities provided in the programme and the contribution they can make to addressing relevant concepts and skills. The degree of challenge can then be gradually increased as students move through the key stage.

There will be times when an issue such as diversity needs exploring directly – how might it feel to be discriminated against? There will also be times when it is woven into other themes – would everyone feel like you? Who might hold different views from yours? The same would be true of 'risk'.

The content of the programme (the 'what') and the teaching styles you adopt (the 'how') will *both* contribute to supporting students develop the qualities, understanding and skills you set out to impart.

Part 1

1.1 The resources in this book

The Smith family (page 52)

Health for Life 11–14 page 19 introduced the Smith family and this resource continues to follow their progress. Once again, although we have created these characters and a family background and put them into a variety of situations, it can be much more fun and more relevant if students create their own family and characters. The Smiths are offered only as a starting point, with a range of relationships that can be pursued in any session where you judge it to be constructive.

The action planners and content boxes (pages 57 and 121)

The action planners are built up from 'content boxes' and arranged in themes. They are the building blocks of the programme. Each content box is the basis of a session plan: it provides a structure for discussion; an opportunity to see what students know that you can reinforce and celebrate; what they think they know that might be wrong; and what they don't know that would be a good idea to teach. There are far more content boxes in the action planners than most schools could use, and the intention is for you to pick out the ones you feel are most appropriate to you and your students.

The suggested themes and pathways (pages 55 and 119)

Although the content boxes can be 'picked and mixed', we have suggested themes and pathways. The headings of the themes reflect those in the action planners. The pathways are possible routes through the themes and offer one way of linking boxes together to make a coherent programme. You can devise your own pathways that best suit the needs of the students you will be working with.

The sessions (pages 66 and 131)

As you think about the content boxes, it is likely that you will have your own ideas on how these could be developed further. Each content box offers a structure for a discussion session and you would only need to arrange students into groups with large sheets of paper to have a workshop session. We have, however, developed some pathways and sessions to show how, by using the students' responses, the content boxes could be more deeply explored. We have not done this for all the content boxes.

The invitations (page 195)

All invitations from *Health for Life 11–14* still apply to the 15–16 age range and some have been repeated in this resource. The new invitations included here for students to think about and respond to could also be used in the 11–14 age range. They can act as:

- a means of helping students 'pin down' their thinking during a session
- a research activity, if students are willing to share their responses, providing you with information about how they make sense of an issue
- a further teaching resource by discussing the collective results once analysis has taken place
- tools for evaluation.

The knowledge frames (page 218)

The knowledge frames reinforce and build on those in *Health for Life 11–14*. Knowledge frames are intended to help identify what critical knowledge we believe students should have about a particular issue. They are not definitive and you should feel free to add to them in order to fit your local context.

The recording frame (page 54)

The recording frame is a simple grid to help you keep track of your planning. Because this resource is also published in an electronic form, we suggest you simply cut and paste your programme. Each sheet will hold three content boxes, a space to include relevant factual information, target language, and any 'pre-teaching' or tasks that you want the students to do in preparation for the next session.

Focus on ... (pages 262–279)

Part 4 of this resource considers different themes within PSHE, each with a title beginning 'Focus on ...' They include ideas applicable to virtually any session, along with suggestions for questions that encourage or deepen enquiry or reflection.

Where is all the factual information?

We cannot make rational choices without accurate information, and an important skill for students to develop is fact-finding and research. The knowledge frames contain the broad knowledge that we believe students should know about a variety of topics. However, this resource deliberately does not offer lots of facts. This is not because we don't think they are vitally important, especially at this age. Our reason is more pragmatic; factual information goes out of date very quickly and local factual information, such as the location of local support services, will be unique to your school. In any case, we couldn't hope to include all the factual information you may need.

As you work through the content boxes, there will be many opportunities to offer factual information, but it is then critical to ask the students how knowing this changes what they feel and how their decisions might change as a result. It is vital that we internalise factual information and connect it to what we already know and think, rather than simply receiving a list of 'raw facts'. Questions to ask include the following:

- What do you already know that will help you make a decision?
- How confident are you about what you know – do you really trust it to be full and accurate?

- Is there anything you feel confused about?
- What more would you like to know or have clarified?
- If you now know (the newly acquired information), has it made you feel any different?
- How might this change your decisions, your advice to others or your relationships with others?
- Now, if you want to behave differently, what do you need to be able to say and do?
- What might be the consequences of this, and how do you feel about them?

What is the relationship between personal, social and economic wellbeing?

Health for Life doesn't separate personal, social and economic wellbeing. Virtually all the issues explored in PSHE impact, in some way, on all three subjects. It is more a question of getting the balance or emphasis right.

For example, an unintended pregnancy or drug dependency is likely to have a significant impact on our personal, social and economic wellbeing. While many products are marketed on the possible benefits to our personal wellbeing, for example mobile phones, or our social wellbeing, for example fashion labels. These have an effect on our economic wellbeing also. The effects of a criminal record are not limited to the personal and social, but may have a significant impact on our career prospects and thus our future economic wellbeing.

Our personal identity, especially a poor sense of self-worth, may limit our future career aspirations regardless of our success in gaining qualifications. Equally, our determination to achieve may help us overcome significant financial obstacles. Financial capability, careers education, enterprise and work-related learning all support one another and contribute to our overall economic wellbeing; however, they are not the same thing. An outstanding careers programme or work experience placement may have little impact on a student's personal financial capability.

Questions that can help explore the financial implications of an issue might include:

- What might be the financial cost/gain? Now? In the future?
- Is it worth the financial cost?
- Is the expected financial gain sufficient?
- Will the cost be a 'one off' or will someone need to keep paying?
- Who will pay? Is that fair?
- If there is a financial cost, might someone need to go without something? Now? In the future? Is this OK? Is this fair?
- Where might they get the money from?
- Will they need to earn it, borrow it, sell something to pay for it?
- If money has to be borrowed, will there be interest to repay? How much and for how long? What will be the true cost of paying back the loan?
- How could this help your financial wellbeing in the long run?

How does it all fit together?

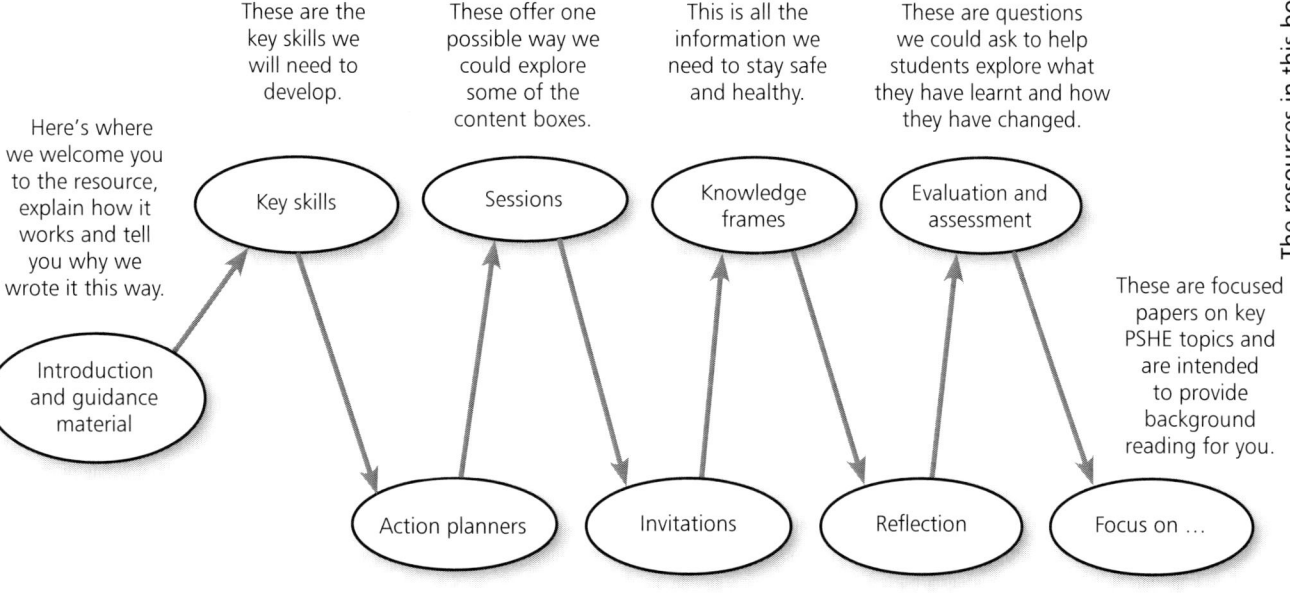

These are the key skills we will need to develop.

These offer one possible way we could explore some of the content boxes.

This is all the information we need to stay safe and healthy.

These are questions we could ask to help students explore what they have learnt and how they have changed.

Here's where we welcome you to the resource, explain how it works and tell you why we wrote it this way.

These are focused papers on key PSHE topics and are intended to provide background reading for you.

These are the building blocks of my PSHE programme.

Each block has a code:
G – General
H – Health
L – Learning
D – Substances
W – Work
E – Work experience
R – Relationships
K – Risk
P – Parenting
M – Moving on
S – Stress

These are open ended activities – some link directly to a session (they have a code that makes the link), whilst others could be used for lots of different issues. Some could be used for research or helping us evaluate how we have changed.

This just helps to pull each session together at the end.

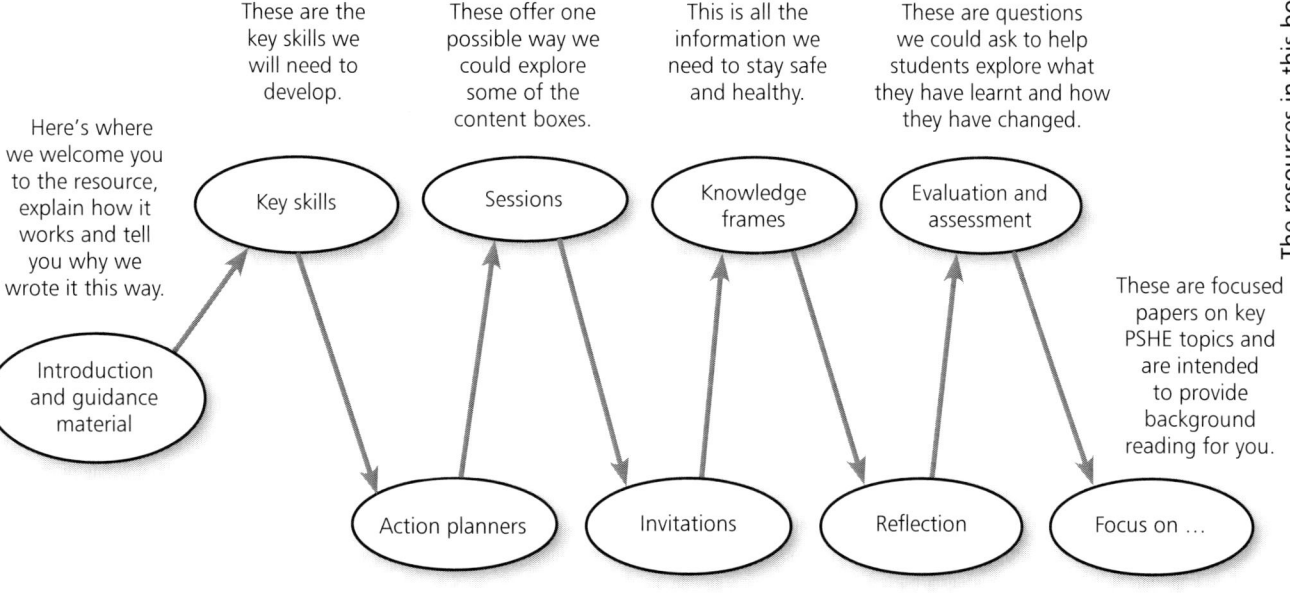

The resources in this book

1.1

How to get the best out of the resources

As both teachers and authors, we are always wary of 'one-size-fits-all' resources, where the authors' agenda predetermines the programme and dictates the learning. Every young person experiences their life from their own unique viewpoint. Consequently, we need to have the confidence to work flexibly. Because the emphasis is on structured questions, this helps keep inside the students' perceptions of reality.

Planning

While it is important to retain a flexible approach to the timing, factual content and the focus taken to explore any issue, it is vitally important not to depart from our general 'student-centred' approach to teaching PSHE. Use the following checklist of tasks when planning your programme.

1   Start by considering the students you teach and begin to select the themes and pathways you believe should make up the outline of your programme.

2   Check how your plans relate to the key concepts and key processes in the PSHE Education Programme of Study, and any local requirements or guidance. If necessary, adjust the content boxes.

3   Using a blank copy of the recording frame, insert the content box numbers into column 2 along with any amended text.

4   With reference to the knowledge frames, consider what key factual information and target language you feel would be appropriate to include, and place these, or references to them, in columns 3 and 4 of the recording frame.

5   Where we have illustrated ways of teaching the content blocks within the pathways, consider our approach and, if necessary, modify it to fit your context.

6   Check to see if there is any pre-teaching or preparation that students could do in order to enrich the next session. If so, record these in column 6 of the recording frame.

7   Consider if the session would benefit from some reflections (summarising questions) and a 'future pacing' activity, and build these into your session planning.

Approaching an issue

1   If you are uncertain about whether an issue is a priority, or exactly what approach or aspect of an issue you should emphasise, consider finding out the students' views. Begin by discovering their current knowledge and beliefs, by using one of the 'invitations' worksheets.

For example, if you wanted to explore 'bullying in school' but were unsure on what to focus, you could use Invitation 2: Bus stop people (page 205) and ask the students to imagine a group of students from the school have met at the bus stop on the way home. Tell the students that the people in the group are all talking and thinking about 'bullying in school'. Ask students what they think the people at the bus stop would be saying to each other and thinking to themselves. If they were listening and the group asked for their opinion, what would they be saying, thinking and feeling?

2   Now consider the students' responses using the bullets below to guide you:
   ● What do they indicate they already know and understand?
   ● What is misunderstood or wrong?
   ● What strategies do they have that you feel are appropriate and what strategies do they offer that might not be such a good idea?
   ● What is missing that you feel should be there by their age? (For example, is homophobic or racist bullying mentioned?)
   ● What do you feel could wait and what can't?
   ● Might there be implications for the school's bullying policy and support strategies?

   It is important to 'check out' your findings by taking them back to the students. You need to be careful about 'surface knowledge' or an 'acquired vocabulary' that can give the appearance of expertise. Deeper questioning can sometimes reveal only a superficial understanding of a topic or issue. For example, many students can name a great many drugs, but this does not mean they understand the implications of using them.

3   Next, consult with local professionals who have relevant national and local knowledge that could inform your planning, for example relating to bullying.

4   Now consider whether parents, carers, senior management and school governors might have a view about the topic or issue.

5 Finally, informed by all this, look for further content boxes that give you a route into where you feel you now need to go.

Remember that in any consultation process, each participant brings their own perspective and, in many cases, that perspective will have been influenced by the media and by local or personal experience. Sometimes, in order to meet the needs of students, others may need to have their own thinking challenged.

No single resource offers a complete programme. It is likely that you will choose to supplement this resource with events, classroom visitors and other teaching material. Whatever you use, always select material that supports the above principles. No matter how seductive a resource appears, it must offer concepts and language appropriate and relevant to your students. Does it give them the opportunity to share what they feel? Does it demonstrate respect for them and their experiences and opinions? Does it challenge them, when necessary, in a constructive manner, helping them move forward rather than putting them down?

Keeping the end in mind

This planning framework recognises that it is vital to pursue a PSHE programme that helps students to clarify who they are and to develop a wide range of transferable concepts and skills. PSHE can also act as a focal point, stimulus and catalyst for exploring and developing how they feel about broader issues that span other areas of the curriculum.

Realistically, in the time available, it is not possible to cover every issue or topic in the depth we would wish. We have to be selective and prioritise, using what we know about our students and what they tell us of how they are experiencing and making sense of a changing world. The value of a safe classroom climate is not only that it allows students to discuss sensitive issues safely and constructively, but because the future will require 'fearless thinkers' who are practised at looking below the surface of issues important to them. Though helping students shape clear and realistic aspirations will help them to engage more realistically with the immediate curriculum, more importantly it will be a habit they will value throughout their lives.

The core values and aims of *Health for Life*

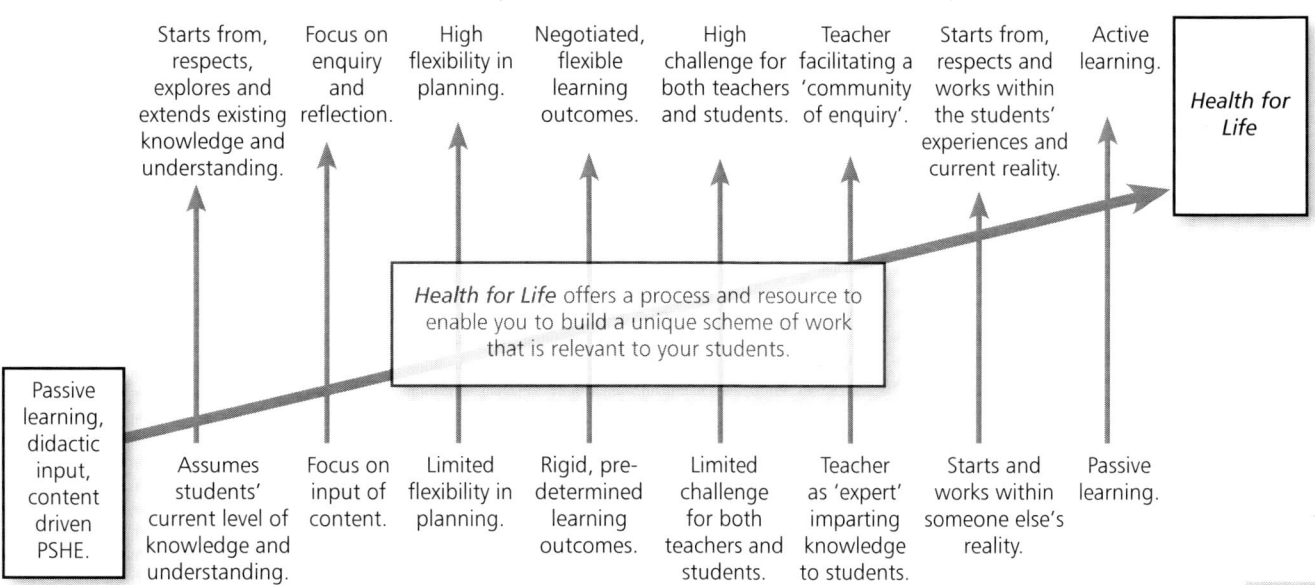

How to use the resources in your PSHE programme

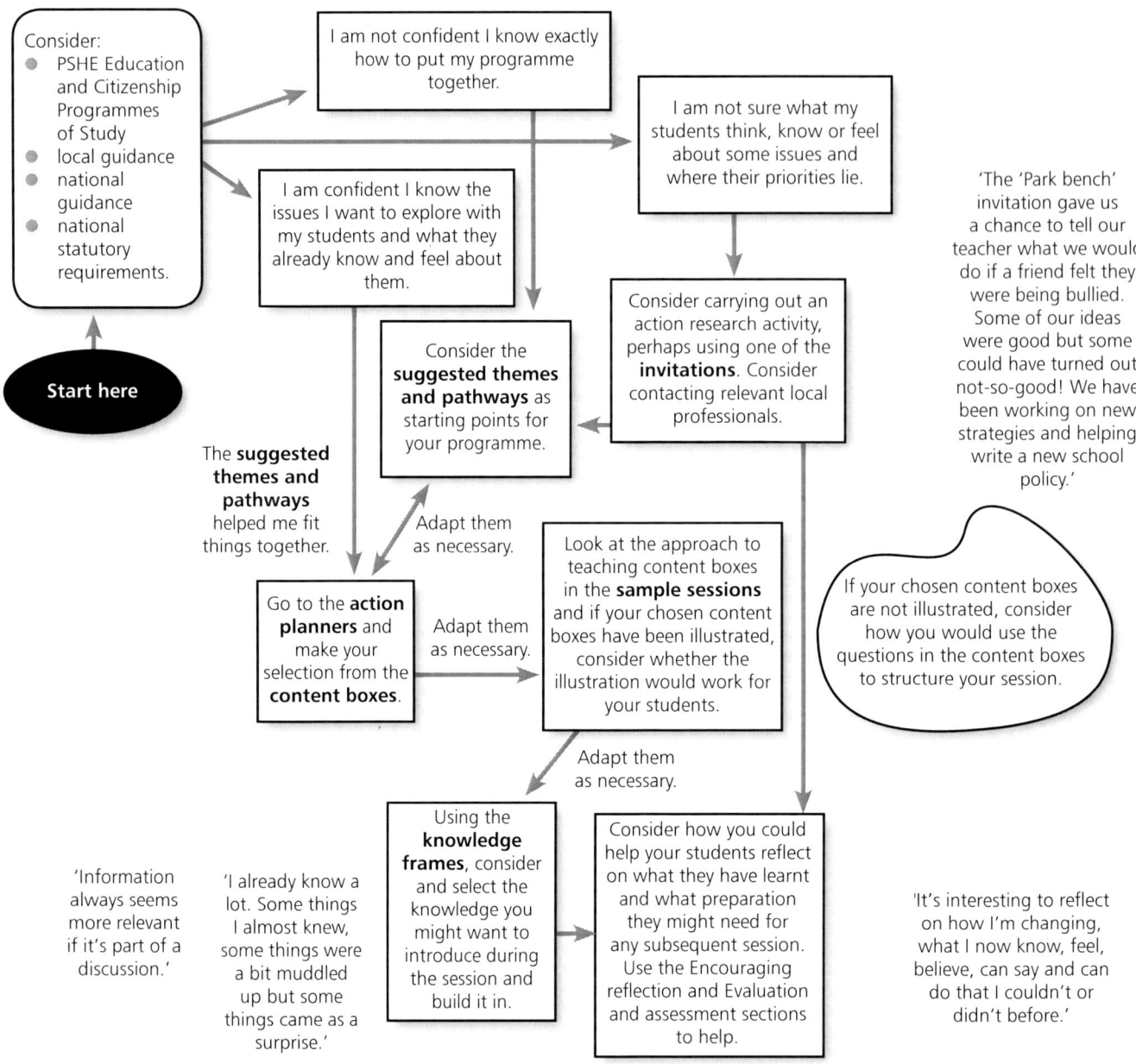

Consider:
- PSHE Education and Citizenship Programmes of Study
- local guidance
- national guidance
- national statutory requirements.

Start here

I am not confident I know exactly how to put my programme together.

I am confident I know the issues I want to explore with my students and what they already know and feel about them.

I am not sure what my students think, know or feel about some issues and where their priorities lie.

'The 'Park bench' invitation gave us a chance to tell our teacher what we would do if a friend felt they were being bullied. Some of our ideas were good but some could have turned out not-so-good! We have been working on new strategies and helping write a new school policy.'

Consider carrying out an action research activity, perhaps using one of the **invitations**. Consider contacting relevant local professionals.

Consider the **suggested themes and pathways** as starting points for your programme.

The **suggested themes and pathways** helped me fit things together.

Adapt them as necessary.

Go to the **action planners** and make your selection from the **content boxes**.

Adapt them as necessary.

Look at the approach to teaching content boxes in the **sample sessions** and if your chosen content boxes have been illustrated, consider whether the illustration would work for your students.

If your chosen content boxes are not illustrated, consider how you would use the questions in the content boxes to structure your session.

Adapt them as necessary.

Using the **knowledge frames**, consider and select the knowledge you might want to introduce during the session and build it in.

Consider how you could help your students reflect on what they have learnt and what preparation they might need for any subsequent session. Use the Encouraging reflection and Evaluation and assessment sections to help.

'Information always seems more relevant if it's part of a discussion.'

'I already know a lot. Some things I almost knew, some things were a bit muddled up but some things came as a surprise.'

'It's interesting to reflect on how I'm changing, what I now know, feel, believe, can say and can do that I couldn't or didn't before.'

The value of critical reflection

The ability to conduct critical reflection means having *internal* resources available to 'watch over' real-life activity and events. Having these resources raises self-esteem and is life-affirming. Critically reflecting is a subtle but significantly different strategy from one such as 'Stop! Think! Act!', which is entirely appropriate for young children, and which depends on them recalling advice received from a grown-up and acting on it *rather than going their own way*. Critical reflection, by contrast, is learning to *become* the advisor and the guide, to muster resources from within. To have critical reflection available is to carry a helpful positive parent and an objective adult with you at all times. The key difference is that the parent and adult carried are your own, not simply recalled advice from someone else.

Critical reflection is both a skill and a habit. In reality, many of us have this skill but may forget to actually apply it at the required time and only reflect in hindsight, often with thoughts such as: 'How could I have been so daft'; 'I can't believe I said/did that!'; 'I *wish* I'd said ...'; or 'I should (never) have listened to ...'

Recognising when it is OK to be impulsive and when we need to pause and think is a skill in itself. Students are bound to meet situations where their first impulsive thought is to act in a particular way. From a structural point of view, in order to foster their critical reflection skills, we need to address two key tasks: to support the development of the rational, analytical capacities of their *adult*; and to help them explore and understand the moral and ethical standards and values, and society's laws and expectations, that their *parent* will then be able to apply. If we can convey our recognition of their personal autonomy and, at the same time, seek to develop their ability to conduct themselves wisely, they can have justifiable confidence in their own judgement, with critical reflection being the key skill that underpins it.

We can support the development of the habit of 'pause, think, think a bit more, now decide if you *can* decide' by building critical reflection into our sessions. This can be as part of planned, reflective pauses during a session and within evaluation.

It might be helpful to think of critical reflection as having two directions. We can ask ourselves questions to critically reflect outwards on what we have heard, seen, been offered or received, or inwards on how what we have heard, seen, been offered or received has impacted on us.

Outward reflection

If we find or are offered a source of information, we could critically reflect on that source:

- Is this information accurate?
- Can I trust this source of information?
- How do I know?
- How can I judge this?
- Am I getting balanced information or advice? Am I getting the 'whole picture'? Is someone selecting what they will and will not tell me or show me? If so, why?
- Is there another source that I can compare it with? How can I be confident that this is any more accurate or reliable? (If they are the same, they still might be wrong. If they are different, you know at least one is definitely wrong – now you have to work out which, or whether it's both!)
- Does the person or organisation really know enough about this to make a safe decision on my behalf – how could I be at least reasonably confident this is the case?
- Does the person or organisation offering information or their opinion have my best interests at heart?
- Who will benefit if I accept this advice or information? Is it me, someone else (perhaps the person offering the advice or opinion), my family, my community?
- Am I being offered accurate information or someone's opinion? If it is the opinion of lots of people, does it mean it's factually accurate or true? (Look for statements like 'they say ...' and challenge with 'who, exactly?')
- Am I being offered someone's factual knowledge, someone's opinion, or someone's beliefs and values?

Inward reflection

This could involve a rational reflection:

- What do my past experiences and trusted, received wisdom tell me?
- Do I now know enough to make an informed choice?
- What might be the consequences to me and others of making decisions and actions based on what I have heard or experienced – now/soon/in the future?
- What can I do/say to help/make things better?
- Am I sure I know what I'm doing – or do I need help?
- Do I still have questions or doubts?
- How can I check these out?
- Who/what could help me?
- Am I being sensible, or am I being silly?
- Will I later regret I did/said this?
- Will I later be glad I did/said this?

It could also involve a values/constraints/imperatives reflection:

- What should/ought/must I not do?
- What is expected of me?
- What will be frowned upon – and by whom?

or an emotional reflection:

- How is this knowledge, opinion, experience making me feel? (Secure, confident, uneasy?)
- Do I have mixed feelings?
- Have my feelings changed?
- Are my feelings the same but now even stronger?
- What are these feelings encouraging me to do?
- How will this change my future decisions or behaviour?

Critically reflecting on our feelings is vital. How we feel is usually a more powerful motivator than our reason. If we do choose to follow our reason, it is usually because we feel it is the right, best or expected thing to do. Students may benefit from the idea that the *adult* is the best of their voices to be in control. While taking into account the shoulds, should nots and permissions of the *parent* within, and the youthful exuberance, natural caution and other emotional responses of the *child* within, the adult within *uniquely* has the ability to weigh everything and make rational judgements. In the scenarios we offer throughout this resource, Sara and Emma commonly appear.

Sara is impetuous, has a strong-willed child within, a weak parent within who doesn't manage to curb the child very well, and an adult ready to help make good judgements, but who often isn't consulted. She could benefit from strengthening both parent and adult voices.

Emma is more naturally cautious, with an internal parent easily able to curb any impetuous tendencies of the internal child, and an adult whose sound judgement is often overruled by the parent voice! She could benefit from increasing her parent's readiness both to encourage and to permit her child more freedom, whilst continuing to listen carefully to her rational adult contribution voice.

Tip: You may want to encourage students to try making their own assessments of more of the characters in the soap, or other well-known characters from TV, film or literature.

1.2 The use of language in PSHE

The broad principles of effective practice in PSHE lessons or sessions are well known. They include: starting from where students currently are; encouraging active involvement in learning; balancing knowledge and understanding with value clarification; and the development of thinking and interpersonal skills. Because PSHE works inside students' personal experience, inside their own heads, working alongside them to help them make sense of their own world, we would argue that our teaching language needs to be as carefully crafted as any other aspect of session planning.

Health for Life presents a particular model of PSHE: we think of it as school-based management training, in terms of learning to manage ourselves and others. We know, however, that there is a world of difference between knowing something theoretically and acting on that learning in a social context. Sports coaches, for example, have long known that the emotional state athletes are able to access when they need to perform is critical to their ability to access the resources needed to achieve their desired outcomes. On the way home from an interview where our brains have gone blank, how many of us have suddenly known exactly what we should have said?

As teachers, we know never to label a student in a negative way because we know how damaging this can be. For example, we would not tell a student that he or she is stupid because this is labelling their *identity*. We might challenge their *behaviour*, for example by saying 'You are really clever, yet you chose to …' The reverse is also true: using affirming language can be just as powerful in a positive way. Saying to someone, 'You are confident and competent' is not a substitute for them actually acquiring those skills and strategies, but supports students in accessing those skills and strategies.

Critical and 'crunch' moments

The learning we acquire in PSHE may need to be accessed and applied in 'crunch' moments. This is the minute or even second when we are confronted with a choice or dilemma that requires both a decision and action. Many 'crunch' moments are heralded by 'critical' moments when perhaps earlier and easier decisions could have been made and acted on. If we had an opportunity to explore these 'critical and crunch moments' in advance, we could consider:

- what we know and feel about what we know
- who we might be with, how they might be feeling, how we feel about them and their possible reactions to our choices
- what others who are important to us might feel and hope for us.

Without this opportunity we may have to 'wing it' at a time when activity in the emotional part of our brain may inhibit the rational part of our brain. This is why, when under pressure, we make an unwise or regretted decision and later find ourselves thinking or saying, 'I can't believe I said/did that'. This is why the *Health for Life* model places so much emphasis on the emotional dimension.

Ethical dilemmas have always been at the core of PSHE teaching. Is the role of PSHE to enable students to make and act on their own informed choices, regardless of what those choices are, or is the purpose of PSHE to support students in making the right or healthy choice according to *our* judgement? It would seem to be a balance between the two: on the one hand, we have a duty of care to promote or prevent a particular behaviour; on the other, we have a duty to give students the knowledge or criteria they need to make up their own minds.

Using language patterns

The language patterns below can be surprisingly powerful and, if you choose to use them, they must be used ethically. The 'holy grail' of PSHE is to construct a learning experience that enables us effortlessly to access the language, skills and strategies we need in the critical moments and, if all else fails, the crunch moments.

Because our brains work on connections, we can help this process by taking students into possible 'crunch moments' and help them install and rehearse the language and skills they may need to access. We then 'anchor' these skills to the situation in which they believe they are most likely to need to access them (see How to use the case studies and timelines on page **38** and Future pacing: imagining your future on page **250**). Because this is going to be unique to the individual, we need to work inside the imagination of each individual student. Ideally, we want students to recognise when a critical or crunch moment is happening, and connect with and access their pre-installed learning.

Using positive messages

Our language can help or hinder this. We need to use every technique available to us. Our basic behaviour management has long recognised that we ask students for what we want not what we don't want. Simple examples are to say 'please walk' rather than 'don't run'. We word classroom agreements in positives: 'respect one another's right to learn' rather than 'don't disturb other people'.

The reason for this is that the brain can't handle deletions. It is a bit like 'don't think right now of a pink elephant'. You have to do it in order to not do it. Much of what we learn happens unconsciously, for example through actions modelled by others. We need to be careful in PSHE that we avoid clumsy language. If in doubt, cross out all negations and you reveal the unconscious message. So the unconscious messages in these statements become depressingly obvious:

- Don't take drugs.
- Don't drink too much alcohol.
- Don't have unprotected sexual intercourse.

Our language should always offer a positive message.

Using embedded commands

If we are empowering students, it can be helpful to use language like, 'If we choose always to use protection, we are choosing to protect ourselves and those we care about from …' At first sight this looks helpful, but it also sends the message that if we succumb to the pressures of others and find ourselves reluctantly agreeing to something we really didn't want to do it was our choice. Therefore, it is our fault for being weak.

This sort of statement could therefore be followed with the question: 'If you want to make this choice, what could help you, what might try to prevent you and what do you need to learn to be able to say "I will overcome this"?' Notice the embedded commands, 'If *you want to make this choice*, what could help you, what might *try* to prevent you and what do you need to learn to be able to say *"I will overcome this"*?'

The following is not a script, but is offered to illustrate some points for consideration.

Today we are going to explore …

This states clearly the area we are going to consider.

What we are going to learn is …

This is an early embedded command. We are already installing the message that learning is going to happen. With practice, it is possible to use a technique called analogue marking, which means slightly altering the pitch, tone or volume of your voice at the 'command'.

In pairs, what do you already know about …? Try to come up with as many things as you can.

Collect some examples, then …

Out of all of this knowledge we have shared, what do we feel is the most important thing that we already know? How would we justify our choice to someone else?

The use of early questions is really important. Apart from drawing you into the learning, it forces us to go to those areas of our brains where our previous experiences are stored and draws these to our attention. It will help us connect new learning to existing learning. For example, if you are asked, 'What is the capital of England?' it is almost impossible not to find that 'London' comes into your mind. It also supports us in recognising how much we already know, which can help us feel more positive about the coming learning. The second question deepens the process by requiring some processing.

Imagine a group of students of about your age meeting together in the place where they normally meet.

'Imagine' is a great word. It is liberating because it gives you permission to go where you like and think what you like. The use of the words 'about your age' begins to pin down that they are students like you. The use of 'where they normally meet' is known as 'clean language'. It is important to avoid using specific words like 'park'. When we hear a story, most people form images in their heads that are relevant to them. By keeping our language 'clean', we avoid disrupting that process and each individual can construct the story in the way it is most relevant to them.

Using uptime and downtime

Uptime is when we ask students to be present in the classroom, perhaps listening to us or talking with another. Downtime is when we ask students to go inside their heads and imagine something. As human beings, we do this all the time, moving our attention from the outside world to the inside of our heads. When we ask students to move into 'downtime' and use their imaginations, we need to be particularly careful about our language, as in 'downtime' we are more susceptible to it.

After a while, one of the group begins to pass around some pills. They are offered to one of the group, who hesitates.

Narrative is also powerful. We generally like stories, even short ones. The use of story with fictional people also allows us slightly to distance what could be a sensitive issue from the learners.

How do you think they are feeling right now?

This can trigger two levels of thinking: one, how might someone else be feeling? (which is still being generated by me); and, two, how would I feel if that was me?

What might those feelings be encouraging them to do?

This is important. We are suggesting that our feelings may influence our choices and behaviour and that what we feel may be more influential than what we know. It is also possible to add in bystanders. For example:

Imagine someone who loves them very much is watching. How will they be feeling? What decision might they hope this young person will make?

Again, ethically, this is interesting. The person 'who loves them' may offer the 'sensible/safe/healthy' choice – what you know you should do, not what you might want to do. They could offer the voice of reason or even conscience. One issue to explore is why different people's perspectives might generate different thoughts and feelings. Of course, even someone who loves them may be capable of giving poor advice, or imposing unreasonable constraints. Another issue is the need for students to recognise that they do not have to choose between obeying *or* rebelling, conforming *or* diverging, all of which are responses from their internal child. Rather, the more mature response is to receive and take account of any messages from outside, and then ensure their internal adult draws from its own knowledge and experience, makes its own decision, and understands the need to be ready to be held accountable for it.

Imagine you are there but invisible to the entire group except the person who is being offered the pills. Everything freezes and the person being offered the pills asks you, 'What should I do?'

This technique aims to move the student into the situation gently and more safely. They can now be invited to offer their advice and we will assume the advice they offer is to refuse. It is possible that the advice they intend to offer openly in the class might be different from the feelings in their heads. We need to push this a little.

The young person listens to your advice and then asks, 'Why?' Do you know enough to make a convincing argument?

Now, if necessary, we can offer new information. We can introduce this by saying:

It would be useful for you to have some factual information about ... You now know [add the information here] ... Is this changing/reinforcing [choose which is appropriate depending on what has come before] how you feel about ...? Is this helping you to better inform someone else?

Ethically, this technique is a little questionable. There is a powerful installation here. It doesn't allow you to dispute the facts, it simply states, 'You now know ... to be true' and quickly moves you into applying this knowledge. This is quite different from, 'Imagine I told you ...' which is open to challenge.

Would it surprise you if I told you most students choose ...?

This is where national or local data is useful. It is an opportunity to reinforce the fact that most students make either healthy or safe choices and, if they do decide to adopt a risky behaviour, often have strategies to minimise that risk. This begins to challenge a possible perception that 'everyone is doing this except me'. This then leads to ...

Why do you think most students make this choice?

This gives students a chance to draw from the reasons that they feel are relevant to them. This gives you the opening to offer other possible reasons that they, perhaps through inexperience or immaturity, might not have considered.

The young person is convinced by your argument and agrees to refuse the pills. They now ask you how?

This really pushes the discussion into the language, strategies and skills we need to assert our wishes over others. We could also explore the consequences of this action but, again, this is best done in a question.

What might be the not-so-good things that happen next?
What might be the good things that happen next?

We can then work the timeline by exploring what might happen tonight, tomorrow, next week, next month or next year? Is it still OK? Does the student feel any different about their decision if moved forward in time?

Moving into the first person

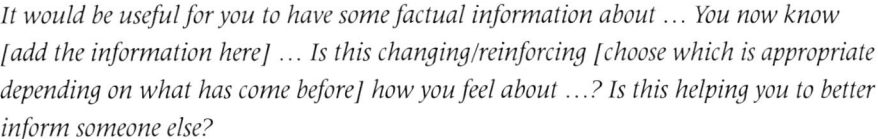

There may come a time when you want to move from the third person into the first person. This needs sensitive handling. Moving into the first person alters brain activity. As we imagine events in our own heads, we may see images, experience feeling and hear remembered or imagined sounds. If we do this in the first person (known as 'associated'), it can trigger physiological changes in us. With a vivid imagination, we literally live the imagined event. The brain doesn't seem to react in the same way if we imagine ourselves watching others (disassociated). This is why we need to be very careful when we take students into the first person. Only use a first person, associated position if you are certain no one is going to be taken back to an unpleasant experience and re-live it. When planning a PSHE session, it can be helpful to think in 'zones'.

- 'Imagine this is happening to someone' is remote but can still generate feelings. You might think of this as a 'cold' or 'cool' zone.
- 'Imagine this is happening to someone of your own age' is getting warmer.
- 'Imagine this is happening to a friend (or best friend)' is even warmer.

- 'Imagine this is happening to you, right now' is the hot zone. Only go 'hot' when you are totally confident it is safe and appropriate for your students (not when you just think it may be). For example, you need to be cautious that you are not opening recent wounds, or focusing on a current situation that is painful for one of your students.

Imagine that you are with a group of people of your age, wherever you normally meet together. You might imagine who you could be with, and where you might be.

Imagine that a similar event is occurring. Imagine you are being offered the pills. Imagine them in front of you and the people around you. What are you feeling right now? What do you feel you want to do next? What decision do you want to make? Now what might you say and do to get the outcome you want?

Now we might move into a paired exercise where we test out our language and strategy with an observer, perhaps feeding us opening lines and offering feedback. We need to find out whether the words we thought would work in our imaginations will 'fit into our mouths'. What we imagine ourselves being able to say and what we feel comfortable actually saying can be very different. When we have the words and strategies that fit, we need to 'future pace' them. This might involve a guided fantasy taking the student back into their imaginations in the first person and running the scenario, applying the language and strategies and noticing what is happening and how they are feeling (see Future pacing: imagining your future, page **250**).

A reflection at the end of any learning is useful to draw it together. In any session there is likely to be a small number of critical pieces of core, transferable learning you want students to take away from a rich overall experience. See Evaluation and assessment on page **44** for questions to help structure this.

At the end of any learning it is important to pre-teach the next (notice how many television programmes offer a taster of 'next week on …' or 'next time on …'). This can be combined with the courtesy of thanking them for participating.

Thank you for all that you have contributed to our learning.

I wonder if you are curious to know more about … well next week we will explore …
I wonder if you, like me, are fascinated by why … Next time, we are going to look at …

This can be extended in the form of a key question for students to ponder or investigate. Anticipation of a good lesson to come brings students who are already curious and motivated.

1.3 Skills development in PSHE

The *Health for Life* series helps students develop and rehearse the following key skills:

- Understanding the differences between fact, fiction, myth, opinion, hearsay and rumour. Being able to find out which is which by enquiry and consultation.

- Understanding that perceived 'social norms' may not be shared by everyone, nor always reflected in their behaviour.

- Recognising the 'critical moment' when a simple or easy decision could be made to take events in a new and better direction.

- Recognising when you have missed the 'critical moment', and having the strategies, language and skills to manage the 'crunch moments'.

- Recognising when the 'feelings part' of us is trying to take over or when it *has* taken over from the 'thinking part' of us, and how to respond to this – is it helping or hindering good management? What can we do about it if it's hindering us?

- Recognising who is in charge, my inner 'parent', inner 'adult' or inner 'child', and managing this.

- Trying to 'put ourselves in another's shoes', recognising the nature or strength of their feelings and understanding that their viewpoint, opinion and experiences are valid, even when they differ from ours.

- Being aware of risks to our own and other people's bodies and feelings; being able to assess those risks, manage them positively, or avoid them.

- Recognising and dealing with pressure both from:
  - within us through our beliefs about 'social norms', 'unwritten rules' and/or our own need for approval
  - outside us in the form of individual, peer group or family pressure or through our response to the media or others in society.

- Finding things out for ourselves and being able to judge whether a source is well intentioned and reliable, well intentioned but unreliable, or just unreliable (or even malicious).

- Being able to work and learn constructively with others and being able to critically reflect on how we could do this even better.

- Emotional competence, which we have divided into:
  - emotional awareness – being aware of our feelings, the comfortable and the not-so-comfortable
  - emotional literacy – having a wide vocabulary for feelings to help us to 'pin them down' and communicate them to others
  - emotional empathy – being able to recognise feelings in others and relate these to our own feelings
  - emotional intelligence – being able to recognise when a feeling is encouraging us to do something good or not-so-good; knowing when, and being able, to follow our feelings or ignore them. Understanding the internal source of our feelings, for example the child in me might get upset when I'm asked to do something demanding, frightening, inconvenient, etc. while my adult knows the request is reasonable. Being aware that our behaviour can create feelings in others.

- Knowing when our life is in balance, when it is not and what actions we need to take to get the balance back. It could be balancing leisure and work or balancing what we feel we want to do against what we know would be more helpful or constructive. Knowing that, like individuals, relationships also need a balance: the skill of recognising when a relationship is wobbling and what words or actions are needed to restore it.

- The skills of:
  - prediction – being able to 'fast forward' to a probable outcome
  - imagination – being able to imagine how we will feel and how we see and hear ourselves managing this likely outcome
  - assessment – being able to assess whether our predictions or imaginings are over optimistic, over pessimistic or balanced.

- Reflecting analytically on our immediate and longer term learning:
  - What do we know now that we didn't know before?
  - What can we say or do now that we couldn't before (or now say or do more confidently)?
  - How do we feel about what we have learned, and how have we changed?
  - What is still missing, confused or in need of further development or practice?
  - How can we apply our new learning?

1.4 How to use the action planners

The purpose of the action planners, which build on those in *Health for Life 11–14*, is to help you put into practice an interactive programme in PSHE that is easy to work through, that is flexible and adaptable, that is able to incorporate other programmes and interventions, and that students will want to try out to help them develop their skills. It should be a programme that the school itself will see as a core activity, and which parents, families and the community will want to support.

Years 10 and 11 present a particular challenge for PSHE. The students, particularly in Year 11, increasingly need to access and apply the skills and information acquired through their PSHE programme, but exams and an often shorter year can put great pressure on the time available. Since there will be far more content than you can possibly cover, it is essential to be pragmatic and choose the topics that are most relevant to your students and which will continue to develop their core skills. One way of planning or reviewing your programme is to start with your priorities for Year 11, backward mapping into Year 10, and then ensuring continuity and progression from your Year 9 programme.

FAQs about the action planners

What are the action planners for?

The action planners in Part 2 contain numbered content boxes, each of which can be used to provide a session outline or workshop. Each box is a little like the paint in a paintbox. The final picture you paint will be a unique combination of different boxes, and some can be blended together to make your own new boxes. All are included on the CD-ROM for you to cut, paste and edit.

Why are the content boxes in the form of questions?

By listening to how students answer the questions, you can celebrate what they know, correct what is almost known and teach what is missing. The questions can also be used to help students evaluate their learning by asking them to reflect on how their feelings about the questions have changed.

Why is there some duplication in boxes?

Just as real life doesn't fit neatly into distinct boxes, so the content boxes allow an issue to be approached in a variety of ways. An approach relevant to one school may be inappropriate for another. In addition, some critical issues and key messages covered in depth in Year 10 need briefly revisiting and reinforcing in Year 11 to reconnect students to their prior learning.

Do I have to use a box in its intended year?

No. Use the content boxes flexibly to address the needs of your own students. Because of the likely range of maturity in Years 10 and 11, the majority of the questions in the content boxes will be appropriate to both years. Any real difference will lie in how the students respond to the questions rather than to the questions themselves. If you feel that a content box is inappropriately timed for your school, you should move it, but do this because:

- you have evidence that your students are not ready for it, rather than because adults feel uncomfortable with the content
- you have evidence that your students, or the context they are living in, require the work to be covered earlier
- it clashes in some way with your programme's organisation, for example the timing of work experience placements.

We frequently underestimate how much students already know or believe they know sufficiently well to make a decision. In evaluating PSHE, we have consistently found that students find our timing in teaching the topics is generally too late. Viewing the range of television programmes students watch, and reading magazines targeted at students, tend to reinforce this opinion.

Some students may overestimate how much they really know. We should not assume that even comprehensive knowledge of health issues acquired through the media translates to actual experience or having the maturity or management skills required to safely manage a possible future experience.

We also need to be aware that students have a tendency to overestimate the actual behaviours of their peers. This is reflected in comments such as, 'Everyone of my age is doing it/has tried it/has done it except me!' Many students feel a real pressure to conform to a perceived, but actually fictitious, level of peer behaviour for fear of missing out or being left out.

What are the key themes?

The action planners have been grouped into three strands:

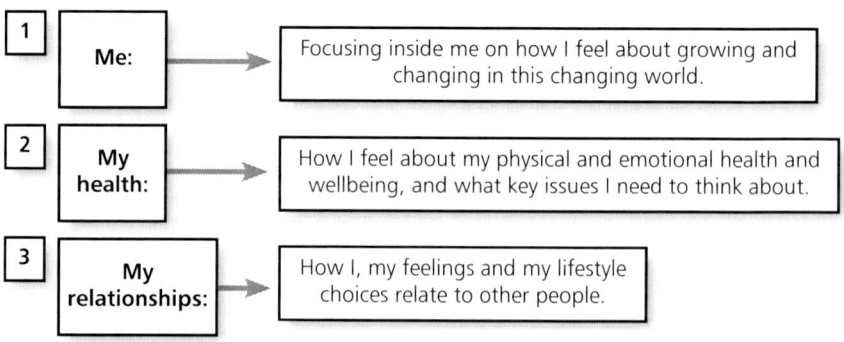

Each strand has been sub-grouped into different 'focus' areas:

- Focus on me as a learner.
- Focus on relationships.
- Focus on physical and emotional health.

Some of these have been grouped to an even tighter focus on:

- relationships and sex
- assessing risks and keeping safe (including in Year 10 cyber-bullying)
- the use and misuse of substances.

In this resource we have added four new strands:

- Focus on economic wellbeing and the world of work
- Focus on work experience
- Focus on being a parent
- Focus on 'moving on'.

Content boxes covering work experience have been placed in Year 11, but these will be relevant to Year 10 if your school operates a Year 10 placement.

Why is there little focus on factual content?

As we said in the introduction, factual information goes out of date very quickly and local information, such as the location of support services, will be unique to your school. The knowledge frames on pages **218–249** provide a comprehensive framework of the broad knowledge we believe students need. Local agencies and professionals can help you with current factual information, help you to target specific local priorities, and provide specific local information. There is also a wealth of websites that can help provide you with more general information.

What about inclusion?

Because the approach we encourage you to adopt takes into account of, and works within, each young person's reality, we believe that the resource will enable all students to equally participate. Each content box offers a variety of possible foci. For example, the content boxes on bullying could be focused on homophobic bullying, or the content boxes on exploring and celebrating difference could be focused on anti-racist work.

How do I go about choosing a topic to explore?

Look at the key themes listed on page **55** (Year 10) and page **119** (Year 11). Each key theme or focus has suggested pathways, from which you can decide on the most relevant to you and either follow or adapt them. You then select content boxes to fit, using the recording frame on page **54** to keep track of them. You might want to blend some together to create your own unique boxes.

You may find that you begin with our suggested themes and pathways but, over time, adapt and modify them to fit your school's unique context and culture.

1.5 How to use the sessions

As with *Health for Life 11–14*, this resource has developed some of the content boxes into sample sessions.* Since schools have different allocations of time for PSHE, you may need to edit these suggestions to fit your available time. However, it is important to preserve the broader session structure and retain the principle of working from the students' own understanding and starting points.

Times have not been allocated to activities within individual sessions. Based on experience, different groups will move at different paces, wanting to put greater emphasis on different issues within a session.

The format of the sessions

Each session explores one of the content boxes, and follows a common format:

- The **rationale** for the session: this is principally our notes to you as the facilitator with our thinking about why we feel this is important.
- The **purpose** of the session: to share with the students and clarify what will be explored. It also includes a brief piece of dialogue to act as a further stimulus for the session.
- **Focusing activity:** to draw students quickly into the session.
- **'Into action':** the core activity of the session.
- **Reflection:** the essential plenary that draws together and summarises the key learning covered during the session. It is important to allow sufficient time for the plenary.

Because the case studies are also on CD-ROM, you can adapt or edit the sessions to suit your purpose. You could also use an interactive whiteboard to project the scenarios, key questions or key factual information to the group.

You may wish to add a simple activity at the start of a session to access and connect briefly with existing or prior learning. For example, if the topic is new, in pairs:

Quickly find four things you already know about …
Share your four things with another pair and see what you have in common and what is different.
We are going to be exploring …, what two questions would you really like answered?
What if you could only have one question, which would it be? Why?

Or, if reconnecting to a previous session:

What is the single most important thing you remember from the last session and why do you think it is the most important? Quickly share it with the person beside you and see if you agree.

---

* Many of the remaining content boxes and those not developed in *Health for Life 11–14* are to be found in the *Real Health for Real Lives* series.

Alternatively, invite the group to connect with the new session with a fast activity such as:

Quickly share one thing you already know about/think about ... with the person beside you.

Write a few responses on the board, then start the session.

At the end of a session, you might want to use a few of the summarising questions listed in 1.7 Encouraging reflection (see page **42**).

How do I construct my own sessions?

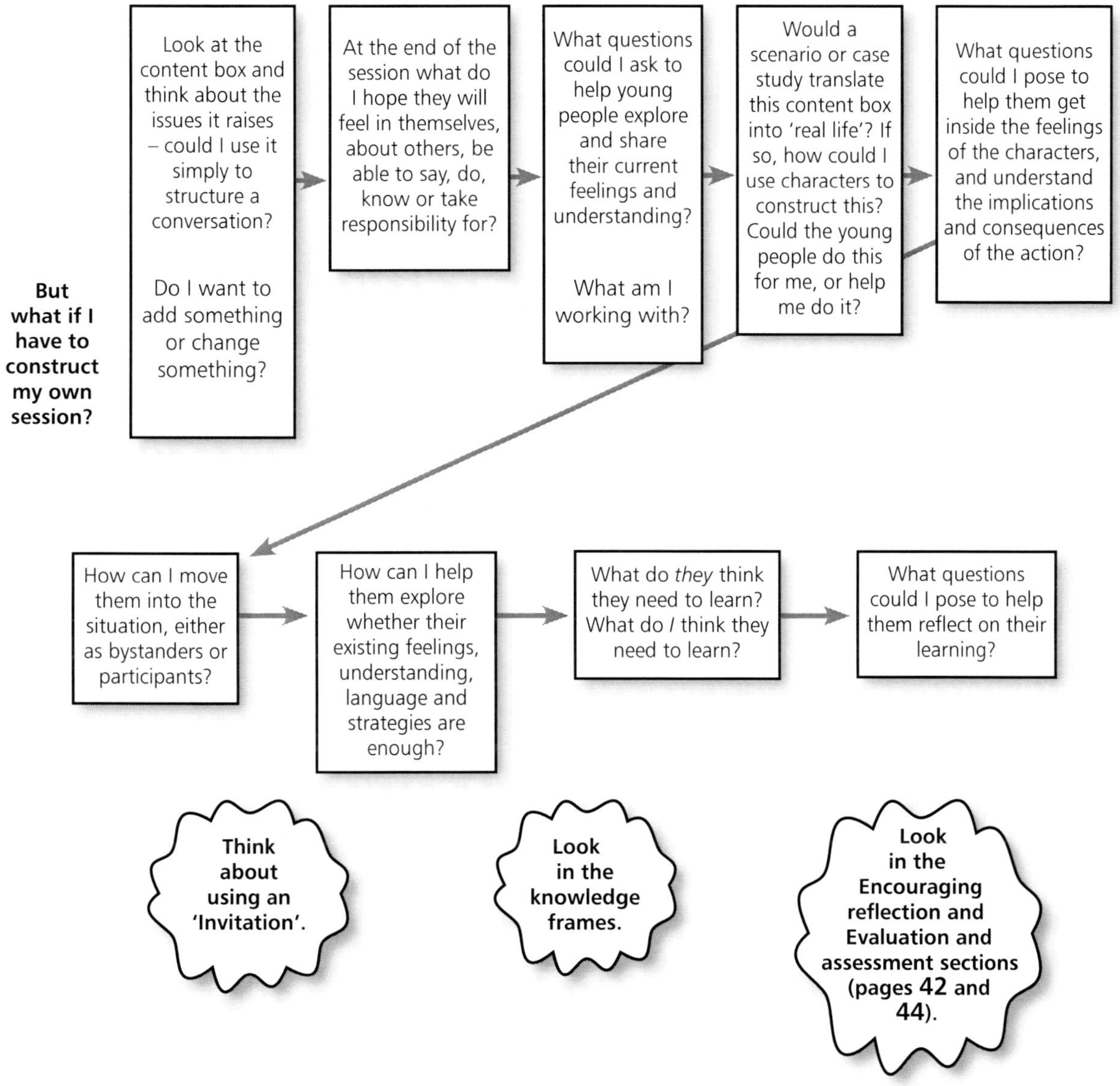

But what if I have to construct my own session?

Look at the content box and think about the issues it raises – could I use it simply to structure a conversation?

Do I want to add something or change something?

→

At the end of the session what do I hope they will feel in themselves, about others, be able to say, do, know or take responsibility for?

→

What questions could I ask to help young people explore and share their current feelings and understanding?

What am I working with?

→

Would a scenario or case study translate this content box into 'real life'? If so, how could I use characters to construct this? Could the young people do this for me, or help me do it?

→

What questions could I pose to help them get inside the feelings of the characters, and understand the implications and consequences of the action?

How can I move them into the situation, either as bystanders or participants?

→

How can I help them explore whether their existing feelings, understanding, language and strategies are enough?

→

What do *they* think they need to learn? What do *I* think they need to learn?

→

What questions could I pose to help them reflect on their learning?

Think about using an 'Invitation'.

Look in the knowledge frames.

Look in the Encouraging reflection and Evaluation and assessment sections (pages 42 and 44).

1.6 How to use the case studies and timelines

Each session starts with a case study to set the scene. It is likely that you will have alternatives to the scenarios, perhaps drawn from a preferred story or situation more immediately relevant to your students.

The use of timelines to explore case studies is encouraged. They are a way of relating what is happening in the present to what happened in the past and to what may happen in the future. You could think about the scenarios as 'the present' and often at the 'crunch' moment – the moment when we need all our skills, belief and knowledge about ourselves in order to make and act on a difficult decision.

If a case study was a DVD, we could press the pause button, literally putting the world on hold while we think about what to do next. The fun of a timeline is that you can fast forward to try things out, rewind and try something new, fast forward months again to see how things turn out in the more distant future or rewind months to change things to make crunch moments less likely to occur or more easily managed.

Exploring the present

We can explore the present through questions:

- How do you think they are feeling right now? Could they be having lots of different feelings at the same time?
- Do you think what they are feeling and thinking is different from what they are saying and doing? Why?
- What do you think their feelings might be pushing them to do?
- Which part of them is in charge right now – their 'adult' or thinking self, their 'child' or feeling self, or their 'parent' or ought to self?
- If you were invisible and watching from a safe place, what would you be feeling?
- If someone who really cared for them was watching them now, what would they be feeling? Is it different? Why?
- If someone in authority was watching, what would they be thinking?
- Imagine that suddenly they can see you, but the rest of the world is still on pause. They ask your advice. What would you tell them to do? They think for a minute and then ask you 'Why?' Could you convince them? What more would you like/need to know to really convince them?

Exploring the future

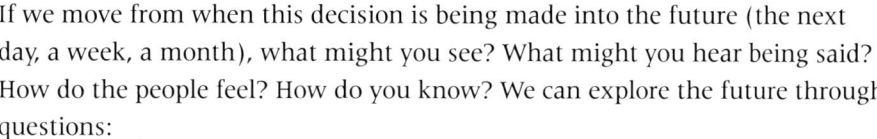

If we move from when this decision is being made into the future (the next day, a week, a month), what might you see? What might you hear being said? How do the people feel? How do you know? We can explore the future through questions:

- What do you think will happen next? Is that good or not-so-good?
- Is anyone at risk, could someone get hurt? Their body? Their feelings?
- Could anyone not actually in this present situation still end up getting hurt later? Who? Why? How? In what way?
- What could be going really well?
- What specifically could be good or not-so-good about the likely outcome?
- What do you think might happen tomorrow, next week, in the future if this decision is made?
- Who else might become involved in the future?
- What might others feel and say now, soon, in the future? Is that good or not-so-good? Are things getting better or worse? If they are getting better, will it stay better?
- Can you think of better/healthier/safer ways this situation could develop?
- If you can, what has to be said or done differently? Who has to do it? What might push them forward? What might hold them back?

Exploring the past

We can explore the past through questions:

- If we could turn the clock back, what do you think might have happened before this situation?
- Could there have been a critical moment when someone could have said or done something different that could have stopped this situation from happening?
- Would it have been easier to have said or done something then, rather than now?

Making it personal

If we feel it is appropriate, we can then take the group into the situation described in the case study.

What if it was you?

- Could we ever imagine this happening to us?
- Where might we be? Who might we be with?
- What would we be feeling, saying, doing?
- Can we have more than one feeling in a situation like this?
- Might our feelings conflict with one another? Could they be encouraging us to do different things or even opposite things?
- What would be the risks for us, now, tomorrow, soon? How do we feel about this?

- Do we think you know enough to make a good/healthy/safe choice? One we would be happy to live with tomorrow, next week, the future? If not, what would we like to know?
- Could we have made decisions earlier that would have stopped us getting into this sort of situation? What would they have been?
- Suppose things didn't go according to what we intended and we realise we have made a bad choice. Who could we talk to about it?
- Imagine we could see into the future and change it. If we could see ourselves in this situation, what would we say and do differently now?
- Imagine we could split ourselves into two and take an invisible 'us' with us. What advice would we give ourselves?
- Imagine we could take anyone we want with us invisibly – someone who you know would be really good in a situation like this. Who would it be? You don't have to say – but you know who it is. Your best friend? A member of your family? A character you admire from a book/film/soap (they don't have to be real)? A favourite musician, singer or sports person? (Perhaps even your pet!) What is it about that person that gives you confidence in them? What are they like? How do they see things? What can they do? What advice would they give you to say and do?
- Could we be held responsible/accountable for anything? Who might hold us responsible/accountable? What might be the consequences of that responsibility?

If you do take students into the future, especially if it is sensitive, it is important to bring them back into the present. Try:

Of course, right here and now in the classroom that isn't really happening. However, you may find it helpful to keep with you some of what you have learned in that imaginary situation you have been exploring. It may be helpful in real life in the future.

If you want to use this opportunity to increase or reconnect students with factual information, it is important to use appropriate language. First say, 'Let's stop the story at this point and let's add something …' Then use one of the following, each of which is subtly different:

1 *You now know, or perhaps you already knew …*

2 *Imagine you have just discovered … and now you say to yourself 'I know …'*

3 *Imagine telling yourself 'I know …'*

4 *Imagine I told you …*

5 *Imagine someone you trusted told you …*

6 *Imagine you read …*

In points 1–3, the language is 'clean' and encourages thinking that begins 'I know …', which can be very powerful. Ethically we should consider using this type of language very carefully. In points 4–6, the emphasis is on the credibility of the source of the information.

If you are confident that all students in a group are making unwise or dangerous choices, it would be appropriate to ask:

- Now you know … how will this change what you are going to say or do?

If you are not certain, then a softer:

- Now you know ... does this change what you might say or do?

The latter is much safer since it allows students with safe or healthy strategies to retain them.

Exploring students' perceptions

You could also use these scenarios to explore students' perceptions about the behaviour of their peers. As stated in the introduction, students' perceptions can be highly inaccurate yet may act as powerful influences on their thinking and subsequent behaviour. It is therefore really important to challenge any incorrect assumptions you discover:

- Do you think this type of situation happens often?
- What do you think most students would want to do in a situation like this?
- What do you think most students would actually do in a situation like this? (Is there a difference and, if so, why?)

You could open up the issue more widely:

- Do you think that many students of your age (or a little older than you) are making these choices?
- What decision do you believe most students make?
- How common do you think this type of behaviour is among students who are [specify age]?
- What made you think this? (Peers' stories? Overheard conversations? Media?)

Now, if appropriate, offer information or data that may support, clarify or challenge students' perceptions.

- Do you think there might be a difference between what people say and what is really happening? Why?
- Consider this information/data from ... source. Are you confident it is a credible source? Why?
- If you now know ... is the real situation (for example only 'x' per cent of students your age use/do/have ever done/have ever tried ...). How do you feel now? Are you surprised? Reassured? Is this encouraging you to rethink your own choices?
- Knowing most students actually choose ... why do you think they make this choice? Are there reasons that you would agree with/support? Are there some you would challenge?

1.7 Encouraging reflection

The final element of every session or series of sessions should be a series of questions that encourage students to reflect on how they feel about their learning. In order for this to be constructive and for students to feel comfortable about responding, the ground rules and climate will need to be conducive to openness without fear of ridicule. When the pattern of this final activity has become established as a routine and the students expect it, it is more likely to be well used by them and need not take longer than a couple of minutes.

If there is time, invite students to think individually, then share their thoughts with a partner, then perhaps in groups of four. Finally, invite any contributions from the whole class. If not, once the climate is supportive, you may want to move straight to open feedback in the plenary.

The prompts listed below make good starting points, though the content and experience of each session will tend to suggest its own direction for your prompts. The aim of this swift activity is to elicit comments and observations from students, rather than begin a dialogue. It is sufficient simply to thank each student for their comment. However, you may want to note any significant feedback, both as evidence when you come to reflect on or evaluate the session or programme, and as a reminder to follow up any problems or difficulties expressed by individuals.

Inviting feedback

For this heading, your questions only need to be general prompts to invite feedback about the session and the learning that has taken place. This can be a simple way of pinpointing some of the learning both in terms of outcomes and process. If a student says 'I learned …', the very expression of this can crystallise, and effectively reinforce, what has been learned.

One way to streamline the process could be to display a wall poster listing 'standard opening prompts' such as the following:

- Today I learned …
- I already knew …
- I can now …
- I am better at …

Other questions may suggest themselves naturally, and these suggestions are offered simply as examples.

Follow-up questions

- Who had a 'got it!' moment – one of those times when something confusing suddenly makes sense? What did that feel like?
- How useful do you think what you have learned today will be to you? Now? Soon? In the future?
- Who is feeling differently about something as a result of this work?
- Who would offer someone different advice now than they would have done before?
- Who learnt something really surprising – perhaps something they didn't expect? How does that feel?

Identifying problems

- Who got stuck? What did you do next? What does it feel like to get stuck, because we all get stuck every now and again? Getting stuck is great – it means you are just about to learn something new! (*Staying* stuck is the problem!)
- Who felt like giving up? What stopped you from giving up? Who helped you? What did they say or do?
- Who made a real mess of something? Was it the type of mess that you can only clear up, apologise for and try to do it differently next time, or was it the kind of mess that you can go back to and put right?
- Who still has a question that they haven't been able to answer? Who is still wondering or curious about something?
- Does anyone wish they could go back and change something they said or did today?

Support to or from others

- Who has worked with someone else? How did you get on? What did they do that helped you? What did you do that helped them?
- Who has helped someone else to learn something today? What did you do that helped?

1.8 Evaluation and assessment

Evaluation in PSHE education is notoriously difficult. It is easy to test a person's knowledge, but knowledge alone may have little impact on beliefs and behaviour; skills and attitude of mind are more crucial factors. Assessment is slightly different from evaluation, in that it is more a judgement of how well we are doing.

Evaluating the success of your sessions

Technically, it is impossible to 'evaluate' meaningfully unless you know what you are setting out to achieve. This means the session purpose needs to be clear to both you and your students. One way of doing this is to start with some statements of intent. Although a little contrived, the following statements 'Walt', 'Tib', 'Wilf' and 'Oli' can be useful:

- **W**e **a**re **l**earning **t**o …
- **T**his **is b**ecause …
- **W**hat **I** am **l**ooking **f**or is …
- **O**ur **l**earning **i**ntention is …*

While we may not want to start each lesson mechanically with these questions, it is reasonable for both the teacher and the learners to be clear about the intended purpose of the session, even if it subsequently takes on a direction of its own.

We, as teachers, also need to reflect on the impact of our work, and receiving feedback from our learners is essential. What we can glean from the simple observation of students is limited; a fuller and more valuable impression about their skills, feelings, beliefs, attitudes, values and sense of identity can only be gained if we also consult them and listen carefully to what they are willing to tell us.

Sometimes a single lesson, or even a moment (the *ah-ha* moment) in a lesson, can have a profound and immediate effect on an individual's thinking. Sometimes change is the result of an accumulation of a number of different experiences that gradually build skills or personal qualities. Change can also be a combination of the two, a gradual accumulation of experiences or influences with a final experience that triggers significant change.

* Devised by the Gillingham Partnership Formative Assessment Project under the leadership of Shirley Clarke.

The most important people to reflect on what they are learning and how they are changing are the students themselves. The invitations provided in this resource offer one useful tool to enable this to happen. Simply looking at what you thought, knew or felt before a session or module and what you think, know and feel after can be illuminating.

- Have I learned a lot or a little?
- Has the 'lot' I learned been significant for me?
- Has the 'little' I learned been a critical piece of learning, the one thing that could really make a difference?
- Have I been reminded of things or strategies I already knew but have forgotten, previously thought irrelevant, or not realised that they might be transferable to this new situation?

If students are to be asked to evaluate their own development, they need help to assess their starting points. Surprisingly, simply asking people to put themselves on a scale can offer an insight into their perceptions of their existing skills and knowledge. (Note: Because this is a personal assessment against personal criteria you can't compare different people's rankings.) As we learn, our assessment of ourselves may prove overly optimistic, accurate or overly pessimistic.

- If I asked you, on a scale of 1–10, how confident you feel you are to deal with …
- If someone asked for your advice concerning … would you feel very, reasonably, a little, or not at all confident that you could accurately advise them?

If someone initially finds this difficult, try, 'If you *did* know where on the scale to put yourself, where would it be?'

At the end of a module or session, simply invite the students to see whether they feel they have moved on the scale. Moving down the scale is not always negative; it may mean students have had a sudden insight into the real complexity of an issue they had previously thought simple.

One of the simplest evaluation tools used in the 'invitations' is a sheet of clouds, or 'think bubbles', each containing a prompt. These prompts could include a selection from those that encourage internal reflection:

- One thing/Things I know now that I didn't know before is/are …
- One question/Questions I still have is/are …
- Something(s) I want/need to find out more about is/are …
- One thing/Things this session has made me think about is/are …
- Something(s) this session made me think about again, reminded me of is/are …
- Something(s) I will remember to do/say is/are …
- One thing/Things I feel differently about is/are … because …
- One thing/Things that have really shocked me/surprised me is/are …
- One thing/Things I would want everyone else to know is/are …
- One thing/Things I am now concerned about is/are …
- One thing/Things I would like to change in myself, my school, my community, my world is/are …
- One thing/Things I am going to do/say differently now is/are …
- One thing/Things I really enjoyed is/are …
- Something(s) I will say now that I wouldn't have said before is/are …

- Something(s) I now feel more confident about is/are …
- Something(s) I will now do differently is/are …
- Something(s) I would like to learn more about is/are …
- Something(s) I feel clearer about is/are …
- Something(s) I now feel confident I could advise others about is/are …

Some prompts can encourage reflection on what we feel willing to share and what we want to keep inside ourselves:

- Something(s) I am happy to share with others is/are …
- Something(s) I want to keep private to me is/are …

If group work was involved, some prompts reflect on the process:

- Our group worked well together because …
- Our group could have worked better if …
- I contributed to my group by …
- Next time, I would encourage our group to …
- It was really helpful when … did …
- I found it hard to express disagreement with the group's view about …
- I felt safe enough to express my opinion, even when I thought everyone else in the group wouldn't agree …

Finally, some prompts offer feedback on the learning to the teacher or facilitator:

- If I could have changed something in this session, it would have been … because …
- One thing I would like the session leader to know is …
- I really found … useful/helpful/interesting
- When we did … it really helped me to …

Many evaluations simply reflect on a single lesson or module and only look back, rather than reflect on what has happened in order to help shape the future. The critical questions are, 'How, through learning this, am I changing?' and 'What will be the difference as a result of this change?'

As time goes by, it is also interesting to offer students an opportunity to reflect on their own reflections, for example at the end of a term, year, or even years later. Do they still feel the same? Did they make new decisions or answer their questions? Did they say and do the things they said they would? Are they still confident?

Assessment

Assessment looks at how well students are doing, and the questions above can help with this. Others might include:

- Did I get all I needed from this session or module?
- Am I as good as I need to be at this skill?
- Can I imagine myself being able to do/say this when I need to?
- Do I think I need to work harder at …?
- Do I really know enough about …?
- Do I have the confidence I need in order to …?

There are many ways of recording work in PSHE education. The purpose of building portfolios of work is, however, to help students reflect on how they are changing and developing.

Although PSHE education is a valuable way of helping improve literacy skills, it is important that assessment focuses on personal and social development. It is better to encourage rich reflections, even if poorly written and spelt, than responses that, while grammatically correct, fail to capture the students' reflections adequately.

It is important to gather this data together in order for teachers to be able to reflect on the quality of their PSHE provision:

- Did we provide what we said we would?
- Were all students actively engaged? If not, who wasn't?
- Does feedback from the students tell us they have felt involved and active during the sessions?
- Have the students appreciated the opportunities the sessions have represented?
- Did I cover the pathways I had planned for this term/year?
- Does feedback from the students confirm the relevance for them of the sessions that were conducted?

A similar line could be taken with sessions conducted by visitors.

External review and feedback

While self-evaluation and self-assessment are at the core of PSHE, opportunities to discover how others perceive us and how they feel we are growing and changing are required. This external feedback can be from adults such as teachers, youth workers, parents/carers or from a young person's own trusted peers.

Peer feedback is very powerful and has the potential to be damaging, and so it needs a clear structure and ground rules. The first rule is that the recipient must be willing to receive it. There also needs to be clarity about the exact focus of any feedback. The peer offering feedback needs to be insightful and considered in their views and opinions about their fellow student, and sensitive and supportive when offering feedback. As a general rule, feedback should either validate the positive or offer positive alternatives to areas that could be developed. However, sometimes it is important to know when our comments or actions have challenged someone (which may be a positive outcome) or distressed them (which may be less so). The following tips may be useful.

Tips for giving feedback

● **Start with the positive.**

Launching straight in with even gentle criticism may be hard for the receiver to take, and may make them feel defensive.

● **Point out things that can be changed, and give examples.**

There's no point mentioning things the recipient can do nothing about – like their height, or where they live! Mentioning a specific example can help focus on behaviour that might be improved or usefully reflected on. Try to say in what way something was (supportive, unhelpful, thoughtless, etc.) rather than just 'good' or 'bad'.

● **Offer alternatives.**

Suggest other ways of dealing with a situation where possible.

● **Own the feedback.**

Be open that it's only the giver's opinion – not necessarily everyone's view.

● **Leave the recipient with a choice.**

There's little point issuing orders – instead, suggest changes in a way that puts the receiver in charge of deciding what to do, perhaps exploring likely consequences of repeating the behaviour or following suggested alternatives.

The following prompts can help:

● I found it helpful when you said …
● I found it helpful when you did …
● Your presentation was helpful because …
● I would have found your presentation even more helpful if you had …
● I would like to have known more about …
● I found it really interesting when you said/asked/did …
● I found it challenging/difficult when you said/did …
● When you said/did … I noticed … happened afterwards.
● I felt you were becoming more …
● When we work in groups, I find the way you … is helpful.
● I think you demonstrated this skill when you …
● I think it might have been more helpful if you had …

Tips for receiving feedback

● **Listen!**

Feedback, particularly criticism, can feel uncomfortable, but it may be useful to listen carefully rather than jumping in with a defence or argument. If the giver seems mistaken, you'll have a chance to say so. If necessary, ask the giver to explain and expand so you are first clear what they are saying (and seeing).

● **Check it out!**

OK, so it's one person's view. Checking with others can help you discover whether your giver's feedback is a minority view, or is generally shared.

● **Ask for what you don't get.**

Want feedback on something particular? Ask for it.

- **Decide what to do.**

  If any criticism you get seems right, decide what to do about it. Can you change?

- **Thank the giver!**

  If you have had honest feedback, genuinely given and meant, thank the giver, even if it was hard for you to hear. They may offer you feedback again. If you seem not to appreciate it, it may be harder to get feedback the next time you need it.

Involving students in assessment, recording and reporting

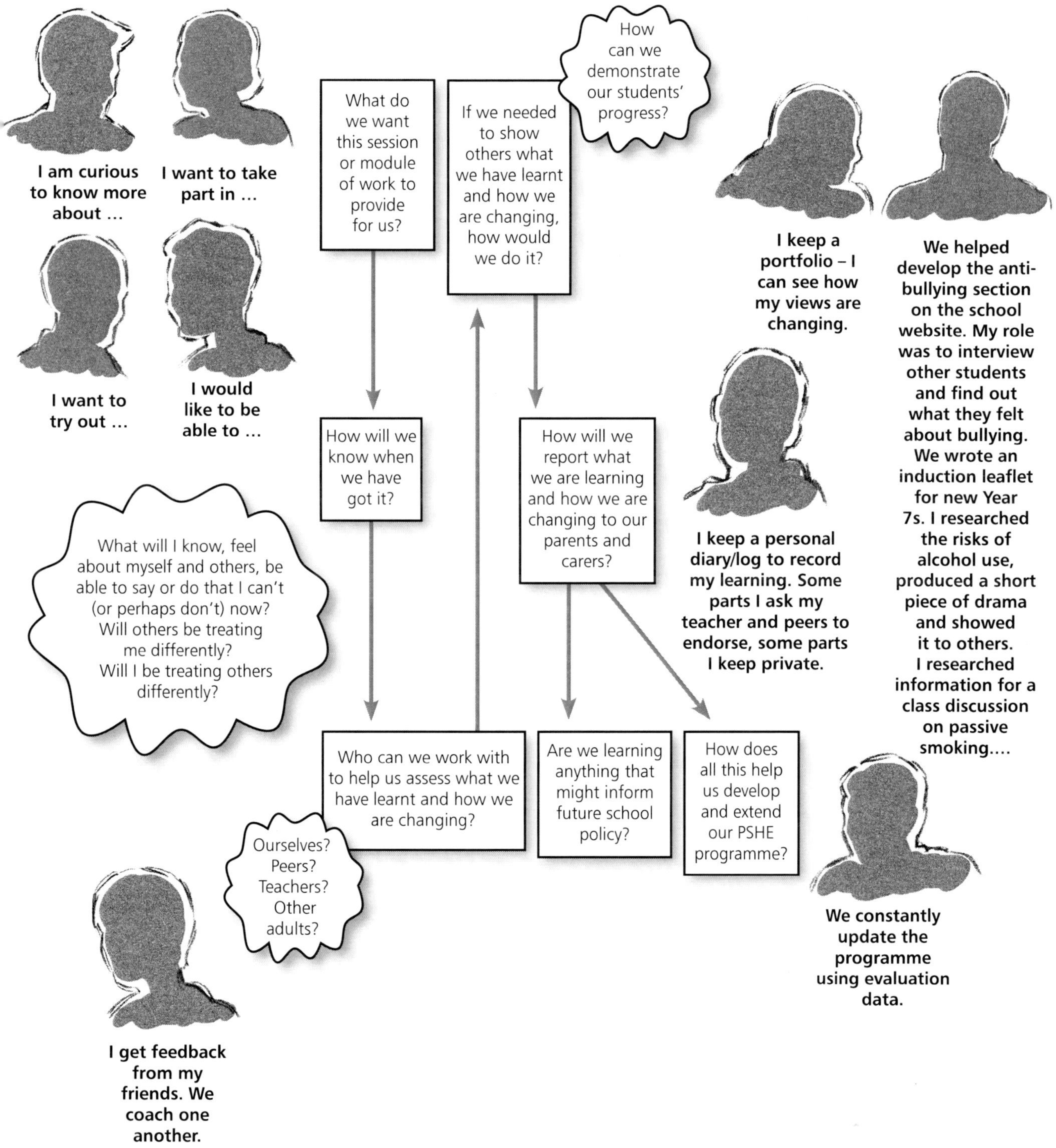

I am curious to know more about …

I want to take part in …

I want to try out …

I would like to be able to …

What will I know, feel about myself and others, be able to say or do that I can't (or perhaps don't) now? Will others be treating me differently? Will I be treating others differently?

What do we want this session or module of work to provide for us?

If we needed to show others what we have learnt and how we are changing, how would we do it?

How can we demonstrate our students' progress?

How will we know when we have got it?

How will we report what we are learning and how we are changing to our parents and carers?

I keep a portfolio – I can see how my views are changing.

We helped develop the anti-bullying section on the school website. My role was to interview other students and find out what they felt about bullying. We wrote an induction leaflet for new Year 7s. I researched the risks of alcohol use, produced a short piece of drama and showed it to others. I researched information for a class discussion on passive smoking….

I keep a personal diary/log to record my learning. Some parts I ask my teacher and peers to endorse, some parts I keep private.

Who can we work with to help us assess what we have learnt and how we are changing?

Ourselves? Peers? Teachers? Other adults?

Are we learning anything that might inform future school policy?

How does all this help us develop and extend our PSHE programme?

We constantly update the programme using evaluation data.

I get feedback from my friends. We coach one another.

Part 2

2.1 Using the Smith family in your PSHE sessions

Health for Life 15–16 continues to follow the Smith family. As in the previous resource, the characters in this fictional family take students into situations where members of the family will witness or face dilemmas or choices.

The use of these characters places a little distance between a sensitive situation and the students. As before, and if appropriate, that distance can then be gradually reduced by taking the student into the scenario, initially as a third person who can offer advice, 'Supposing they asked you "what should I do?", what would you say?' and eventually into the first person, 'Now imagine this is happening to you.'

The first critical questions to ask about a scenario might be: 'How do you think they are feeling right now?' and 'What do you think those feelings might be encouraging them to do?' These questions offer a starting point for exploring the events that might have led to this moment and what might happen next, soon, and in the future.

Changing the names and family structure

In this family, Emma and Josh will continue to be in the same year as the students and their older brother and sister, Hannah and Jack, will once again be confronting issues that lie two years ahead. If you think students may not relate to this family, either in terms of personality, dilemmas, choices or structure, you can change it, editing the names and family structure to suit your own context. For this reason, the family is included on the CD-ROM, which you can edit.

Each session starts with members of the family facing a situation or choice. Once again, all these scenarios are included on the CD-ROM, so that you can edit them to ensure that they are relevant to your students' context.

The Smith family tree

All names and the family structure in this family tree are suggestions only. You may well wish to change them to ensure that they are relevant to young people or, even better, constructed by the young people themselves.

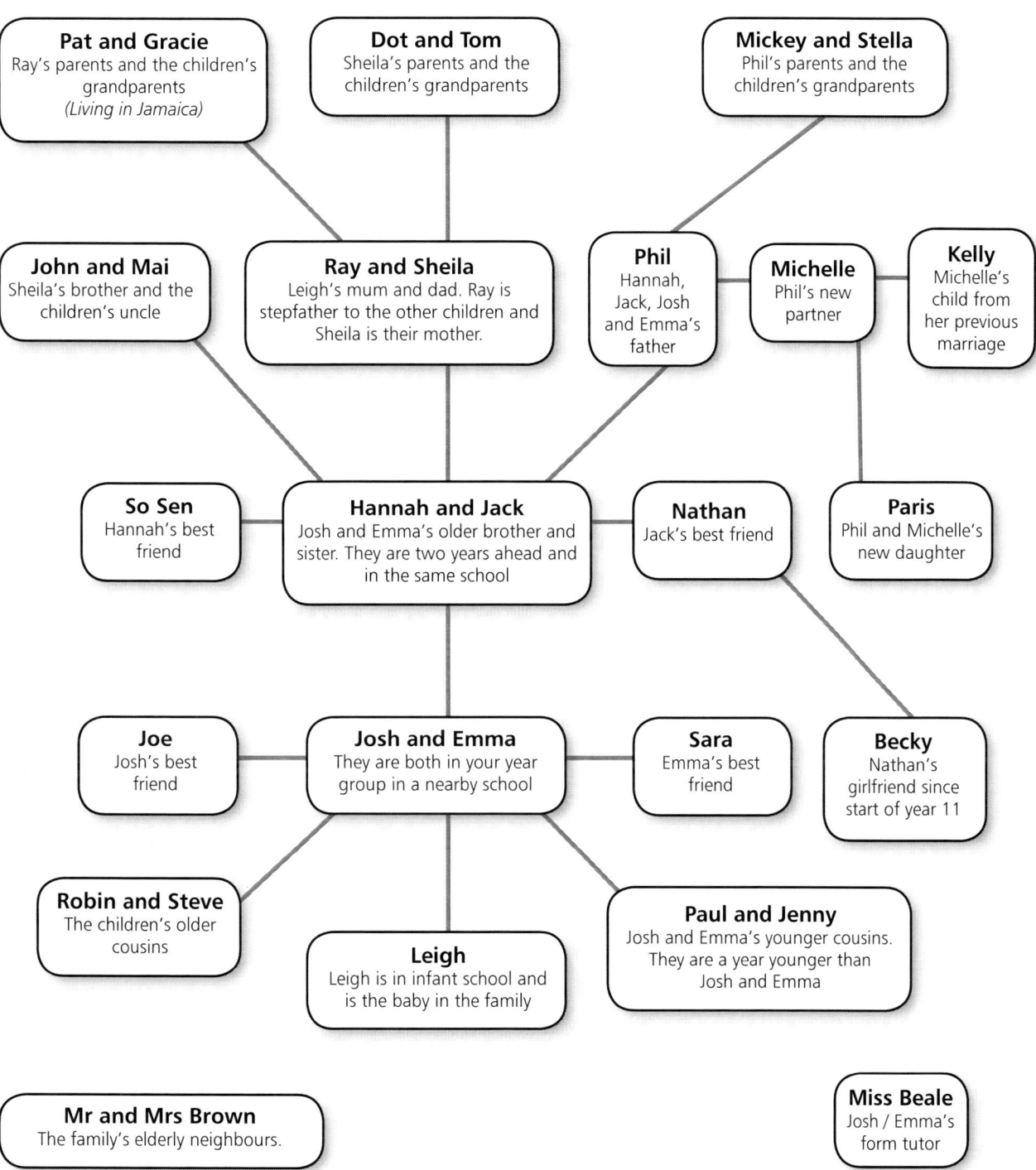

Pat and Gracie
Ray's parents and the children's grandparents
(Living in Jamaica)

Dot and Tom
Sheila's parents and the children's grandparents

Mickey and Stella
Phil's parents and the children's grandparents

John and Mai
Sheila's brother and the children's uncle

Ray and Sheila
Leigh's mum and dad. Ray is stepfather to the other children and Sheila is their mother.

Phil
Hannah, Jack, Josh and Emma's father

Michelle
Phil's new partner

Kelly
Michelle's child from her previous marriage

So Sen
Hannah's best friend

Hannah and Jack
Josh and Emma's older brother and sister. They are two years ahead and in the same school

Nathan
Jack's best friend

Paris
Phil and Michelle's new daughter

Joe
Josh's best friend

Josh and Emma
They are both in your year group in a nearby school

Sara
Emma's best friend

Becky
Nathan's girlfriend since start of year 11

Robin and Steve
The children's older cousins

Leigh
Leigh is in infant school and is the baby in the family

Paul and Jenny
Josh and Emma's younger cousins. They are a year younger than Josh and Emma

Mr and Mrs Brown
The family's elderly neighbours.

Miss Beale
Josh / Emma's form tutor

Recording frame for session planning

Dates	
Content box Which content box(es) do I want to focus on?	
Concepts What concepts am I introducing or developing?	
Skills What key skills am I developing or rehearsing?	
Content What content/key factual information am I introducing or revisiting?	
Target language What vocabulary do I want students to acquire or practise using?	
What curriculum opportunity am I providing? How am I organising the learning?	
Pre-teach for next session What do I want students to be thinking about, researching and/or bringing to the next session?	
Reflection and evaluation How did this session go? Do I need to make changes? What will I do differently next time?	

Year 10 themes and pathways

The content boxes shown in bold have been expanded into suggested sessions.

Theme 1 – Focus on changing relationships

Pathway		Content boxes					
1	How am I now?	G1	G2	G4	G5	G6	G9
2	Me and my friends	G7	G13	**G14**			
3	Me and my skills	**G3**	G10	**G15**	**G17**		
4	Me and my responsibilities	**G11**	G12	G8	G16		

Theme 2 – Focus on me as a learner

Pathway		Content boxes				
1	Me in focus	L1	L2	L7	L10	
2	Managing interruptions	L9	L12			
3	Looking ahead	L3	L8	L11		
4	Making it count	L4	L5	L6		

Theme 3 – Focus on economic wellbeing and the world of work

Pathway		Content boxes				
1	What it's all for	W1	W10	W3	W2	
2	The financial deal	W5	W7	W8	W9	
3	Worth thinking about ...	W4	W6	W11	W12	

Theme 4 – Focus on health and healthy futures

Pathway		Content boxes				
1	Making the most of healthy me	H1	H2	H3	H4	H12
2	Being OK, staying OK	**H5**	H7	H8	H10	
3	Knowing and feeling	H6	H9	H11	H13	

Theme 5 – Focus on managing my health, risk and keeping myself safe

Pathway		Content boxes					
1	Risky feeling	**K1**	K2	K3	K16		
2	Weighing it up	K5	K6	K7	K14	K15	
3	Cyber health	**K8**	**K9**	**K10**	K11	K12	
4	In my defence	K4	**K13**				

Theme 6 – Focus on drugs

Pathway		Content boxes					
1	A view of drugs	D1	D2	D3	D6	D7	D14
2	The facts and so much more	D5	D8	**D9**	D10	D16	D17
3	Let's consider others	D12	D15	D18			
4	In the long term	D11	D13	D19			
5	Help!	D4	D20				

Theme 7 – Focus on relationships and sex education

Pathway		Content boxes					
1	Reality check	R1	R2	R3	**R7**	R17	R18	R27
2	I've never felt this way before	R4	R5	R6	R19	**R20**	R25
3	Avoiding the avoidable	R9	R10	R11	R12	**R13**	**R15**	R16
4	The issues are so complicated	**R21**	R22	R23	R24	R27	
5	So what else should I know?	R8	**R14**	**R26**			

Theme 8 – Focus on managing stress

Pathway		Content boxes					
1	Know thine enemy	**S1**	**S2**	S3	S5		
2	Can I manage?	**S4**	S6	S7	S8		

Becoming everything I can be	Enriching a healthy and safe lifestyle	Managing my changing relationships

Focus on changing relationships

Becoming everything I can be	Enriching a healthy and safe lifestyle	Managing my changing relationships
G1 Is there anything about me I want to leave behind as I move into the senior part of the school? Are there changes I want to make in me, things I want to do differently?	**G9** Has my view of a healthy lifestyle changed? How would I describe a healthy lifestyle? Can I learn from examples of healthy and unhealthy lifestyles in those around me? How do I rate or rank my lifestyle? How do others rate it?	**G12** Do I believe everyone, including me, has a right to feel physically and emotionally safe? How much responsibility do I have in this?
G2 How do I think others see me? What do others think I am good at? How do I feel about what they think? Are there parts of me I think I should change, or things I should do differently?	**G10** How do I manage communication technology? What are the advantages of communication technology? How would my life change if it all stopped working? Are there any disadvantages? (For example, cost, being always 'available', use of webcams and the ease of being online.)	**G13** How do I feel about my friendships? Am I part of a group or 'gang'? Do my friends expect me or others to behave in certain ways or do certain things to be accepted by, or remain part of, the group? What are the possible good and not-so-good consequences to me of doing these things? Am I OK with this? If I am not OK with this, what can I do about it?
G3 Do I recognise that I have an inner 'parent' who can make judgements and tell me what I *ought* to do? Do I recognise that I have an inner 'child' that can tell me what I *want* to have or do? Do I recognise I have an inner 'adult' that can make sense of these child and parent voices and help me decide when to listen to them, when to ignore them and when to mediate between them?	**G11** What do I know about my rights and responsibilities? As I become older, what rights do I have? How do I feel about complaining when I feel I have been treated unfairly? Do I have the skills to express my rights assertively when they are abused, or not recognised?	**G14** How good am I at negotiating a friendly outcome with people I speak to or challenge? How good am I at standing my ground when it would be easier to just go along with a suggestion or idea I don't like?
G4 How am I becoming more independent? What can I do now that I couldn't do last year?		**G15** Can I recognise when I am putting myself, or others are putting me, under pressure to obey 'unwritten rules' or social norms? Can I recognise when it is appropriate to follow a group or society's 'unwritten rules' and when following them could put me at risk?
G5 Am I meeting more people? Am I spending more time on my own or with my friends?		
G6 How would I describe my personality? (For example, risk taker, cautious, friendly, empathic, submissive, assertive, aggressive.) How might these characteristics affect my relationships with others?		
G7 Do I have a strong network of people who can help me? Do I need to expand this network to include new people?		

Becoming everything I can be	Enriching a healthy and safe lifestyle	Managing my changing relationships
G8 Do I have someone who I know I can talk to and who will be able and willing to support and help me, no matter how bad things might become and no matter what I might have done? Am I willing to help friends who need support? What do I need in order to be able to do this well? Can I put a friend in contact with professional help if needed?		G16 As I become more independent, what responsibilities do I have towards others? How will I feel if others I am with encourage me, dare me or all decide to do something that I suspect or know is criminal? How will I feel if I am caught? What would my friends or family feel? If I don't want to, what could I say and do? What if they all agree to do something I don't want to do or feel is wrong?
		G17 How do I feel about sudden changes in my relationships? How do I feel about loss or bereavement that might happen or will happen in my future? How well have I managed past losses and bereavements?

Focus on me as a learner

L1 Am I still learning as well as I can? Do I need to change anything in the way I learn? How is my organisation? Am I still motivated or are other things distracting me? Can I make compromises between my leisure interests and my school work? Do I see what I am doing at school as relevant to my future?	L7 Is my style of learning changing? Are new sources of information becoming available to me? How am I accessing, evaluating the value of and using different sources of information? Am I able to think up my own questions and carry out research on my own? How do I organise my time, especially on coursework?	L10 How good am I at managing my work/life balance? How good am I at knowing when I need to adjust the balance, for example in the run up to examinations or important coursework?
L2 How good am I at receiving constructive feedback? How good am I at ignoring inappropriate criticism or put downs? Am I able to ask questions when I don't understand something? Am I able to keep asking until I do understand?	L8 How do I feel about examinations? Am I able to manage my emotional state to make sure I can perform to my full potential in examinations?	L11 How am I getting on when working with other people? Do I get on well with others? Can I work well as part of a team? Can I take responsibility within a team? Can I take a leadership role? Can I provide constructive feedback to others? Can I compromise with others? Can I help others who disagree with one another to reach a compromise? Can I follow others' instructions? How do I feel about working with others who I may not have met before? Can I tell them when I don't understand?
L3 What am I trying to achieve? Are my goals or aspirations changing? What am I really good at? Are my strengths changing? What choices will I have this year? What choices do I think I will make and why? If I make those choices, what might be the long-term consequences or benefits?	L9 Do I know who I can talk to and when, where and what to say if I feel stressed about my work or anything else that might be worrying me?	L12 How good am I at managing others who try to disrupt my learning, either individually or as part of a group?
L4 How do I organise my approach to any coursework or modular tests? How do I plan my time? How good am I at keeping to my time plan?		
L5 How is my expertise in studying and revising effectively continuing to develop? Am I able to motivate myself to study and revise? How good am I at recording, recalling and applying what I have learnt?		

Becoming everything I can be	Enriching a healthy and safe lifestyle	Managing my changing relationships
L6 Do I need to make changes in my approach to learning or revising as a result of mock or practice examinations? Do I need to change my focus; do I need to alter my priorities?		

Focus on economic wellbeing and the world of work

W1 What am I looking for in a future career? What is important to me? Do I want a challenge and, if so, what type: safety; rapid change; or stability? Do I want to work on my own or with people, doing the same thing or different things? How do I balance having an enjoyable career with the rewards it brings? Are there areas of work I want to know more about?	W5 Do I know how to set a personal budget? Do I understand the difference between 'gross' and 'net' pay? Do I understand the term 'stoppages'? Do I understand 'income tax' and 'national insurance'? How do I feel about budgeting? Do I know who can help me if I need accurate, trustworthy support and advice with managing my finances?	W10 What do I understand by the terms 'enterprise', 'employment', 'career', 'job', 'profession', 'self-employment' and 'voluntary work'?
W2 What am I prepared to do to get the type of future employment I want and/or the rewards it brings?	W6 Do I understand my rights as a consumer? How do I feel about exercising those rights?	W11 What qualities do I have that make me employable? What skills and qualities can I clearly demonstrate to others? What skills or qualities do I need to develop? How will I market myself in an application or interview for a future college place, career or job?
W3 Is it OK if I don't yet know what I want to do when I leave school?	W7 Do I understand the full range of risks of getting into debt? Do I know how to evaluate a potential source of a future loan? Do I understand what happens to people who cannot repay their loans?	W12 If I need help with exploring future career choices, do I know who can offer information and guidance?
W4 What experiences and skills do I have, what responsibilities have I held that might give me a competitive advantage over others applying for a similar position in employment or further education? What could I do to increase these? In school? Out of school?	W8 Do I understand the term 'credit rating'? Do I understand how my credit rating can affect my life?	
	W9 Do I understand how apparently small differences in interest rates can have huge implications on the cost of borrowing money and the time it will take me to repay a debt?	

Focus on health and healthy futures

H1 What new choices do I have? What new opportunities and responsibilities do I have for myself? What if these choices relate to the use of drugs, sexual activity or other risky activity?	H6 How good am I at judging whether a source of health information is accurate or reliable? How can I be confident that a source of information can be trusted, and to what degree?	H11 Do I know how to access my doctor, a nurse or a clinic? Do I know how to book an appointment?
H2 What do I understand by 'self-esteem'? Who or what helps to build my self-esteem; who or what lowers it? To what extent am I responsible for my own self-esteem? How can I build, restore and reinforce it? Am I attractive? How can I find out?	H7 Do I understand the impact of being both over and under weight on my physical, emotional and social health? Do I know what would be a healthy weight for me? Does it matter if I am not exactly my perfect weight? Is it OK to be a little under or overweight?	H12 How are the images from the media influencing me and my health choices? Do I understand how images of people in magazines can be manipulated to be attractive but actually unrealistic and unachievable? Am I being manipulated into deciding what 'attractive' means?

Becoming everything I can be	Enriching a healthy and safe lifestyle	Managing my changing relationships
H3 What do I understand by the concept 'self-image'? How do I see myself? How do I think others see me? How do I feel about my self-image? What or who influences my feelings? Do I compare myself to others? Who? Why? How do these comparisons make me feel?	H8 Do I understand the difference between a 'balanced diet' and 'dieting'?	H13 How do I feel about mental illness in other people? Do I understand the most common mental illnesses? Do I understand what they say and how they behaviour is related to their illness and may be beyond their control? What do I feel when I see or meet people with mental illness?
H4 If I want to change my self-image, how do I balance what is achievable and what isn't? How do I feel about this? Is looking after or changing my self-image making me feel good or miserable? How do I feel about getting help if I (or I feel someone else) need(s) support?	H9 As I get older, what medical check-ups do I need to have regularly? (For example, the dentist, optician, health screenings.) How do I feel about these check-ups?	
H5 Do I understand the importance of sleep – especially at my age? Do I understand that lack of sleep will influence my moods, my physiology and my ability to learn and recall? How do I feel about staying up later? How do I feel when others encourage me to stay up late? How do I feel when my parents or carers want me to go to sleep?	H10 Do I know where I need to take a prescription for a medication to be made up? Do I understand how important it is to follow the dosage exactly and, if appropriate (in the case of antibiotics), to complete the full course of the treatment even if I now feel completely recovered?	

Focus on managing my health, risk and keeping myself safe

K1 What are my feelings about risk? How are they changing? Do I feel more confident about doing things I haven't done before? How do I assess risk? When do I find risk exciting? Do I understand that I can take risks with both my body and my feelings? How do I balance this with my need to stay safe?	K5 What new opportunities do I have? Do these bring any new risks that I need to think about? To what new places am I going? Do these bring new risks? What sensible precautions do I take to stay as safe as I can?	K13 Why do I think some people carry weapons when they go out? How do I feel about people carrying weapons? What are the risks to themselves and others if they choose to carry a weapon? Have I ever felt the need to carry a weapon?
K2 Do I think about how others might feel about risks I might be taking? Is it OK for them to feel like this? Do I have a responsibility to protect their feelings?	K6 How do I feel about the difference between 'dangerous', 'risky' and 'challenging'? As I get older and have more skills, knowledge and control, are the risks of some activities decreasing or increasing? How realistic is my assessment of my knowledge, control and skills? Are some decisions or activities still just as dangerous?	K14 When I go out alone or with others, during the day or during the evening, how do I plan to manage any possible risks?
K3 Am I still sensitive to the early warning signs my brain and body give me when I need to pay attention to people or situations that might hurt my body or my feelings? (For example, 'butterflies' in my stomach or a raised heart beat.) Do I know when it is important to follow these feelings and when it may be necessary to manage or overcome them? Can I avoid or manage stressful situations?	K7 How do I balance the possible benefits or rewards against the risks? Are some risks worth taking because of the potential benefits or rewards?	K15 Am I 'tuned in' to developing risks around me? How good am I at assessing how serious the risks around me are to me physically or to my feelings, and how good am I at finding ways to avoid them before they become dangerous?
	K8 Do I understand how I might be at risk from my own use and other people's use of communication technology? Do I understand that once material, including images, is uploaded to the internet, it can be there for ever? How do I feel about this?	K16 How are my assertiveness skills developing? Can I find the words I need when I want? Can I balance what I want with what others want in a way that makes me feel comfortable? Can I walk away when a compromise would leave me feeling worried or uncomfortable?

Becoming everything I can be	Enriching a healthy and safe lifestyle	Managing my changing relationships
K4 How do I balance the really serious things that are perhaps unlikely to happen with the less serious things that may be more likely? (Big risk, small risk, serious risk.)	**K9** Do I understand how to use webcams safely? Do I understand how to use online communication safely, especially communicating within online communities – 'social networking' sites? Do I understand the risks of physically meeting people only previously 'met' online? **K10** Do I understand the term 'cyber-bullying'? Do I understand how technology, for example texting, telephone calls, e-mail, chat rooms, instant messaging, personal websites and blogs, pictures and video clips captured on mobile phones can all be used for bullying? Do I think this is the same as, or different from, any other type of bullying? Why? How might people feel who experience bullying like this? What might they do? Who would be responsible? What do I feel about this type of bullying? Do I know how to get specialist support if I experience cyber-bullying? K11 Do I understand how my 'identity' can be 'stolen' by others using information technology? Why do I think people might do this? How do I feel about this? If I think that this has happened to me, do I know where and how to get help? If someone's identity can be 'stolen' and be used and abused by others, how do I feel about any information about a person that might be on the web? K12 Do I know that internet 'providers' record all the websites people visit? Do I know that downloading or sharing some material or images is a very serious criminal offence and can lead to prosecution? (For example copyright material, terrorist material and pornographic material, especially child pornography.)	
Becoming everything I can be	Enriching a healthy and safe lifestyle	Managing my changing relationships

Becoming everything I can be	Enriching a healthy and safe lifestyle	Managing my changing relationships

Focus on drugs

D1 What do I remember from previous education or learning about drug use? How do I feel now about the use of drugs, especially when tobacco, alcohol and illegal substances are the cause of so many health and social problems?	D5 Do I understand that medicines contain drugs that change what is happening inside us? Do I understand how to use prescription medicines and over-the-counter medicines safely? Do I understand why a course of antibiotic medicine should always be completed? Do I feel confident I know when to accept medicines and when it may be sensible to reject them?	D14 What do I think others around me feel now about drug use? Do I think people of my age are using alcohol or tobacco more regularly? What do I feel about this? Am I right? How can I find out? Are my views on the consequences changing? Do I think anyone of my age has tried any illegal drugs or solvents? What do I feel about this? How can I find a true picture?
D2 Are my views changing? As I get older am I revising my view of new risks and consequences for my own drug use? Am I confident that I know enough to be able to manage invitations to go out with others to places where drinking alcohol and other drug use might be involved?	D6 What new questions do I have about alcohol and drug use? How do I feel about non-medicinal drugs being easily available? Can I recognise the most commonly available drugs, their effects on people's physical systems, and the social and legal consequences of their possession, dealing and use?	D15 Do I know how the use of alcohol can change people's behaviour? Do I know how this could affect or be a risk to them, to me and my relationships with others, including my friends, family and school?
D3 Why do I think we hear so much about illegal drugs in the media, on the news and in films?	D7 What might be the possible health and social risks of using performance enhancing drugs in sports? What do I feel about drug use in sports?	D16 Do I understand how my own and others' use of alcohol, cannabis and other substances can seriously affect my ability to keep myself and others safe?
D4 If I, or others close to me, experienced problems with drug use, do I know who is available to support me? Do I know what will happen if I get support? Do I know what can be and can't be kept confidential by different sources of support? How do I feel about getting support if I need it?	D8 What do I know, or remember, about alcohol? Do I understand the effects alcohol has on my brain and the health and social risks I might be running as a alcohol drinker in the short and long term?	D17 Do I understand that many substances affect our ability to assess the effect they are having on us? Do I know that if we use substances, we can be affected and not realise? Do I understand that very small amounts of many substances can affect our ability to make safe judgements and split-second decisions, especially those involved in driving a car, riding a bike or crossing the road? Do I understand that our ability to make judgements and split-second decisions can be impaired by some substances long before it becomes obvious to anyone, even the person who has consumed the substance?
	D9 What do I understand by the term 'binge drinking'? Why do I think some people choose to binge drink? Do I understand the health and social risks to my personal safety of binge drinking?	D18 How will I manage if I am offered a lift in a car or on a bike being driven by someone who I believe might have consumed alcohol or drugs?
	D10 What do I understand by the term 'drink spiking'? Do I know how to guard myself against someone who might spike my drink?	
	D11 Do I know that mixing drugs, including using drugs with alcohol, can be a potentially lethal combination?	

Becoming everything I can be	Enriching a healthy and safe lifestyle	Managing my changing relationships
	D12 What are my responsibilities when younger pupils ask about drugs, alcohol or tobacco? D13 Do I understand that future employers may have strong policies on employees' recreational drug use, both in the workplace and outside the workplace, and that recreational drug use can have a serious effect on my future career prospects? Do I know that a prosecution involving illegal substances can stop me ever visiting some countries?	D19 What might I feel, how will I manage, and what will I say and do if I am in a situation where I am offered something suspicious or something I don't want to consume? What if it is offered by a friend or someone I really like? D20 If I thought a friend was having difficulties with their drug use, what would I do? Would I know enough to advise them? Would I know how to get them help if they asked me for it?

Focus on relationships and sex education

R1 How are my feelings about relationships changing? If I don't yet have a boyfriend or girlfriend, what do I expect having one will be like? How important is it to have one? Do I feel anxious that 'I can't be attractive' because I don't yet have a boyfriend/girlfriend? R2 What do I feel about what others say they have done or are doing? Do I believe them? How does this affect what I think and do? What do I think about the way relationships are portrayed in the media? Do I think they are realistic? Do I think that I am missing out or that something is wrong? R3 Do I understand that, although it may seem like everyone else is having sex (or is saying they are), in fact most are still not? Do I understand that the number of young people of my age who have experienced sexual intercourse is still low and that, if I haven't, I am normal? R4 How do I talk to someone new that I really like? How do I ask out someone I really like for the first time?	R9 What do I already know about contraception? What questions do I have? What more do I think I need to know? What do I feel about the use of contraception? R10 Do I know how and where to obtain contraception? How do I feel about contraception and how do I feel about obtaining it? Do I understand how to use contraception? Do I understand the difference between methods of contraception that only prevent pregnancy and barrier methods that also minimise infection? R11 What do I already know about sexually transmitted infections? Do I know that some are easy to cure if caught early, while others can only be treated but not cured? What do I know about how to protect myself, reduce the risks and stay healthy? R12 Do I know how to use a condom to ensure I don't put myself or someone else at risk? Would I know what to do if I feared that a condom hadn't worked, and that I or someone else might have been at risk?*	R18 How do I, or others, feel when friends are making new relationships? How does it feel to be the odd one out? R19 How long or well do I have to know someone before I feel it is OK to go out alone with them, allow them to hold my hand, kiss me or touch me more intimately? R20 How do I decide when a relationship is right for me? How do I decide if it isn't? R21 Do I know that I have a right to only do what I feel comfortable with? Do I know that I have a responsibility to protect others' rights to be safe and feel comfortable? R22 If I have been going out with someone for a while, do I know I can always do only what I feel comfortable with? How do I feel if my girlfriend/boyfriend wants to do something I don't feel comfortable with? Am I able to be assertive in order to stay comfortable?

* **Note to teacher:** While condoms are normally an excellent barrier to pregnancy and STIs, they can fail if not used properly, or (rarely) if they are faulty.

Becoming everything I can be	Enriching a healthy and safe lifestyle	Managing my changing relationships
R5 How do I feel about being rejected? How do I deal with embarrassment? How does it feel when others know I really like someone? How does it feel when others know I have been rejected? R6 How do I feel about caring for someone? How do I show that I care for them? How do they show that they care for me? R7 How are my feelings about having a sexual relationship changing? Are they getting stronger? How might my feelings affect what I do? What else could influence me? How do I know when I am ready to begin a sexual relationship with someone, and what does this mean for me? R8 What questions do I still have about sexual behaviour? Are there some things I am not clear about? Are there things I overhear that I want clarified? Do I feel able to ask about what I don't yet know?	R13 Do I feel able to negotiate the use of contraception with a partner? How do I do that? Do I feel able to refuse a sexual advance from someone who refuses to use contraception? R14 What do I know about how the use of alcohol and other drugs might make me vulnerable to others, or change my own ability to make decisions and keep myself safe? R15 Do I know where to obtain 'emergency contraception'? How would I feel about approaching someone to ask for emergency contraception? Do I understand issues of confidentiality? Do I know how quickly emergency contraception has to be used in order for it to be effective? Do I know who to get support and advice from if it has been left too late? R16 Do I understand that no method of contraception is guaranteed to be 100% effective? How would I feel if I felt I should use emergency contraception but my boyfriend didn't feel it was necessary? How would I feel if I felt my girlfriend should use emergency contraception but she didn't want to or feel it to be necessary? R17 What do I remember about the law around sexual activity? Do I believe the law protects me? Do I know my rights? Do I know my responsibilities?	R23 If I feel I have gone too far for me, how do I feel about saying 'no' next time? How would I feel about talking to someone if I was worried? Who would I choose to talk to? Could I trust their advice? Do I understand that I may need help quickly? Do I know how quickly, and why? R24 How do I feel when relationships require compromises? What will I not compromise about? R25 Do I expect relationships to go on, to change or to stop? How do I feel about breaking up with someone I care about? How would I feel if someone I cared about or still care about now wants to be close to someone else? R26 Do I know who I can go to in order to get reliable help and advice about sex or my relationships? How do I know I can feel confident in the advice they offer me? How do I feel about approaching someone to ask for help or advice, especially if they are a professional I have not met before? Do I understand that counsellors will not advise, but will help me find my own way forward? R27 How does my family feel about me becoming an adult and forming new types of relationships? What do they expect from me? Do other people or groups have expectations about how I should behave? How do I feel about that? Do I agree?

Becoming everything I can be	Enriching a healthy and safe lifestyle	Managing my changing relationships

Focus on managing stress

S1 Am I aware of what can cause me unwanted stress (stressors) and how this can affect me? Do I know that stress is something common that affects everybody in some way, and can have both positive and negative effects?	**S4** Do I know how simple changes in my breathing and body posture can actually change the way my brain and body respond to stressors, and help me feel less stressed?	
S2 Am I aware of how this affects me personally? How good am I at recognising unwanted stress in myself (and others)?	**S5** Do I know how important it is to allow myself time to relax and to balance that well with work time? Do I know enough healthy ways to relax?	
S3 Am I sensitive to the early warning signs my brain and body give me when I face potentially stressful situations? (For example, 'butterflies' in my stomach or a raised heartbeat.) Do I know when to follow these feelings and when to manage or overcome them?	**S6** Do I know that physical activity can help me feel less stressed by releasing 'feel-good' chemicals called endorphins, and that it can also reduce some of the health risks of destructive stress?	
	S7 Do I know that, as well as having physical benefits, sufficient rest and healthy eating can also help me feel less stressed?	
	S8 Am I worried about how an important relationship is going? Do I worry about raising sensitive issues with someone who might be able to help me?	

A question of 'parent', 'adult' and 'child'

> **G3**
>
> Do I recognise that I have an inner 'parent' who can make judgements and tell me what I *ought* to do?
>
> Do I recognise that I have an inner 'child' that can tell me what I *want* to have or do?
>
> Do I recognise I have an inner 'adult' that can make sense of these child and parent voices and help me decide when to listen to them, when to ignore them and when to mediate between them?

To the teacher

This is an important session that should be built early into your programme, since the principles will apply in subsequent sessions. As it is quite long and may not fit into one lesson, consider splitting it into two lessons rather than shortening it.

Health for Life 11–14 had a recurring model similar to traffic lights but with two ambers. These stood for *stop, think, think a bit more, now decide. Health for Life 15–16* introduces the model of 'parent', 'adult' and 'child', drawn from transactional analysis. Both of these models may be useful throughout Key Stages 3 and 4.

The idea that the 'parent' *judges*, the 'adult' *considers* and the 'child' *feels* is an over-simplification, but offers a possible model to help explain a young person's conflicting thoughts. You may want to refer to, or distribute, copies of this model (see page **70**) at a suitable point in the session.

Another useful model for talking about feelings is 'redefining' – when we distort the world around us to make it fit what we want to see or do – and 'discounting' – when we deny evidence that doesn't suit us. This session fits well with the sample sessions on unwritten rules (Year 10, G15, page **73**) and groupthink (Year 11, G11, page **135**).

An alternative approach would be to use recorded television material from a drama to illustrate the 'parent', 'adult' and 'child' roles.

To the students

Have you ever been in a situation where you really want to do something, but something is holding you back? Have you ever been in a situation where others want you to do something that looks like fun but that you are uncertain about?

Have you ever made a choice that you knew deep down was risky, but you did it anyway and hoped for the best? Have you ever been aware of a risk, but a voice inside has said 'never mind that, just go for it'?

In this session, we are going to explore two 'models'. A 'model' isn't real, it is just a way of thinking about something that can sometimes help to make sense of what is happening. Think about this scenario; perhaps you have been in a similar situation or found yourself thinking in the same way.

'You know sometimes you can be a real pain,' said Sara. 'You only ever see all the things that could possibly go wrong!'

'No, I don't. I'm just more cautious than you,' Emma replied. She hated it when Sara wanted to do things Emma was fairly certain were risky.

Sara always put having fun right now over 'the possible risk or consequences later'. Mostly, things didn't go wrong or perhaps they had just been lucky and got away with it. There were times when Emma told herself to 'go for it' but another voice told her not to. Was she just sensible enough, or perhaps <u>too</u> sensible? She was a bit afraid that she was too sensible and that she might miss out on lots of things.

Was Sara right, Emma wondered? Was she always seeing risks that either weren't there or were really unlikely? Trouble was, Sara always told everyone she didn't care about the risks right up to the moment when things actually did go wrong. Then Sara would burst into tears and moan about how stupid she had been and swear to the whole world that she would never do anything so stupid again!

Of course she always did.

'You are frightened of getting into trouble, aren't you?' said Sara, standing with her hands on her hips and giving Emma one of her looks. 'Everyone else is up for it. It will be fun!'

'I want to but what if something happens?'

'Not a chance! Are you coming or what?'

Focusing

Everyone can find a 'parent' voice, a 'child' voice and an 'adult' voice inside them if they try. And these voices don't necessarily say the same thing! Both the 'parent' and the 'child' have helpful and unhelpful sides. The 'parent' learns (usually from adults) what it considers 'good' and 'bad'. These judgements *may* not be very sound, though. The 'child' is where feelings live, and the child may want us to rush in, or run away, without much thought. The 'adult' is where a person's main rational thinking takes place, and is where our soundest decisions are made.

Can you identify the loudest voice Emma hears when she decides what to do? And for Sara, is her loudest voice her 'parent', 'adult' or 'child'? It's the adult who is best placed to make decisions, although the adult may have limited knowledge, or may naturally want to be ultra careful. Even so, it's usually better not to allow either the child or the parent voice to dominate. Their advice (caution, exuberance) may or may not be helpful. The adult can consider the evidence.

into action

In pairs, ask the students to think about themselves. Do they recognise 'parent', 'adult' and 'child' voices inside themselves?

- *Is there one voice they generally listen to? Are there any consequences of this?*
- *Does one voice seem louder at different times? For example, is it easier to listen to our 'parent' voice when we are on our own and our 'child' voice when we are with others?*
- *Is it difficult to listen to and act on our 'adult' voice if everyone else we like (and want to like us) is listening to and acting on their 'child'?*

Introduce the ideas of 'redefining' and 'discounting'. Ask students to find if there is evidence of these in the scenario above.

In pairs, consider the following:

- Do you think Sara is redefining or discounting anything?
- If we see a risk others want us to discount or deny, how might they behave towards us?

Look for:

- People acting aggressively towards us (especially shouting – point out how some people think shouting 'I am telling you IT WILL BE OK!' very loudly will, as if by magic, make all the risks and consequences disappear).
- People telling us we are wrong and that it will be OK.
- People being exasperated with us.

In pairs, explore why people might act like this.

- Does the way they behave towards us actually change the risks?
- If not, how could you respond?

If Sara's 'adult' voice could be heard, what do you think it would say? What might Emma's 'adult' say? Why isn't Sara listening to her 'adult'? What do you think she could do about it (if she wanted to)? Collect some suggestions for the 'adult' voices.

Explain that the three voices can consult together. The 'parent' can quieten the 'child', giving the 'adult' a chance to use its knowledge and judgement to decide what to do. The 'adult' can take into account the 'child's' recklessness, or nervousness, the 'parent's' view of what is OK and what is not, and can decide what to ignore and what to act on, adding its own (growing) understanding and experience of the world. Only the 'adult' can decide whether the 'parent' and the 'child' have got a point or not. In some situations, getting the 'parent' to quieten the 'child' for long enough for the 'adult' to take charge is a vital skill.

Think about these possible responses from Emma:

- *'Oh all right then, if it makes you happy, I'll come along.'*
- *'Now look, I think this is really risky, I am not going to go and I don't think you should do it either!'*

If Sara is in the role of 'child', what role is Emma taking in each of the responses above? What is likely to be the consequences of each?

- What are the risks of two people in 'child' roles managing a potentially risky situation?
- How might a person who is in 'child' role react to someone moving into a 'parent' role?

In pairs, explore how we could respond to Sara by staying in 'adult'. Ideally, we need a win-win outcome – therefore strategies that will keep both of them safe and happy – but, failing that, strategies that keep Emma safe.

If it makes it easier, think about what could be happening and build a quick 'back story'. For example, imagine where they could be going and what they might be going to do.

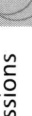
Alternative

This is an opportunity for group discussion or even role play (but it is important that each person plays all three roles).

Offer some risky but potentially fun situations and explore them in groups of three.

Examples might be:

- *Going for a drive with someone who drives very quickly.*
- *Going on a date with someone you hardly know (or even a 'blind date').*
- *Going to a party when you only know a few people who are likely to be there.*

- What might the 'child' voice be saying?
- What might the 'parent' voice be saying?
- What might the 'adult' voice be saying?

The 'child' will have strong feelings, but may not be a good judge. Perhaps it's keen, or frightened.

The 'parent' may have plenty of judgements to make, but may not be able to weigh the risks against the opportunities very well.

The 'adult' has to balance the two, and add knowledge and experience, perhaps deciding how to take safety precautions without losing out.

Now offer a situation which may feel risky but carries little or no danger (for example going on a ride at a theme park or going for an interview). In this scenario, the 'parent' might be the encouraging voice and the 'child' the dissenting voice. Again the 'adult' must listen to the voices and try to add some calm understanding in order to come to a balanced, informed choice.

Finally, remind the class that a good 'adult' may not be a killjoy. The 'parent' says, 'I'd better not go out dressed like that!' The 'child' says, 'But I want to!' The 'adult' says, 'I think I will. I know how to take care of myself.'

Reflection

In pairs, talk about one thing you have learnt from this session.
Think about your own relationships – what role do you most naturally take? Do you feel able to 'listen' to all three voices, and then allow your 'adult' to have the final say?

Either:
Over the rest of the day, watch and listen to other people and try to work out which voice is dominating and what is happening as a result of this.

Or:
Watch a soap opera tonight and try to spot when the characters are predominantly in 'parent', 'adult' and 'child' roles. Watch how others react.

The parent/adult/child model

Everyone has a 'parent' voice, an 'adult' voice and a 'child' voice. The model sets out some of the characteristics of each. The diagram shows *one* person.

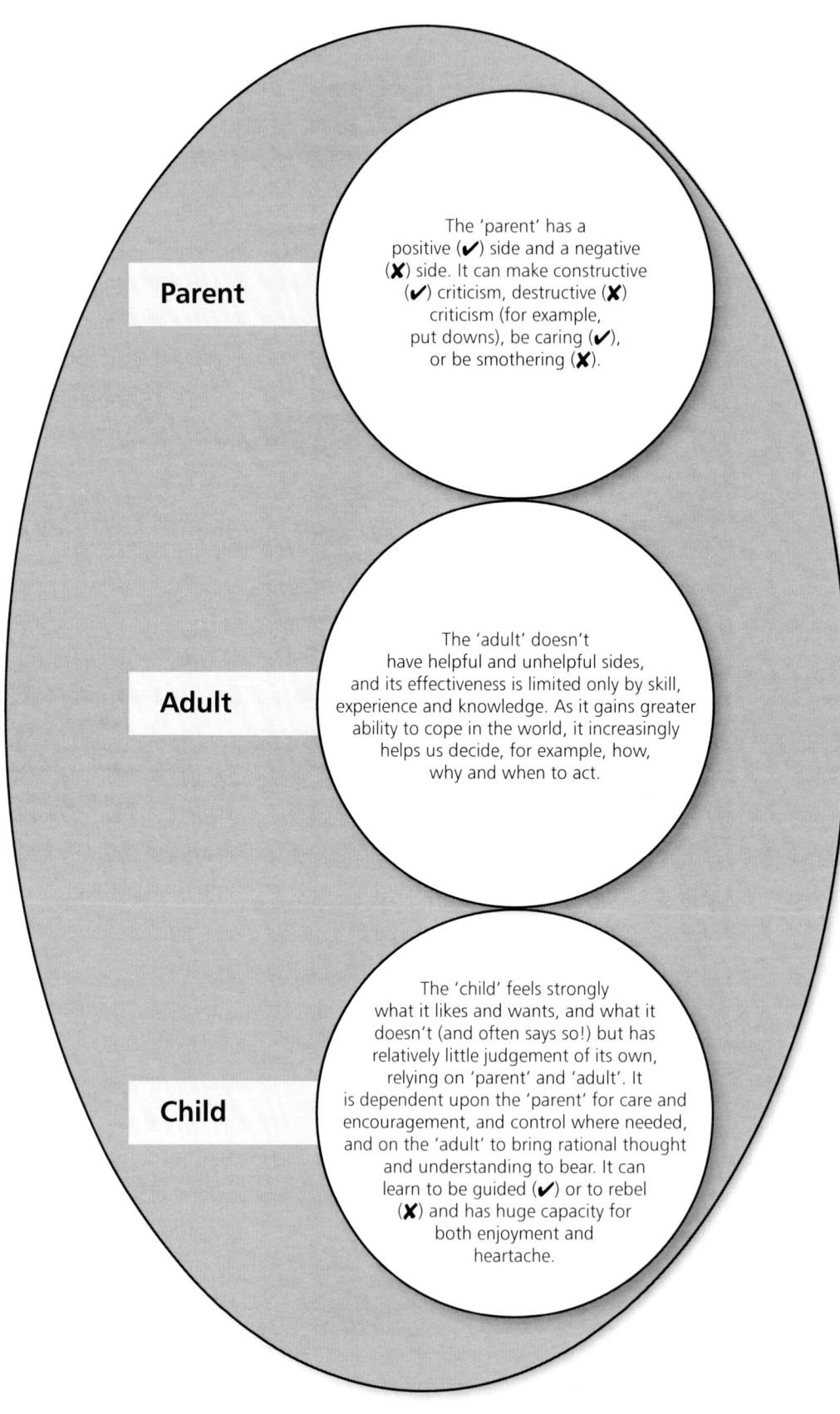

Parent

The 'parent' has a positive (✔) side and a negative (✘) side. It can make constructive (✔) criticism, destructive (✘) criticism (for example, put downs), be caring (✔), or be smothering (✘).

Adult

The 'adult' doesn't have helpful and unhelpful sides, and its effectiveness is limited only by skill, experience and knowledge. As it gains greater ability to cope in the world, it increasingly helps us decide, for example, how, why and when to act.

Child

The 'child' feels strongly what it likes and wants, and what it doesn't (and often says so!) but has relatively little judgement of its own, relying on 'parent' and 'adult'. It is dependent upon the 'parent' for care and encouragement, and control where needed, and on the 'adult' to bring rational thought and understanding to bear. It can learn to be guided (✔) or to rebel (✘) and has huge capacity for both enjoyment and heartache.

A question of negotiation

> **G11**
> What do I know about my rights and responsibilities?
> As I become older, what rights do I have?
> How do I feel about complaining when I feel I have been treated unfairly?
> Do I have the skills to express my rights assertively when they are abused, or not recognised?

> **G14**
> How good am I at negotiating a friendly outcome with people I speak to or challenge?
> How good am I at standing my ground when it would be easier to just go along with a suggestion or idea I don't like?

To the teacher

This session picks out the issue of negotiation from these two boxes, and focuses on the process of negotiation, when two or more parties are keen to come to an agreement.

Negotiation means finding a way to get as close as possible to a win-win outcome – one where everyone is content with the outcome and feels that their views and rights have been aired and considered. If negotiation is to lead to a settlement, then both (or all) sides need to feel sufficiently positive and motivated to stick with the agreement.

The formal process of negotiation involves a process of 'chunking'. To begin with, the question is asked of each party, 'what do you want?' This is then 'chunked up' using the question: 'and if you had that, what would this give you?' The aim is to reach a point where the chunk size is so large there is agreement.

The next step is to 'chunk down' back to a day-to-day level using the question: 'what stops you from getting this?' The process gradually 'chunks down' until a point is reached where there is a disagreement, this is known as a 'sticking point'. The focus then needs to be on resolving this issue so the 'chunking down' can continue.

In reality, it is often far messier than this. For this reason it can be helpful for a neutral negotiator to be asked to facilitate the process.

To the students

This session will help us focus on what can be done when two (or more) people have different views, needs or rights, and want to come to a mutually acceptable agreement.

'Cinema!' Sara said.

'Ice skating!' Emma replied.

'Cinema – great film!' Sara said.

'Ice skating – great fun!'

'Cinema – everyone says it's great!'

'Ice skating – loads of the others will be there!'

'Cinema – we saw the first one, this is the sequel. We have to know what happens next!'

'Actually, I think I can cope without knowing what happens in "Attack of the Chainsaw Wielding Maniacs from the Underworld 2".'

'It was good! Especially the bit when …'

'Yes, except I was almost sick down the back of the neck of the person sitting in front of me! Ice skating!'

'Cinema! Oh, go on, please, pretty please, you know you want to. Right, that's settled. Cinema it is. Let's go!'

Emma sighed. I suppose I can always shut my eyes, she thought. Great. Pay to sit in a loud dark room with my eyes shut …

Focusing

How many of you can recall feeling upset or unfairly treated (or both) when a decision (where to go, what to do, when to meet, etc.) doesn't seem to have gone your way? Why is this? Sometimes it can feel easier to go along with others' ideas, or even keep quiet while they decide.

Into action

In pairs, discuss what we can do to make sure our ideas and opinions are heard, and taken account of, in joint decisions.

Look for:

- Assertive statements of your wants and needs.
- Be ready to listen to others' views.
- Be prepared to say why you feel as you do.
- The need to practise ways of saying (to anyone wanting to ignore your opinion) you don't agree and have a different view you want to be considered.
- Be ready to insist, compromise, give in, as seems appropriate.
- Try to avoid picking a quarrel or simply arguing.

Situations like these can involve one or more people, and be at home, at school or anywhere. However, perhaps they share a common factor – they are not about very important issues.

Ask for examples of important issues where agreement is vital, and disagreement would be a serious problem. Collect some ideas. In such cases, is it acceptable to 'go with the flow' or just give in, in order to avoid a row?

Introduce the idea of supported negotiation. What could sabotage this from the outset? (Two angry people ready to fight; either one not prepared to give an inch, still less negotiate; half-hearted agreement to negotiate). This will only work if two (or all, if there are more than two) people are committed to making it work, being open and honest, and staying in the 'adult' position rather than letting their 'child' or 'parent' voices dominate.*

* This sentence refers to the issues of 'parent', 'adult' and 'child' addressed in the sample session (Year 10, G3, page 66).

Introduce the 'chunking' model of negotiation. In pairs, ask the students to construct examples of fictitious, but really important, issues, two characters, where it's vital both people come to an agreement, and something that makes agreement hard for them. Ask for pairs to volunteer to come forward and play the parts of these characters, with someone else playing the role of negotiator, to support each and explore the sticking points. You may find the class elects you to this role. Emphasise that it is the issue that is important. Sticking points are often less so, and may even be trivial: 'You always get to decide!'; 'But I want to watch EastEnders tonight!' Nevertheless they might be very important also: 'I don't want to – I don't feel ready!'; 'I promised my parents I'd be back by 10.30 – that's when me Dad leaves for night duty!'

Discuss how successful the model has been, and how appropriate it was in the instances chosen.

Reflection

What have I learned about:

- myself and assertiveness
- the importance of my wants, needs and rights
- the importance of the wants, needs and rights of others
- the value of negotiation
- the process of negotiation?

A question of unwritten rules

> **G15**
> Can I recognise when I am putting myself, or others are putting me, under pressure to obey 'unwritten rules' or social norms?
> Can I recognise when it is appropriate to follow a group or society's 'unwritten rules' and when following them could put me at risk?

To the teacher

This session could be expanded into a longer piece of work. It concerns the 'unwritten rules' we either consciously feel under pressure to follow or, more worryingly, follow unconsciously and without challenge. Sometimes these rules have become established over time to keep us safe, sometimes they arise from the peer group to establish or maintain the group's identity. Frequently, they are not planned but arise over time; they become 'the way we do things here'. When an individual challenges the unwritten rules, even if they seem risky, this can be seen as a threat to the group (see Year 11, G11 sample session on page 134). The value of the unwritten rule is often in protecting the cohesion of the group, rather than the outcome of following the rule itself.

The format of this session is slightly different; it invites students to offer a definition before outlining the session purpose.

Further work could extend this session in a new direction, offering a deeper exploration of their or others' expectations of minority groups, different cultures, etc., the appropriateness, origin, legitimacy and consequences of these expectations in our own behaviour and the reaction of others to that behaviour. Because of the likely richness of this extension, it is recommended that this is treated as an entirely separate session. It could also provide a lead in to work in SRE, looking at expectations in relationships or work on issues such as alcohol.

To the students

Have you ever heard the term 'an unwritten rule'?

Emma and Josh were talking.

'I am getting really annoyed. There seems to be a whole set of rules that people expect me to follow. I don't know what they are, no one seems to know where they are written down but you get nagged, left out or just odd looks if you don't follow them.'

'Ah,' said Hannah. 'Welcome to the world of unwritten rules!'

The purpose of this session is to begin to look at unwritten rules and how they might be affecting your choices without you even noticing.

Some rules in society are agreed and written down, for example legal laws, school rules or club rules. There are others that people carry in their heads and that we learn over time. It could be thought of as a way of behaving that somehow just becomes a rule within a family, a group, a club, a gang or even society.

Often no one knows when it became a 'rule'. It can be there to keep you safe; it can be really odd (just why do men wear ties?); it can help others to feel that you agree to their rules or values, and are therefore similar to them; or, sometimes, they can put pressure on you to do something really risky.

You usually know you are near an unwritten rule when you hear people say:
- 'Well, you just have to don't you?'
- 'Everyone does it!'
- 'Don't say that round here.'
- 'We all wear them.'
- 'You just don't do that, do you!'
- 'Well, if want to look really stupid ...'
- 'You have to ...'
- 'People expect you to ...'
- 'You can't go out looking like that.'

Unwritten rules give you a clue about people's expectations. The purpose of this session is to explore some of the effects 'unwritten rules' might have on us, even without us knowing.

Focusing

In pairs or groups of four, explain what the term 'unwritten rule' means to you. Collect a few definitions and write these on the board.

Each group takes one of the following (or construct a list that you feel is appropriate to your group):

- *Friends.*
- *Teenagers.*
- *Girlfriends or boyfriends.*
- *Young men.*
- *Young women.*
- *Adults.*
- *Men.*
- *Women.*

- How do you (or other people) expect these groups or individuals to behave? Be as honest as you can.
- Can different groups have conflicting expectations (for example our parents and our friends)?

Extension questions

- Think about any pressures these expectations bring with them. Are they helping the individual to be safe or accepted, are they helping others to feel safe or powerful, or are they possibly putting someone at risk? How?
- Where have these expectations come from?
- What happens to people who don't follow these rules? How do we treat them or behave towards them?
- How might this encourage them to behave towards us?
- How do you feel when you suddenly get the feeling you have broken an unwritten rule? What does that feeling encourage you to do?

Do a 'marketplace' activity inviting the class to circulate, explore others' thinking and draw up some results.

Reflection

Think about the unwritten rules we have explored today. Will you be able to identify them more easily now?

Which unwritten rules might put you under pressure to conform to others' expectations? Pick a couple, perhaps ones you feel a little uneasy about.

- When you notice the unwritten rules are operating, who are you with?
- How do their expectations of you make you feel?
- If you decide you want to fulfil their expectations, what are the consequences to you?
- If you decide you don't, what are the consequences to you?
- How might you challenge them, and whose support (in the group) might you seek?

A question of loss

> **G17**
> How do I feel about sudden changes in my relationships?
> How do I feel about loss or bereavement that might happen or will happen in my future?
> How well have I managed past losses and bereavements?

To the teacher

Helping students to manage their feelings involving sudden changes in relationships makes up part of most schools' planned curriculum, perhaps in PSHE or in other subjects such as RE. Bereavement can take many forms, including death or the break up of family. Many students cope remarkably well with the death of a family member or friend, but many report the break up of a family as even more painful.

Although there is a recognised process of following bereavement or sudden unwanted personal change – denial, anger, bargaining, depression, acceptance (Dr Elisabeth Kübler-Ross, *On Death & Dying*, 1969) – it is a generalisation and should be treated only as a guide. Each individual will feel, and has the right to feel, their own unique set of emotions.

This session does not attempt to set itself within any faith system. It focuses only on offering students a chance to consider their own recollections or anticipations. It is vital that this session is planned with sensitivity and with an awareness of the group's (including any adults') recent experiences. Without this, a session to explore grief, loss and change could leave a recently bereaved individual feeling very upset, vulnerable or exposed. It is almost impossible to explore change or bereavement without remembering our own experiences. This does not mean we should not explore the subject, because the alternative is just to leave students to cope as best they can.

Sometimes, just understanding that our reactions are 'normal', that we have a right to …, that it is OK to …, that it may be very appropriate (and that we can give ourselves permission to) feel whatever we feel, can be a help. Most schools maintain a policy and protocol for managing incidents of bereavement and this session should take account of these, especially letting students know of sources of support. It would be essential to revisit the group's 'groundrules' prior to starting this session, and to use or edit the scenarios offered as you feel appropriate. The first two scenarios below focus on family breakups and the third bereavement.

To the students

The only thing we can be very certain about in life is that we will experience lots of changes. Some changes are really great and cause us to have fantastic feelings, some are difficult or challenging and may cause us a real mix of excitement and stress, while others are just dreadful and bring horrible feelings. Sometimes we look forward to a change because we want it, sometimes change happens very suddenly, perhaps unexpectedly, and we definitely do not want it. We are going to think about the sort of changes people might experience where they might need support and changes that we ourselves might encounter.

Situation 1

Kelly, Emma and Josh's stepsister, was staying over. After the initial shock of their father having a new partner, they were surprised to find they got on really well together. They had just heard that one of their friends' parents were breaking up and they were thinking about what they had felt.

'I hated that time,' Emma said. 'I got so angry. I didn't understand how it could happen. Dad had just always been there.'

'I just couldn't believe it,' Josh replied. 'I thought it would all go back to the way it was.'

'I was scared. I knew mum had met someone new and really liked him, but after my dad died I didn't think there would be anyone else. I thought it would just be the two of us,' Kelly said. 'I think I gave Phil a bit of a hard time. I know he made mum happy, but I didn't think we needed anyone else. I was scared stiff about meeting you two in case you thought it was my fault!'

'I remember thinking I was to blame, that I must have done something. I remember offering to do lots of things if Dad wouldn't go,' Emma said.

'I don't think it was until Paris was born that I finally believed it wasn't going to go back to how it was. I mean I knew deep down it wasn't but … I guess I just didn't really believe it,' Josh said.

'Do you know, I felt exactly the same when Leigh was born,' Emma replied. 'I guess feelings can change over time.'

Situation 2

'It was so sudden. Do you know what our first thoughts were?' said Mickey. Josh and Emma were talking about their friend with Mickey and Stella, their grandparents. 'We panicked that we wouldn't see so much of you all.'

'That's silly, why wouldn't you?' Josh and Emma asked.

'Well, we were lucky. Sometimes when families break up it can be difficult for grandparents to visit,' Stella said.

'Why?' Josh asked.

Situation 3

'Something really awful has happened,' Sheila looked dreadful. 'It's your grandma Gracie. She died early this morning.'

Josh and Emma had only met their grandmother Gracie twice, once when she had come to their home and once when they visited hers. They had liked her immediately, a fun-loving woman who seemed to laugh all the time.

Ray came in. He was very quiet and it looked like he had been crying.

'I'm so sorry, Ray,' Hannah said.

Josh and Emma didn't know what to say.

'I can't believe it. It's not fair!' Ray said.

Focusing

From one of the scenarios, pick a character and ask the group why the person might be, or has been, having those feelings. Collect a few ideas on the board. Try to collate them into groups that will reflect the six stages below.

Into action

Begin this section with a 'mini lecture'. Explain that people may go through a series of stages when they have experienced a really difficult change.

1 **Shock**: initially people may be so shocked that they feel nothing, their thinking literally shuts down.

2 **Denial**: it is perfectly natural to try to pretend the change isn't happening or hasn't happened. 'This isn't happening'; 'It can't be true'.

3 **Anger**: people can be angry with themselves, angry with others, especially those they love, angry with the person who has left or even died (and with God or the universe). 'It's not fair'; 'Why did they leave me?'; 'How could they hurt me like this?'

4 **Bargaining**: this is also very natural and involves some form of 'deal'. Perhaps in the case of a breakup: 'If I promise to …'; 'Can we still be friends'; or in the case of a bereavement, more irrationally, 'If I promise … let it not be true.'

5 **Depression**: this can be a mix of emotions as the certainty of the change begins to become accepted. It can be a mix of sadness, worry or fear about future uncertainty and regret. Asking 'what if …?' is quite common, which can involve feeling guilty or blaming oneself for things said, not said, done or not done.

6 **Acceptance**: we accept what has happened and, whilst not forgetting, are able to move to new things.

How long it takes to move through the stages is different for everyone, and they don't always follow in order. Some people can manage to progress through the stages themselves with little or no support, others need more help. We call this emotional process the process of 'grieving'. Some people use the language 'letting go' and 'moving forward' or 'moving on' but many people need time before they can do this. It can take months, or even years, to grieve for the loss of someone close.

Read the three scenarios above again. Can you see evidence of the different stages within them? Did anyone find it hard to 'let go' and 'move on'?

Talk about:

● Is it OK for people to feel whatever they are feeling when they are going through a difficult or unwanted change?

● When people are really upset, do you think they really mean all the things they might say?

● If we can't change things back to how they were, if we can't 'put things right', how can we support people who are going through an unpleasant change?

● Think about people at different stages; is there anything particular you could do to support them at these different stages?

This session has focused on the feelings experienced following a family breakup and the death of a loved one. What other unwanted changes might trigger the same process?

Look for:

● Break up of a boyfriend/girlfriend relationship

● Break up of a close friendship

● Being forced to move to a new home (maybe in a new country)

● An unwanted change of school

● Loss of a job

● Death of a pet

● Life not going the way you planned. For example poor examination results or failing to get a part in the school play.

How might the stages of grief appear in these situations? What might people feel, say and do?

Reflection

Take time to reflect privately, or in pairs if you are comfortable to do so. Has this session helped you to think differently about anything? Has it given you some insights that you might not previously have had? If so, what are they?

How might it be helpful to understand that many people experience a similar process when something sad or difficult happens, and that this is quite normal?

How do you think you might support someone going through a process like this? What might they need or appreciate most?

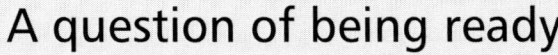

A question of being ready

R7
How are my feelings about having a sexual relationship changing?
Are they getting stronger?
How might my feelings affect what I do?
What else could influence me?
How do I know when I am ready to begin a sexual relationship with someone, and what does this mean for me?

R21
Do I know that I have a right to only do what I feel comfortable with?
Do I know that I have a responsibility to protect others' rights to be safe and feel comfortable?

To the teacher

This session aims to help students reflect upon the factors that influence young people in having sexual relationships, and to consider what it means to be 'ready' for sex. The session explores the notion that feeling uncomfortable or unsafe can be good indicators that we are not ready for something (sexual or otherwise), and to consider the advantages of delaying sex in such circumstances.

This session connects with Year 10, R13 and R14 – the scene below precedes the scene (focusing on different characters) in the sample session provided for R13 and R14. There is a link also with R22.

You may prefer to arrange for the scene below to be read out loud by a group of confident students. You may even wish to use the drama technique where other 'actors' stand behind the main characters and say what they are thinking, before or after they speak (see Focus on pedagogy, page 262).

To the students

What are the 'triggers' that prompt relationships to become sexual, or perhaps become more intensely sexual? What are the thoughts and feelings that tell us when we are ready for something to happen? This is a good question to ask regarding lots of situations in life – not just sexual ones. What happens when relationships start to change? What responsibilities do people in a relationship have to each other? This session explores those questions.

It was Friday night and Katie was really looking forward to her birthday party. They'd had the family celebration last week on her actual birthday but this was different – going out for a meal with her family and getting the money from gran was all right, but this was the proper party. Katie's family were away. She had the place to herself and loads of people were coming, including her friends Emma, Sara and Sara's boyfriend Sean. Sara and Sean were a real laugh – and they could always be relied on to bring plenty of drink. Katie's boyfriend Jay had come round early to help her get everything ready – not that they'd got very far with that yet …

'Come on, Jay,' she said, pushing him away. 'We've got to start getting ready.'

'Yeah, later,' he said, grabbing her again. 'C'mon, we've got the place to ourselves …'

Several minutes later, Katie broke away from him again. 'Look, Jay, we've really got to get ready – people will be here soon.'

*'Yeah, OK – there's always later,' he grinned. 'I'll be staying here when everyone goes – and we can celebrate your birthday **properly**!' Behind the big grin, Jay's heart was thumping – he'd never had an opportunity like this before.*

Katie didn't know what to say 'cos she hadn't actually asked Jay to stay overnight – she'd never even mentioned it! They'd been going out together for a while but they'd never gone that far …

Focusing

Prompt some immediate reactions and discussion by asking these questions:

- What sort of thoughts and feelings do you think Katie might be having?
- Why do you think Jay assumes he'll be staying when Katie hasn't even asked him to?
- Do you think it's a good idea, or not? Why?
- What do you think Jay is thinking and feeling? Do you think he's assuming they'll have sex?
- Do you think these two are ready for a sexual relationship? What tells you this?
- What do you think might happen if Katie does have sex with Jay?
- What do you think might happen if she doesn't?

OK, now we've got your immediate thoughts and feelings about this …

Into action

Divide the class into small groups and hand out marker pens and three flip-chart sheets to each group. Each sheet will have one of three different headings:

Messages for Jay

Messages for Katie

Checklist for being ready

The students' task is to ensure that the evening does not end in a way that could spoil Jay and Katie's relationship, or upset Jay or Katie. Students must try to keep them together as a couple, but with nobody feeling bad, used, or worried or regretful.

Ask each group to discuss what they would say to Jay and Katie to help a 'happy' outcome. Decide what you think Jay and Katie need to hear, including what the other person is probably thinking or feeling. Discuss what to advise them to say and do.

Finally, students create a 'checklist' that tells the couple how they would know when they were both really ready to start a sexual relationship. This might involve thinking about how you know when you're not ready for something, and how to say so.

Tell the students they will have a few minutes to quickly write their ideas on the sheets. The groups will then swap sheets and see if they have anything to add to what other groups have written.

Look for:

- Whether they feel Jay and Katie are both equally keen on having sex or not – and how this is reflected in what to say to them
- Suggestions that Jay and Katie talk to each other
- Any thoughts about Katie feeling pressured or 'bounced' into a situation she wasn't prepared for
- Things Katie could say to Jay if she doesn't feel OK about him staying the night – trying not to hurt his feelings
- Things Jay could say to Katie to help *her* feel OK about not being ready for him to stay overnight
- Questions about Jay's readiness. Is Jay *really* ready to have sex, or might he just be feeling it is what is expected of him, and that he must take the opportunity to be alone with Katie?
- Awareness that 'being ready' might include 'being prepared', for example having contraception/ protection sorted
- How the thoughts and feelings might relate to a checklist for being ready, for example does a feeling of anxiety indicate readiness? Or a thought like, 'I might regret this …'

Discussion

Post the various sheets on the wall and discuss the ideas students have generated, in particular their checklists for being ready. Explore with the class what 'readiness' for a sexual relationship is actually about.

- Is it enough that being with the other person makes you feel sexy – or is there more to it than that?
- Is sexual attraction enough to make a relationship – or is there more to it?
- Do students think it is different for boys and girls – or the same?
- Does it change things if you think how you might feel *afterwards*?

Talk about the way other feelings and thoughts might indicate not being ready – not feeling quite comfortable with the situation. For example, worrying about regretting it, feeling pressured, doing it to please the other person rather than yourself, not having talked about it or sorted contraception/ protection. What do your three inner voices say? Does your 'parent' voice say you should or you shouldn't? Does your 'child' voice want to, or is it frightened? Are you ready to listen to your 'adult's' careful, rational thinking and then act on it? (See Year 10, G3 page 66).

Reflection

How easy is it to tell when you are really ready for something, especially in a close relationship? What influences how you behave in a relationship? *Encourage the class to say what they have learned from this session.*

Privately reflect on what influences *your* relationships.

A question of choice – a question of control

R13
Do I feel able to negotiate the use of contraception with a partner?
How do I do that?
Do I feel able to refuse a sexual advance from someone who refuses to use contraception?

R14
What do I know about how the use of alcohol and other drugs might make me vulnerable to others, or change my own ability to make decisions and keep myself safe?

To the teacher

This session aims to develop students' abilities to evaluate, communicate and negotiate for healthy choices in sex and relationships, and to notice how factors like alcohol and other drugs can affect our abilities. It encourages students to acknowledge that relationships without sex are actually OK, but that if sex is part of the relationship, to recognise also that unprotected sex is highly risky. It is about enabling students to think through options in relationships and how they can influence and change situations.

This session links with Year 10, R15, R26, R7, R21 and R22. The sample session provided for R15 and R26 follows on from this session. You could consider running them consecutively.

You may prefer to arrange for the two scenes below to be read out loud by a group of confident students. You may even wish to use the drama technique where other 'actors' stand behind the main characters and say what they are thinking, before or after they speak (see Focus on pedagogy, page 262).

To the students

This session is about how young people decide how far to go sexually in a relationship, the options that they might have, how they decide what to do or what not to do, and the timing of those decisions. It also addresses what might influence their options, how far they are in control of a situation and how safe they are.

It's a Friday night and Emma and her friend Sara are going to a party at their friend's place. Sara is going to be picked up by her boyfriend Sean. Before they go, Emma and Sara are talking on the phone.

'You're going to look fantastic if you wear that top you bought last Saturday – Sean won't be able to take his eyes off you,' Emma said – just a little bit enviously.

'Never mind his eyes – what about his hands …' Sara laughed.

'Sara!' Emma thought that was just such a typical Sara sort of answer. She was laughing too – but she did worry about Sara a bit sometimes.

'Sara …' she began a bit cautiously – she didn't want to offend Sara. ' … Are you taking anything with you?'

'Yeah, a bottle or two – or three!' Sara said.

'No, I mean – er, you know – um you know …' Emma began to wish she hadn't started this conversation. Then she took a deep breath and blurted out, 'Condoms!'

'No! What kind of a slapper do you think I am?!'

'Look you know I don't,' said Emma, really embarrassed now. 'And it doesn't mean you're a slapper if you carry condoms … and anyway, I worry about you – I'm your best friend, aren't I?'

'More like my mum,' laughed Sara. 'Look, don't worry, nothing's going to happen, we've never gone that far.'

Two hours later, at the party, Sara and Sean have been having a really good time – their friend's parents are away and people have brought loads to drink – and they've had plenty of it. Sara said she felt hot and needed to sit down (probably before she fell down) and Sean had suggested they go into one of the bedrooms instead and lie down. Giggling, Sara had agreed. Now things were getting really hot!

'C'mon,' Sean mumbled. 'You know how I feel about you.'

'Yeah, I do but …' Sara was feeling a bit flustered. Sean was really lovely and they'd been going out for ages and he did make her feel good, but she wasn't sure she was ready for this. 'C'mon, Sara,' repeated Sean. 'You know you want to …'

'No, Sean, we can't – oh, I don't know …' She felt a bit confused and 'fuzzy'. ' … Have you got a condom?'

'It's all right – it'll be OK – I'll pull out in time. C'mon, we can't stop **now** …'

Focusing

Prompt some immediate reactions and discussion by asking these questions:

- What do you think of the phone conversation between Sara and Emma?
- What would you think of Sara if she carried condoms?
- Do you think it was wrong of Emma to ask Sara about condoms like that?
- Do you think Sara would have been wise to take condoms to the party?
- What do you think about the situation with Sean and Sara?
- Do you think they did have sex?
- If yes, why? If no, why not?
- Why do you think Sean wasn't going to use a condom?
- Is there anything wrong with just 'pulling out'?

Into action

In small groups, some working on the scene between Emma and Sara and some on the scene between Sean and Sara, consider the following:

● What are the 'crunch' points where somebody has to make a decision?

● What do you think is influencing how the characters behave? Any 'unwritten rules' at work here?

● Are there any elements of risk or possible problems for the characters in this scene? If so, who for?

Now rewind back in time …

● What, if anything, could have been *said* or *done* differently?

● How easy would it have been for the character to *say* or *do* those things? How easy would it be for you (if in a similar situation)?

● Could anything have reduced the risk and avoided possible problems? If so, what?

● As a group, think of the possible options and write a few lines of script that would make the scene work out better. Ask one person in the group to read it out.

When the groups have read out their alternative scenes, discuss ideas.

Look for:

Decisions, such as:

● whether to say what you're thinking to a friend

● whether (and when) to carry condoms

● whether to drink alcohol and how much to drink if you do

● how far to go in a sexual relationship.

Risks, such as:

● offending your best friend

● getting a bad reputation

● putting pressure on another by *implying* that you are going to have sex, rather than discussing it openly

● upsetting your boyfriend or girlfriend or appearing 'easy', 'obstructive' or even 'frigid'

● feeling like you won't enjoy it

● feeling like you'll regret it – it might spoil the relationship

● getting an STI or an unplanned pregnancy.

Options/different choices, such as:

● Sara could have discussed taking condoms with Emma

● she might have decided then to take some with her

● Sara and Sean could have stayed sober – they could have been more in control

● when Sean said, 'You know how I feel,' Sara could have said something like, 'I do too, but I'm not ready to go all the way'. Or …

● Sara could have said, 'Not unless we use a condom', and she could have had some of her own to use

● Sean could have planned to use a condom. Or…

● Sean could have told her it was OK, he could wait until she was ready

● Sean and Sara could have talked about it.

Discussion

Do you think Sara and Sean were actually ready to begin having sex? Talk about what readiness for sex actually means. Discuss the way Emma was looking out for her best friend and how friends can give us positive support to stay safer. Peer pressure isn't all bad – really good friends can be a positive influence.

Talk about the influence of alcohol on the situation: how alcohol and other substances can cloud people's judgement when making the choice that's really right for them; how alcohol can also hinder contraceptive use. For example, the difficulty of putting a condom on when really drunk, or how throwing up can reduce the effectiveness of the contraceptive pill. In this scenario they may have been too drunk even to negotiate.

Talk about whether Sara and Sean's relationship would still be OK if they didn't have full sex and whether you have to have sex to make a relationship work. Ask whether you have to have penetrative sex to have a satisfying experience. In this case, they might even have enjoyed it more if they'd waited, or done other stuff. Tension and worry about what could go wrong do not make for great sex, and penetration isn't the only way to have good sex.

Discuss the things that can get in the way of us being able to negotiate safety. In a healthy relationship, both people can talk about what they want and need, and also what the other person wants and needs. The best relationships are those where each person takes some responsibility for keeping the other person safe – and feels safe themselves.

Reflection

Privately, think about what you would have done in either of these situations. Would you have done anything differently? Have you changed your mind about anything during this session? Be ready to say what you have learned only if you feel comfortable about doing so.

A question of help when you need it

R15
Do I know where to obtain 'emergency contraception'?
How would I feel about approaching someone to ask for emergency contraception?
Do I understand issues of confidentiality?
Do I know how quickly emergency contraception has to be used in order for it to be effective?
Do I know who to get support and advice from if it has been left too late?

R26
Do I know who I can go to in order to get reliable help and advice about sex or my relationships?
How do I know I can feel confident in the advice they offer me?
How do I feel about approaching someone to ask for help or advice, especially if they are a professional I have not met before?
Do I understand that counsellors will not advise, but will help me find my own way forward?

To the teacher

This session is intended to raise students' awareness, or remind them, of how to access emergency contraception and sexual health advice and help generally. The session also aims to help students explore any concerns they might have about accessing help and to think through how they might approach a situation where they need help. It will be important to have information about local services available for this session, and it would be a good idea to liaise with a school nurse and/or other local professionals/services.

The session uses the Smith family characters and works on the principle of focusing on different possible scenes within one storyline. It allows students to create their own 'take' on the action. There are aspects of the scenario that you might need to adjust to fit your local situation, for example policy about, and procedures for, accessing help during school time or through the school. It will be particularly important in this session to ensure that the material is used in a dissociated and hypothetical way, and that students are discouraged from disclosing personal information about their own experiences.

This session links with Year 10, R13 and R14 and follows on from the sample session provided for those content boxes. Therefore, you might consider running the sessions consecutively.

You may prefer to arrange for the scene below to be read out loud by a group of confident students. You may even wish to use the drama technique where other 'actors' stand behind the main characters and say what they are thinking, before or after they speak (see Focus on pedagogy, page 262).

To the students

This session is about getting help when we need it – getting the right sort of help, what could get in the way and the best ways to go about it. The situation you will explore is specifically about help related to sexual health, and what you might do when you're worried and it's urgent …

It's Monday morning. Emma and her friend Sara were at a friend's party on Friday night. There was a lot of drink as their friend's parents were away. Sara was there with her boyfriend Sean – they were both pretty drunk and Emma had seen them go into one of the bedrooms. Emma has gone to Sara's place to meet her and go to school together. When she arrives, Sara is talking to her mum …

'Sara, are you OK? You seem a bit down? Are you worried about something?' Sara's mum looked concerned.

'No, Mum. I'm all right – don't go on – I've got to go!' Sara grabbed her bag and rushed out the door before her mum could ask any more questions.

'Great party on Friday, wasn't it?' Emma said, linking arms with Sara.

'Yeah, I suppose …'

'Sara, what's the matter? I saw you and Sean disappear – is everything OK?' Emma was anxious now.

'Well, we did it – you know – we'd never done it before but he really wanted me to – and we didn't use anything …' Sara stopped and looked at her friend's face. Emma had suggested she take condoms to the party, and Sara had said she wasn't a slapper and, anyway, nothing was going to happen … 'I know, I know! Don't say, "I told you so!" I'm worried sick. Can you lend me some money to buy a pregnancy test after school?'

'Sara, I don't think a pregnancy test will work yet – I think you need emergency contraception. You'd better see the school nurse.' Emma hardly got the words out –

'But she's not in school till Wednesday!' Sara shrieked at her.

Emma put her arm round Sara to calm her down. 'Don't worry, I'll come with you to talk to Miss Beale – she can contact the nurse – you won't have to say why you need to see her – and if she can't come, you can always get advice from the clinic. Have you talked to Sean yet?'

'No …'

'Call him now on his mobile,' Emma said.

Focusing

Prompt some immediate reactions and discussion by asking these questions:

- Why do you think Sara didn't want to talk to her mum?
- Do you think Sara should have told her mum?
- How do you think her mum would have reacted?
- Is Emma right? Is it too soon for a pregnancy test?
- Why does Emma say Sara needs emergency contraception instead?
- Does Sara have any other choices?
- How do you think Sara is feeling?
- Is Emma being helpful?
- How do you think Sean will react?

Into action

Allocate different aspects of the 'soap' scenario to small groups. Ask each group to choose one of the scenarios below and write a script for a short scene approximately two or three minutes long.

1 Sara *does* talk to her mum.
   What does she say to get help from her mum? How does Mum feel? What does she say?

2 Sara talks to Sean on his mobile and they meet up.
   What does Sean say, and what does this say about how much he cares about Sara? What might Sean say if he felt differently about her? How could Sean support Sara? How might he be feeling about the situation? Might he have been worried too?

3 Sean talks to somebody close to him for support.
   Who might this be? His friend? His brother/sister? His mum or dad? What does Sean say to get help? What does the other person say?

4 With Emma's support, Sara talks to Miss Beale their form tutor.
   What does Sara say? What should she *not* tell Miss Beale? Why? What does Miss Beale suggest? (In *your* school what sort of help could a form teacher find for a student?)

5 Sara meets the school nurse.
   What does Sara say to the nurse? How does the nurse respond? Would she just tell Sara what she should do? Is it a problem that Sara and Sean are under 16 years? Would a nurse be able to get Sara emergency contraception?

6 Sara and Sean go together to get help at a sexual health clinic/her GP/another GP practice.*
   Would Sara and Sean feel OK about going to a clinic? What problems could they face at Sara's GP, or at a different one? For example, how would they deal with a GP's receptionist?

   * Choose the scenario that fits local facilities.

into action

Assist and prompt groups, and supply factual information as necessary. Ask them to practise finished scripts ready to present to the class. Encourage volunteer groups to act out their scenes. Praise contributions and clarify/add any useful factual points. Encourage resulting discussion.

Look for:

Sara and Mum:

- Perhaps Sara could tell her mum how worried she is and how she really needs her help.
- An emotional, as well as practical, response from Mum – she isn't 'impersonal'.
- Telling Mum while Emma was there could have helped give Sara the confidence to talk.
- Sean could offer to go with Sara to talk to her mum.

Sean and Sara:

- Sean might be worried too (they could *both* be regretting what they did).
- He could offer to go with her.
- He could *tell* her he cares. (Supposing he doesn't, what then?)
- He could let Sara know that he'll support her whatever happens.

Sean getting support:

- If Sean talks to somebody, they might point out that if Sara were to have a baby, he's financially responsible.

Sara, Emma and Miss Beale:

- Teachers can't guarantee to keep details confidential, but they *can* get help for somebody **without** knowing the details. Therefore, Sara wouldn't have to tell her all the information.
- Sara could just say to Miss Beale, 'I need to see the school nurse – it's important that I see her today.'

Sara and the nurse:

- Sara would need to tell the nurse that she had unprotected sex on Friday night.
- The nurse could confirm that Sara might be pregnant and that emergency contraception is effective up to 72 hours after sex.
- She might recommend it as an option, but wouldn't just tell Sara she must do it.
- Getting Sara out of school to go to a clinic could be a problem. (How much of a problem, depends on the protocol at the school.)
- The nurse might also highlight the risk of STIs.
- Although Sara and Sean are under 16, they can get contraceptive advice and help. The nurse has to follow some guidelines, like making sure they understand the implications.
- The nurse will raise the issue of future sexual behaviour and contraception.

Sara and Sean getting help:

- They might prefer to use a specialist clinic, particularly if there is a service geared to students. However, that might not be available.
- They might need to be assertive (polite, clear and firm) at a GP practice – being clear that it is **urgent** and that Sara doesn't want to discuss it in reception. This might not be easy to do of course – many adults find this difficult.
- They could ask to see a nurse if a doctor is not immediately available.
- They could have written a note to hand in at reception explaining that Sara needs urgent medical help. That way they wouldn't have to say anything out loud.

Talk about local services where students could get help in this sort of situation, or for other sexual health needs. Discover what the students in your class already know and make sure you have information to give out on: Family Planning Clinics; Students' Clinics; GUM/Sexual Health Clinics, GP Practices; plus any other source of contraception, emergency contraception, pregnancy testing, STI testing, advice and/or counselling.
In discussing GPs be sure you know whether GPs in your area treat patients not registered at that practice – they are meant to do so for contraception – but not all will comply with this.

Reflection

- If you feel comfortable to do so, tell the class one thing you have discovered during this session about getting help.
- What do you think you would have done in this situation, either for yourself, or to help a friend? (You need not share this with the class – **just think to yourself.**) Would you have done anything differently? Would you do anything differently now from what you might have done before?

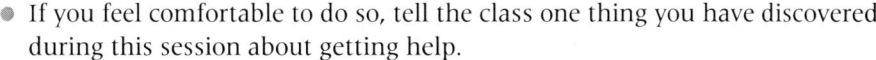

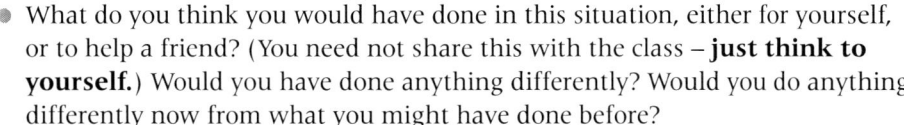

A question of feeling OK – in ourselves and our relationships

> **R20**
> How do I decide when a relationship is right for me?
> How do I decide if it isn't?

To the teacher

This session is about enabling students to understand that some relationships are healthy and feel 'right' for us and that some are not. Students need to learn to identify for themselves the characteristics of healthy/unhealthy relationships. Linked with this, the session encourages students to consider the benefits of strong supportive relationships where both partners are equal. It extends and develops work done in earlier years about what we look for in relationships (*Health for Life 11–14*). You will need to be sensitive to the possibility that, for some people, this activity could evoke feelings about very unhealthy (abusive) relationships they or others close to them have experienced.

To the students

This session is about feeling good in our relationships. It's also about knowing when a relationship feels good and healthy for us and is working well, and how we decide when it isn't.

Focusing

Invite the class to help you swiftly generate a collection of 'features of a good relationship'. Ask students to be as 'ideal' as they like, but to only choose features that benefit both people in the relationship. Write their suggestions on the board, with no discussion (for example reliability, friendship, honesty, both good listeners, sensitivity, etc.)

Ask the class to create in their mind and think about a 'fantasy person' – someone who they would like to know. This could be an imaginary character their own age who they think they could make friends with. Ask students to endow this person with a mixture of characteristics drawn from their imagination (looks, skills and talents, personality attributes, etc.) or from real life, from one or more people they actually know, or people they admire such as celebrities from TV, film or sport. Ask the students:

- Imagine how you would feel about this person.

Perhaps they'd feel admiration, respect, awe, warmth, attraction, etc. Ask them to share these feelings with a partner and, without devoting time to actually describing the person, to discuss briefly some of the ways they'd like to be treated in this 'virtual' relationship, with this amazing, imagined person. Then ask the students:

- How do you imagine this person would behave (or how would you *like* them to behave) if:
  - ○ one day you were upset and needed some support
  - ○ you got angry with him/her
  - ○ you needed to rely on him/her for something very important
  - ○ you wanted him/her to be open and honest with you about a sensitive issue?

How do you imagine (or expect) *you* would behave in the above situations if the 'roles' were reversed? In pairs, can you list the things that would tell you that you were 'equal partners' in your respective relationships?

Ask if any students are happy to share their responses with the class.

Explain that even when what we want from others is reasonable both to give and to receive, and even when relationships feel good, in real life they are seldom perfect. The reality, even in a healthy relationship, may fall short of our best hopes – it may not be as good as the fantasy. But how 'short' is too short? Explain to the class that you now want to help them explore the shortcomings of 'real', healthy relationships.

Into action

Ask the class to think of characteristics they wouldn't like, **but could put up with** *in another person, and to ponder on when unwanted characteristics stray into being unhealthy and unacceptable. For example: 'I could maybe accept someone lying to me once, but never again!; 'I could accept them not keeping an arrangement with me, but if they were going to do it all the time …'; 'I could understand if he didn't listen to me when the football's on, but if he never really listened to me …'*

Ask each pair to generate a list of ways to complete sentences such as these:
- In a healthy relationship, I hope that the other person will *usually* …
- In a healthy relationship, I would *expect* that the other person will *always* …
- In a healthy relationship, I would *require* that the other person will *never* …
- In a healthy relationship, I would *expect* (most of the time) to feel …
- I would consider a relationship *unacceptable* and *unhealthy* if the other person …
- I would consider a relationship *unacceptable* and *unhealthy* if (most of the time) I felt …

Students may choose instead to generate sentences of their own. Tell them that you want them to be specific in what they list. What sort of things would they **see** *if they looked at people in a healthy relationship? What sort of things would they* **hear**? *What would the people* **feel** *like?*

Give students another tip about what to look out for in the relationship:
- What the people feel they can or can't *say*.
- What the people feel they can or can't *do*.

Point out that in a good relationship both people are equally important, and each has *desires*, *needs* and *rights*. Some of the desires of each may be met, but probably not all, and not all of the time. Ask:
- Is it healthy if the *needs* of both people are not met all of the time/some of the time/with negotiation?
- How important is reciprocated giving and receiving?
- What if the rights of one or both people are not met, are ignored or abused?

You may want to use some of the following as prompts during the exercise:

Healthy:

- Both people are able to discuss things, they make decisions together and can both compromise equally if they have different opinions.
- Both people can talk about and listen to each other's feelings, needs and wishes.
- Each can trust him/herself and also the other person. In a healthy relationship you are honest with the other person and yourself.
- Each can do things separately as well as together if they want to – with friends, family or as solo activities.
- When they have disagreements, they do it in a calm way and they sort things out calmly.
- Both people respect each other's sexual 'stopping points' and need for safety.
- Both people feel good about the relationship most of the time.
- They might say that they feel: happy; comfortable; relaxed; energised; cared for; secure.

Unhealthy:

- One person makes all the decisions, controls everything and doesn't listen.
- One person can't say things and so feels unheard.
- You lie to the other person and to yourself – you make excuses for the other person.
- One of you has to justify what you do, where you go, who you see.
- Arguments are aggressive – one person yells, hits, shoves or throws things.
- One person is forced/coerced by the other into doing sexual stuff they don't want to do. For example, they feel scared to ask their partner to use protection (he or she refuses requests for safer sex). Or they are asked to perform acts they don't want to.
- One or both of them feel bad about the relationship a lot of the time: sad; angry; frustrated; nervous; scared; exhausted; insecure; threatened.

Collate feedback and comments.

Now ask the class to consider and say what might indicate a fatally flawed relationship. Feelings are vital indicators of how things are. Ask students to focus on what would take a relationship 'over the line' from healthy to 'unacceptably unhealthy'. Collect ideas, and perhaps ask for the feelings that go with them. Is there general agreement about what would spell 'the end' for a relationship? Students will probably agree on the extremes (for example theft, violence, rape), but is there consensus about more borderline situations?

Invite the class to summarise the conclusions reached so far in this session. The class may agree on some aspects (perhaps about both people being equal, relationships seldom being perfect, everyone has desires, needs and rights), but may disagree about what, precisely, is and is not acceptable, and what marks out a relationship as either 'acceptable' or 'unhealthy' to those involved. They may place the boundaries in different places. Every relationship is unique. People are free to decide who they want relationships with.

At the end of the session you might usefully point out that if people feel bad about a relationship they are in and/or are afraid of the other person, there are people they can speak to. Give information about local sources of support, in school and outside.

Reflection

Invite the class to share whether any of their ideas about relationships have changed or been challenged. Encourage them to say what else they have learned in the session.

A question of sleep

> **H5**
> Do I understand the importance of sleep – especially at my age?
> Do I understand that lack of sleep will influence my moods, my physiology and my ability to learn and recall?
> How do I feel about staying up later?
> How do I feel when others encourage me to stay up late?
> How do I feel when my parents or carers want me to go to sleep?

To the teacher

Certain health choices we make can seem simple, but they actually have a profound effect on our health, relationships and performance. As the old saying goes, 'If you want to be healthy, eat a balanced diet, exercise and get a good night's sleep.' At adolescence, as independence increases, there is often a desire to stay up later and ICT, especially mobile phones and access to personal computers, has made it easier to communicate with friends until the last one falls asleep.

Many students do not understand the consequences of lack of sleep and schools often underestimate the impact of lack of sleep on learning and performance. Gradually, staying up later is a sign of growing up and it can be hard for students to admit they need more sleep. As The Corrs song 'So Young' says:

> *And it really doesn't matter that we don't eat*
> *And it really doesn't matter if we never sleep*
> *No it really doesn't matter*
> *Really doesn't matter at all*
> *Coz we are so young, yeah we are so young, so young now*
> *And when tomorrow comes we'll just do it all again …*

The consequences of staying up late and missed sleep can spiral into many other aspects of life. The effects of too little sleep include:

- missing school
- sleepiness
- tiredness
- irritability and low frustration tolerance
- difficulties with our self-control of attention, emotion and behaviour
- difficulties with focusing our attention
- difficulty in controlling our emotions and their intensity (especially temper, frustration and sadness)
- difficulty in linking the right emotion to our thinking (for example, we *know* it is inappropriate, but we still *feel* irritable or angry)
- reduced learning and consolidating our memories of prior learning
- weight gain (although the reason is not yet clear – it may be through lowered levels of a hormone 'leptin', which reduces appetite and is released during sleep).

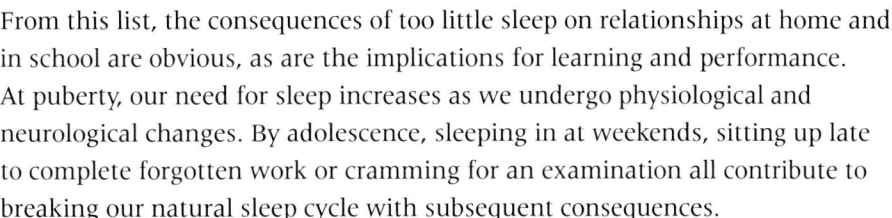

The use of alcohol can exacerbate any or all of these.

From this list, the consequences of too little sleep on relationships at home and in school are obvious, as are the implications for learning and performance. At puberty, our need for sleep increases as we undergo physiological and neurological changes. By adolescence, sleeping in at weekends, sitting up late to complete forgotten work or cramming for an examination all contribute to breaking our natural sleep cycle with subsequent consequences.

It may not be an exaggeration to say that insufficient sleep may be one of the major contributors to poor academic performance and behaviour issues among students.

To the students

Do the people we live with ever have a go at us for staying up too late? How do we feel about having 'early nights'? How do we feel about admitting to others that we are really tired or sleepy?

The purpose of this session is to explore what happens when we don't get enough sleep and how we can make sure that we do.

'You OK?' Josh asked.

'Yes, I'm fine!' snapped Joe.

'Don't bite my head off, I only asked. You look dreadful,' Josh replied.

'Well, I'm fine, OK. So leave me alone.'

Recently, Joe had been really irritable and tired and Josh was becoming worried something was seriously wrong with his friend. During a lesson in the early afternoon Joe had almost fallen asleep, and Josh had had to nudge him with his elbow when their teacher had almost noticed. As they left school Josh decided to confront Joe.

'Look, it's nothing,' Joe said. 'I have just had some late nights talking online to other people. I get carried away and don't get to bed until really late.'

'Is that all it is, I thought you were on drugs or something!'

'Actually, I do feel really weird, but just staying up late can't make you feel ill can it? Perhaps I've got something like flu coming,' Joe replied.

'You online later, Joe?' some others called over.

'Yeah, sure am,' Joe called back.

Focusing

In pairs, discuss what time you generally go to sleep at night.

- Are you staying up later than you used to? Why?
- Has something changed in your evening lifestyle? Is it difficult to be the first to leave a telephone or internet conversation and go to sleep?
- Do you find you sleep in longer at the weekends or at holiday time?
- How do you feel when you get up in the morning? How would you describe it? Do you feel 'ready to face the day' or do you still feel tired?

- What sort of mood are you in first thing in the morning? Do you find yourself getting up at the last minute and rushing? Does how you feel or the lack of time make it difficult for you to have breakfast?
- Do your parents encourage you to go to bed earlier than you want to? Does this cause any problems or conflict?
- Do you feel you have your sleep-time/awake-time balance about right?

Into action

Provide students with the following information:

- Although there are many theories, we still don't fully understand why we sleep.
- We seem to all need different amounts of sleep but, on average, adults need eight hours sleep per night, teenagers nine hours. (Given the chance at weekends and holidays, teenagers can often sleep more than this.)
- Ideally, we should have 'quality' as well as quantity. Something that is worrying us, or the use of drugs such as caffeine or alcohol, can affect the quality of our sleep.
- There is a theory that we can build up 'sleep debt'. If we have too little sleep during the week, we wake later on weekends. If we do this, it may mean we are not getting long enough sleep during the week.

Ask students to discuss in pairs whether they experience any of the following (you could create a quick 'questionnaire' sheet to help their individual reflection, but warn them before they complete them if you plan to ask them to share their responses with others):

- Sleepiness during the day.
- Feeling exhausted even after a long sleep (worrying, fitful, unsatisfying night's sleep).
- Tiredness during the day.
- Irritability, especially if people don't do what you want, if things go wrong or if things take longer than you think they ought to.
- Difficulties with self-control, especially managing emotions and behaviour.
- Difficulties with focus of attention (unable to keep your attention on a task without your mind wandering).
- Not being able to take part fully in learning, or not being able to remember your learning later.

Prompts might be:

If I had to describe myself against this list I would say …

… that's a lot like me.

… that's a little like me.

… that's nothing like me.

If others (my friends, members of my family, my teachers) had to describe me against this list, I think they might say …

… that's a lot like him/her.

… that's a little like him/her.

… that's nothing like him/her.

They could check their choices with their friends, families and teachers, perhaps getting some insights or even surprises.

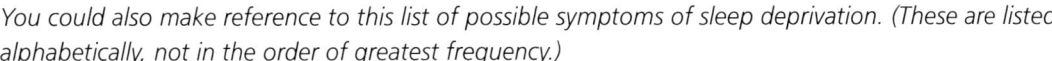

Into action

You could also make reference to this list of possible symptoms of sleep deprivation. (These are listed alphabetically, not in the order of greatest frequency.)

- Aching muscles.
- Blurred vision.
- Clinical depression.
- Colour blindness.
- Decreased ability for the immune system to fight off sickness.
- Decreased concentration.
- Decreased mental activity.
- Dizziness.
- Fainting.
- General confusion.
- Hallucinations.
- Hand tremors.
- Headache.
- Hypertension/hyperactivity.
- Impatience.
- Irritability.
- Memory lapses/loss.
- Nausea.
- Need for daytime naps.
- Nystagmus (rapid involuntary rhythmic eye movement).
- Pale skin tone (looking pasty).
- Psychosis.
- Slowed reaction time.
- Slurred speech.
- Weight gain.
- Yawning.

Invite students to carry out an experiment. For one week, they could keep a sleep diary and record what time they get to bed and what time they get up. Particularly note what time they wake up on Saturday morning.

Then, in the second week, starting on a Monday, ask students to try to get to bed earlier in order to get about nine hours sleep per night. Notice what time they wake up on Saturday. If they wake up naturally at the same time as during the week, this is a fair indicator that this is the amount of sleep they need.

Extension questions

Entering the question, 'How much sleep do we need?' into an internet search engine brings up a wealth of information. Invite the class to explore some of the following questions and add some of their own.

- Why do we dream?
- What can affect the quality of our sleep?
- Why is sleep deprivation considered a form of torture?

Reflection

If we are suffering from any of the symptoms that indicate we are not getting enough sleep, what can we do about it? What changes can we make? What changes are we willing to make? What might be the costs and benefits to me of making some simple changes? Can I create a compromise? What might a win-win outcome look like? For example, could I decide to have a couple of earlier nights each week? Could I negotiate agreement over this with my online friends?

If students say they lie awake if they go to bed earlier or wake up earlier, it is worth mentioning that going to bed earlier may not mean going to sleep earlier. It can take a little time for new sleep patterns to become routine. They may notice a gradual change in sleeping habits at the start of school holidays, where they may slowly settle to steadier and more consistent pattern as the frenetic activity of the term is replaced by a more relaxed period.

A question of balancing risk

K1
What are my feelings about risk?
How are they changing?
Do I feel more confident about doing things I haven't done before?
How do I assess risk?
When do I find risk exciting?
Do I understand that I can take risks with both my body and my feelings?
How do I balance this with my need to stay safe?

To the teacher

This session is intended either to open a module on risk or to reconnect with previous work. It crudely sets out two contrasting extremes. Sara is at one end of a continuum taking every opportunity to do what she wants, regardless of the consequences. Sara appears to live in the present with a 'let's do it!' attitude. Emma takes the opposite position where she analyses every consequence and, as a result, does very little that she wants. Emma lives in the future with a 'what if?' attitude.

The session explores how you manage navigating between these extremes, and some of the other dimensions of risk, such as excitement, challenge and embarking on the unfamiliar or the new. Is it possible to be inventive, creative, make major discoveries, explore the limits and question the orthodox or the 'norms' without taking risks? This session has three parts, a simple self-reflection, an analysis process to help risk management and a brief exploration of risk as an equation.

To the students

Risk is a strange word. In this session we are going to explore what risk actually means. Does risky mean it is dangerous? Does it mean that there is a chance something unpleasant, unwanted or dangerous could happen? We are always being warned about 'risks' but can doing something risky be exciting? Sensible? Unavoidable? Does everything we do involve some risk? Would there be new discoveries, inventions, new ways of seeing the world without risks? What would life be like if people never took any risks?

In this session we are going to explore 'risk'. The purpose is to discover how complex an idea it is, and how people can see it in so many ways.

'I don't understand,' Emma said.

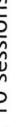

'So, no news there then!' Sara replied.

'Thanks for the first put down of the day,' Emma sighed. She was reading an article in her magazine. 'Seriously, it says here the risk has doubled. I can never understand these news articles. "You have a 14% risk of … The risk has gone up by 10%. If you choose to do this your risk of your head exploding has just doubled!"'

'Where does it say that?' Sara asked, suddenly curious.

'Joking, only joking,' Emma sighed. 'Got your attention though!'

'So?' Sara said. 'What's the problem? Usually it just means if you do or don't do this, there's a chance things will get better; if you do or don't do that, things will get worse!'

'But hang on a minute,' Emma said. 'What if I want to do something really exciting and I know it's risky? Let's say, parachute jumping.'

Sara had stopped and was looking up. 'Right, lots of opportunity round here for that then! Anyway, you get dizzy standing on a chair!'

'It's an example! How do I work out the risk? How do I know if the chances of something going wrong are so high the excitement I would get just isn't worth it? Or if the chances of something going wrong are actually so low it is worth taking the chance and having a great experience?' Emma asked.

Sara was quiet. 'Yeah, I think I followed that … just… Ever thought you think too much? I just see an opportunity to have fun and go for it!'

'Which may explain why you spend so much time crying on the phone to me afterwards telling me how it's all gone wrong, how you are now worried sick, how could you have been so stupid and that you'll never do it again!' Emma said.

'Well, I never said it's a great way of making choices, but I do have a lot of fun!' Sara justified.

'Yeah, and then we spend the next week trying to put everything right! But what if the thing that might go wrong couldn't be put right …?' Emma asked.

Emma was thinking later. She seemed to do this a lot. Sara never seemed to take anything seriously. She seemed to live only in the present, not to see any of the risks, to just go for it and have far more fun than Emma did. But then Sara had to live with far more problems and worries afterwards. Emma, however, always took life seriously, was really cautious especially about her future, could see all the risks and so didn't do half the things Sara got up to, but felt safe and, frankly, spent more time worrying about Sara than she did about herself. The problem was, some of the consequences of Sara's choices could have been really serious. So far she had been lucky!

There had to be a balance, Emma thought. How do you balance having a great time now while still staying safe, so that you can carry on having a great time afterwards?

Focusing

- So, if you had to choose, who are you more like – Emma or Sara?
- Is this all of the time or some of the time? If some of the time, when? What does it depend on?

Is it as simple as always being like Emma or being like Sara? Are there times when you need to be like Emma? Are there times when it is OK to be like Sara? How good are you at judging when it is appropriate to be one or the other?

Into action

In pairs, students discuss:
● What does the word 'risk' mean to you?
● How would you explain it to someone who didn't understand the word?

Collect feedback from the whole class.

Risk means …
Doing something risky means …
The *good* things about risk include …
The *not-so-good* things about risk include …
Ask students to study this risk map diagram. It might be useful to distribute copies to each pair or group of students.

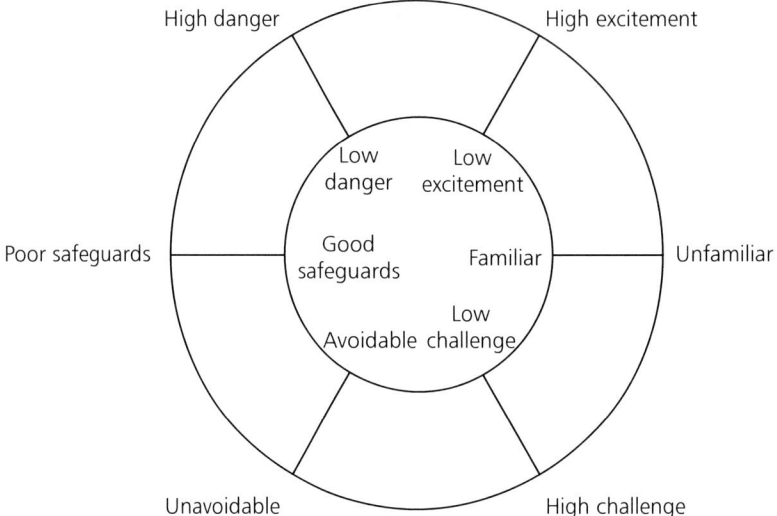

Imagine you have to cross a main street to get to school. There is no pedestrian crossing, crossing patrol, and no subway or alternative route. You might map the risks like this: medium danger; low excitement and low challenge; good safeguards; almost absolutely unavoidable; and very familiar. The map would look like this:

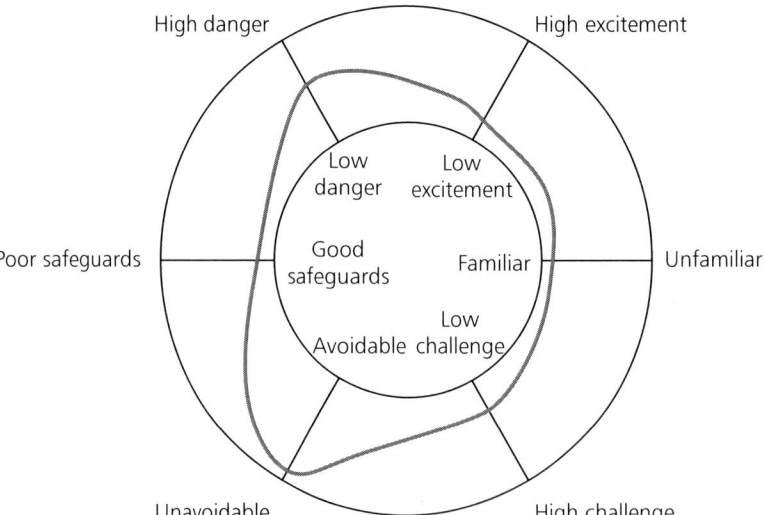

How might the map look if, instead, you had to travel a long distance on your own?

Are there some situations that are easy to map, but others that are more difficult? Would better information help? Information is obviously vital, but it needs to be accurate and comprehensible. Beware of statistical jargon. Suppose you read these headlines in a newspaper:

THE NUMBER OF PEOPLE WHO CONTRACT XYZ DISEASE DOUBLES

To make any sense of this you need to know how many contracted it in the first place. If it was every other person, it would be different from if it was originally one person in a million. In the first case, we would all be infected and, in the second, only two in a million.

THE RISK HAS RISEN BY 25 PER CENT

This usually means the number of people experiencing the problem has risen by 25 per cent. Therefore, if it was four people per 1000 it is now five people per 1000. Unless you know the figure *before* the rise, it is meaningless.

1 IN 6 PEOPLE WILL DIE OF ...

Possibly true, but since we all die of something what does this mean? In what circumstances do these people die? What do they have in common? Is there something risky they all do? If you knew 90 per cent of them were over 75 years of age, would you see it differently from if they were all in their late twenties to early thirties? If you knew they all smoked heavily or used sunbeds regularly for long periods of time, and you do not, would you be less concerned?

Therefore:

- if the risk 'doubles', we need to know what it was in the first place. And what difference does it make if that's one in a million or one in 10?
- if 'the risks go up eight per cent', it's not possible to say how worried we should be unless we have a lot more information
- if there is an 'increased risk', what does this mean? How increased? Risk of what, exactly? Does it mean increased *severity*? Increased *likelihood*? Both?

How convinced are you now about the need for reliable and *helpful* information?

With this in mind, think about the following risks. In pairs, choose one and draw the shape of the risk using a blank copy of the risk map.

- Setting up a new business.
- Going to a new job.
- Regular use of sunbeds.
- Smoking tobacco or cannabis.
- Asking someone out.
- Going somewhere like a club for the first time.
- Meeting someone for real that you first 'met' in an internet chat room.
- Two first-timers (heterosexual) who are about to have sexual intercourse for the first time.
- Unprotected sex.

Into action

After you have drawn the risk-shape, ask yourselves:

- Would you feel better if there was a way to relocate some of the cross-points in the diagram to different places?
- What would need to happen, or what would people need to do, for the positions to move?

In your pairs, explain your risk-shape to another pair. If a shape is being explained to you, are you convinced? Can you see possible risks or factors the other pair hasn't spotted? Or might they have overstated the risks? Tell the other pair how comfortable or uncomfortable you feel about your risky activity.

Draw out this important idea: risk of something bad happening is the result of balancing the *severities* of what could go wrong against the *likelihood* of it going wrong.

For example;

- we might worry about flying because the severity of something going wrong appears great, yet actually the likelihood of it going wrong is very low
- we might not worry about accidents in our home, but actually it is the most likely place for us to suffer an injury.

As human beings we seem pre-programmed to be more fearful about the severity of something going wrong, rather than the likelihood. This can lead some people to make potentially dangerous choices. For example smoking, where the likelihood of serious health consequences is high but the severity seems distant and perhaps unreal. It can also lead to people being over-fearful of situations where the chances of something going wrong are really small. Even if we *know* there is little danger, we still *feel* scared, and our feelings can try hard to overcome our thinking, for example a white-knuckle ride at a theme park. Sometimes it can be the reverse, when we *feel* there is little danger but *know* there is, such as crossing a main road with no pedestrian crossing.

- How can you use reliable information to help you balance the severity of unwanted outcomes (on the one hand) with their likelihood (on the other)?
- How can you get reliable information … and where/who from?
- How can you make sense of what your gathered information means, so that you can use it to assess the risks?
- If there are lots of possible consequences, do they all have equal 'weight'? Might just one possible *unwanted consequence* be more important to your decision than all the others? Might one *benefit* be more important than all the others?
- Could some good and not-so-good consequences happen immediately, or could they only happen in the future?
- How do you decide what to do, once you feel able to gauge the risk?

What does all this information tell you? How well does it help you now decide what to do? There may be further questions you should be asking – of people who are well informed, or have experience of the situation (or both). Process the responses carefully.

Reflection

Take one of the risky behaviours you explored in class and research it more fully. How accurate was the risk-shape you drew in class?

Ask yourself: on a scale of 1–5 (1 = totally able; 5 = totally unable), do I now feel better able to analyse at least *some* of the risks I might face than I felt before?

A question of looking after your image

> **K8**
> Do I understand how I might be at risk from my own use and other people's use of communication technology?
> Do I understand that once material, including images, is uploaded to the internet, it can be there for ever?
> How do I feel about this?

To the teacher

This session on internet safety focuses on protecting our image. Students are now confidently using ICT both for learning and communication, taking it for granted as an essential part of their lives, yet they are often naive about the risks. For example, it is easy for anyone to carry out a fast and cheap check on someone by putting their name into an internet search engine.

It might be useful to team teach this session with a member of the school ICT team. Although we have used our usual approach of a case study, it is possible to work with ICT teachers to set up practical demonstrations to illustrate the risks. See the knowledge frame (page 247) to see further key internet safety considerations.

To the students

Have you ever put your name into a search engine to find out what information or images about you are already on the internet? It can be OK or really scary. Did you know that once an image of you is uploaded to the internet that image can be copied by others and shared with virtually anyone in the world? Did you know that companies sometimes do this to check out an applicant for a job?

The purpose of this session is to explore how we can protect our 'image'.

'Have you heard about Kelly? She is in a terrible state, she has been sobbing all day,' said Sara.

'What happened?' Emma asked.

'Well, she was with her friends when, for a laugh, they put their names into a search engine to see what was on the web about them or other people with their name; see if anyone else with their name is famous or done anything interesting. Anyway, it turns out there were all these photos of her on some really nasty websites,' said Sara.

'How could that have happened?' Emma asked.

'It turns out that, for a laugh, she had, well, you know, flashed her, well, you know, to the webcam in her room to a mate. They were just mucking about. Seems it wasn't much of a mate because they recorded it and, for a laugh, put it on their own website.'

'That's pretty cruel!' said Emma.

'That's not the worst bit. It seems that there are lots of people out there who search for that sort of thing. They copied the images off the site and they are now on a load of other websites in different countries and they have her name on them,' said Sara.

'So what is she going to do?' asked Emma.

'Nothing she can do. They are there pretty much for ever. They could be there for the rest of her life! She is dreading her parents finding out.'

Emma felt a bit worried. She sometimes forgot her webcam was on in her room.

Focusing

In pairs, think about all the ways images of you could find their way on to the internet.

Look for:

- Video material captured on webcams and used for video messaging
- Photographs or video clips captured on a mobile phone camera
- Photographs taken on digital cameras
- Images uploaded personally to a profile on a social network site.

Inform the class that, in 2008, Facebook was the most popular website for uploading photos, with 14 million uploaded daily.

Into action

In groups, talk about how we could protect images of ourselves or those we care about from being available to anyone online.

Look for:

- Take responsibility for not putting ourselves in a position where we could have images captured that we might later regret being seen by others.
- Take responsibility for sharing images of ourselves only with people we really trust.
- We have responsibilities to protect other people's images. Do we have a right to put images of others on the internet, even with their permission, if they don't fully understand the risks?

Write suggestions on the board.

Reflection

What practical steps can we take to protect our image?

Look for:

- Covering webcams or disconnecting them when not in use
- Not uploading images of ourselves to websites unless we are comfortable for them to be available to the public for many years
- Not uploading images of others to websites, even with their permission
- Not passing on images of ourselves to others unless we are sure we totally trust them
- Not passing on images of other people to others without their permission.

A question of being safe online

> **K9**
> Do I understand how to use webcams safely?
> Do I understand how to use online communication safely, especially communicating within online communities – 'social networking' sites?
> Do I understand the risks of physically meeting people only previously 'met' online?

To the teacher

ICT may be a tool for an older generation but it is a way of life for students. The use of ICT is, for many students, their principal means of communication and, through this, students are able to interact with a global community. This is something to celebrate; however, it obviously brings risks. The high level of confidence many students have over the use of ICT can mean they may miss some of the real dangers. In 2006, MySpace already had 160 million users. If it was a country of that size, it would already have been the eleventh largest in the world.

This is one session where it may be best to let students take the lead, unless you are very familiar with the rapidly changing variety of media that they use. It may also be useful to team teach this with an ICT specialist, and offer a context for cross-curricular learning. See also the knowledge frame on the safe use of ICT on page **247**.

To the students

Use a show of hands to see how many of you use technology to communicate with one another. What types of services do you use?

Describe them, if necessary, to ensure everyone, including your teacher, understands them.

Look for:
- Instant messaging services
- Social connection utilities (sites where students can upload information about themselves)
- Chat rooms.

New services and technologies are always emerging.

The purpose of this session is to explore some of the risks that you might be running by using these services. The teacher is probably going to need your help with this subject.

Focusing

In pairs, discuss what information there is about you on the internet. How did it get there? Who do you allow to see it? How can you be sure it is only them?

into action

Ask the class to help you generate a list of all the known social networking websites. They will doubtless mention sites like Facebook, MySpace and Bebo. How many of these networks are class members signed up to? Ask the pairs to talk briefly to each other about how comfortable they feel about the privacy and security arrangements offered by these sites.

Take feedback – how many in the class are less than 100 per cent sure they are protected by these arrangements? Invite anyone in the class who can, to try to reassure the doubters. Are any of the doubters now convinced?

Explain that, as part of a research project on Facebook privacy published in December 2005, two students from Massachusetts Institute of Technology were able to use an automated script to download over 70,000 Facebook profiles from four US universities, including their own. Ask students if they have heard of any other internet security breaches. Did the owners of these sites believe they were secure? What conclusions can the class draw about the security of 'private' personal information stored on websites?

Reflection

Have any of the students ever visited an internet chat room and pretended to be younger, older or a different gender from their own? How easy would this be to do? How easy is it to detect false information?

Reflect on how an unscrupulous, dishonest or malicious person could exploit this uncertainty. What safeguards could students put in place to avoid putting themselves at risk from such people?

A question of 'cyber-bullying'

K10
Do I understand the term 'cyber-bullying'?
Do I understand how technology, for example texting, telephone calls, e-mail, chat rooms, instant messaging, personal websites and blogs, pictures and video clips captured on mobile phones can all be used for bullying?
Do I think this is the same as, or different from, any other type of bullying?
Why?
How might people feel who experience bullying like this?
What might they do?
Who would be responsible?
What do I feel about this type of bullying?
Do I know how to get specialist support if I experience cyber-bullying?

To the teacher

This session assumes that the students have previously explored and defined what the term 'bullying' means to them. If they haven't, it is important to do this first. While bullying using ICT is motivated by the same influences as any other form of bullying, there are two significant additional issues.

Technology, such as mobile phones, can be with us wherever we go and, potentially, 24 hours a day. Students may have their own computers, which can present them with targeted unwanted and potentially abusive, demeaning or cruel messages into their bedrooms, again, potentially, 24 hours a day. This means that it is possible for victims to experience relentless bullying in places where they might have previously felt safe. We suggest this session be team-taught with an ICT teacher or with a police officer who is knowledgeable about the law relating to cyber-bullying.

Attacking someone using ICT also allows otherwise less powerful students to become powerful. It can be a formidable weapon for revenge, especially by those who may have been targeted for bullying by others.

In addition to abusive messages, it is possible for an individual's image and identity to be uploaded to the internet with a fictitious biography containing false, embarrassing, cruel information allegedly about that person. Sites can be located anywhere in the world and support may be needed to have them removed.

We need to teach this session very carefully, otherwise it could teach some students sophisticated methods of bullying others. It is essential that your school has a clear policy over the acceptable use of ICT (and makes reference to cyber-bullying in the school's anti-bullying policy) because school sites can be used to cyber-bully students.

This session should be part of the school's ongoing programme of work on relationships and not taught as a 'one-off'. It is important to give the message that ICT is a medium through which people bully or hurt others, and not project it as something different. Bullying is assault and bullying using technology is no different and will be treated as seriously as physical bullying.

We have used the terms 'victim' and 'bully', but you might like to renegotiate these to 'perpetrator' and 'target'.

To the students

ICT is fantastic – it lets us keep in touch with people anywhere in the world virtually any time we want. In this session we want to explore the way ICT is used by a very small number of people to bully and hurt other people. This is something we, as a school (society), take very seriously and, if it ever happens to you, we want to explore what you can do to help yourself and how we can support you. The police and many companies who provide internet services and mobile telephone services also take this very seriously.

'What's up, Sara?' Emma asked. Sara had been down for a few days and, come to think of it, most of last week. 'It's the weekend, two days off!!'

''Yeah, I know,' replied Sara. 'Great …'

'OK, I know that look, what's wrong?' Emma asked again. This wasn't right, Sara was the strong, tough, lively, adventurous one of the two of them. Emma was the shy, timid one. This is probably why they got on so well. If you put us together, Emma thought, it would make one balanced person! Suddenly, Sara burst into tears and out poured a story.

It had started a week ago with a really nasty text. First, Sara had thought that it was meant for someone else and that she had received it by mistake, but it happened again and this time had her name in it. Whoever had sent it knew her, knew where she went to school and even what she did in the evening. She was getting texts every few hours and sometimes late at night. Next, she had started getting e-mails and messages on her computer. She was frightened to switch her computer on in case there was another.

'I can't get away from them!' she sobbed. 'I need my phone and I have to use the computer for homework. It isn't fair!'

'No, it isn't,' Emma replied. 'It's vicious, cowardly and cruel. Have you any idea who it is?'

'No, but it is someone at school. They know what happens in lessons, but that isn't all. One of the e-mails told me to look at an internet address. Someone had put a picture of me on a site with loads of things about me that aren't true and which I am supposed to have written about myself. What if a teacher or my parents see it?' said Sara.

'We need to tell someone right now,' Emma said. 'We need to get some serious help!'

Focusing

What are all the ways we use ICT – mobiles, texting, chat rooms, messenger services – to talk to one another? Ask the students, in pairs, to come up with as many as they can.

Collate feedback from the class. Now ask the class to suggest any ways ICT could be used to spread information about someone. Again, collate feedback. Ask:

- Who can put this information online?
- Is it possible for false information to be put online?

Into action

Ask what makes ICT bullying different from physical bullying. How might it feel different to the person being bullied? For example, it can happen any time of day/night, so there is 'no safe place'; the bully is not present and may want to hide their identity; it always leaves evidence that can be shown to a teacher or the police; it can be done by small people to big people; bullying and the emotions it causes can extend into homes and other 'safe' places.

Now, ask for suggestions about what we, our school and other people can and should do:

a) to prevent it happening in the first place

b) to support the victim, if it does happen

c) when a perpetrator is identified (caught).

You might divide the class into six groups (two of which explore each issue). Give each group a flip-chart and marker and allow some discussion and recording time.

Collect and display their ideas.

a) To prevent bullying happening in the first place:

Look for:

- Increase feelings of inclusion and make people feel valued at school
- Strengthen the unacceptability of bullying throughout the school
- Publicise and reinforce this climate and associated policies
- Strengthen caring management of mobile phones and computers during the school day
- Reinforce channels for student support (which might benefit potential perpetrators, potential victims, and everyone else).

b) To support the victim, if it does happen:

It is usually relatively straightforward for police to trace the source of information sent or posted online, so remaining anonymous is not easy for a perpetrator unless they consistently use someone else's equipment.

Look for:

- Reassuring the victim that this bullying can and will be stopped
- Encouraging them not to delete any evidence, but pass it to the authorities
- Being sympathetic to how they feel
- Helping them look at their relationship with the perpetrator (if they know each other) to see if there are clues as to why it is happening

- Raising the victim's morale and strengthening or confirming their feelings of self-worth
- 'Catching' the perpetrator and stopping the abuse happening
- Contacting the police, if necessary.

Dealing definitively with dishonest or otherwise criminal online postings may be more difficult, depending upon where the information is stored. If it is on the server of a UK or reputable foreign host, getting it deleted may be straightforward. Ensuring the information and, for example, any photos have not 'got out' and been shared elsewhere on the web may be impossible. See the knowledge frame on Internet safety, page 247.

c) When a perpetrator is identified:

Students may make some suggestions of serious retribution. Sympathise strongly with any feelings of revulsion, anger and wish to punish, but temper these with a need, first and foremost, to act constructively, rather than taking the law into their own hands. A desire to punish may feel natural, but acting on it may do more harm than good.

Look for:

- Make it clear that this behaviour must stop
- Do precisely what the school's anti-bullying policy says for this eventuality
- Try to discover why the perpetrator is acting this way
- Try to discover why the perpetrator chose this victim – perhaps their relationship needs outside help; maybe any difficulties they have can be resolved
- Try to sympathise with any feelings (inadequacy, desperation) that may be causing the person to bully
- Avoid labelling this person as a 'bully'
- Review and strengthen the school's anti-bullying policy, if necessary.

Reflection

Does anything need to be done in school *immediately* to start the process of making cyber-bullying less likely? (Perhaps the School Council needs to take this forward.)

Reflect upon the responsibilities *all* individual students share to make bullying less likely, and to support anyone who is bullied by ICT.

A question of carrying weapons

> **K13**
> Why do I think some people carry weapons when they go out?
> How do I feel about people carrying weapons?
> What are the risks to themselves and others if they choose to carry a weapon?
> Have I ever felt the need to carry a weapon?

To the teacher

The focus chosen here is knives, but the session could be widened to include any sort of weapon. The carrying of knives by young people is a major problem in some areas of the country. Research suggests that, rightly or wrongly, young people believe knife carrying among their peers is widespread. If knife carrying is actually rare in your community, this is an important message to reinforce and you could explore why most young people make this choice. It is important to maintain a sense of balance. If we don't, there is a danger that we might inadvertently reinforce knife carrying as being widespread – encouraging, rather than discouraging, the behaviour.

When asked, most claim it is for self-protection against other knife carrying peers. As institutions increasingly introduce metal detectors, it is becoming easier to be caught carrying a knife and there are legal consequences to face.

No single session, even a long one such as this, can address this issue in full. This session opens up the issue for discussion. If you only have limited time, focus on a few key questions to explore. If you have more time, you may wish to extend the discussion to include defensive measures, such as carrying pepper spray to ward off attacks.

As with so many health and social issues, the knives themselves are not the problem. This work needs very careful planning. It is important to focus on the feelings associated with, and the motivation for, carrying knives and managing, limiting or (better still) avoiding the social situations where they may be used or feared. It is important to keep the focus on how people are feeling and how the presence of a knife influences what happens. There is a danger that focusing on the knives helps them become the modern equivalent of the 'cowboy six-gun' (actually, largely a Hollywood myth).

There is obviously a range of serious risks associated with carrying a knife, from simply being found in possession of one by a police officer, through to serious injury or death if it is used, and the subsequent punishment of the perpetrator or perpetrators and the devastation to family and friends.

In reality, despite the huge physical and legal risks in carrying a knife, it offers little if any protection. A knife attack or mugging is sudden and usually over before we can defend ourselves. Most uses of a knife are a sudden, unexpected slash rather than a fight or exchange of blows. A knife or knives drawn in a verbal exchange usually makes things far worse not better. It is possible one person will back down but, if it becomes a true 'knife fight', both parties usually end up seriously injured. This is because adrenalin can allow a knife fight to continue even after serious, even life-threatening, wounds have been exchanged. It is possible to puncture a vital organ or cause internal bleeding with a very small blade and a very shallow cut. Craft knife blades are easy to conceal and, apart from obvious injuries, can scar for life.

This might be a good session to team teach with a local police officer, or perhaps use as an 'issue raising session' for a subsequent question and answer session with a police officer. This is definitely a session where the established ground rules need to be revisited and, if necessary, renegotiated.

You could also use Invitation 2: Bus stop people (page **205**) and Invitation 3: Adults (page **206**), either within the session or as action research prior to the session. Try this invitation:

> A group of students from our school/adults from our community have met together. They are talking about young people carrying knives. What do you think they are saying and thinking? Draw yourself in the picture. What would you be saying and thinking?

If you do use an action research approach, it is essential that the students are clear as to who will eventually see their responses.

To the students

There are often news reports about young people carrying weapons, including knives. In this session we are going to explore whether or not you believe this to be true, and what the immediate and longer-term consequences of making a decision to carry a knife might be to ourselves and to others. If appropriate, this might be a good time to feed back the results or key messages from any action research.

The purpose of this session is to explore why a small number of young people carry knives and what we feel about this.

'Have you seen what Jason's carrying?' asked Joe.

'Err … hang on, let me guess. Bag? Magazine? Something really valuable that belongs to someone else that he is "borrowing"?' Josh replied.

'Yeah, very funny, just not a lot. No, he has got a knife,' said Joe.

'With or without the fork and spoon?'

'Will you stop being a complete idiot! He's got a knife, a seriously large knife!' exclaimed Joe.

'Why?' Josh asked.

'How should I know? He's just the sort of idiot that might use it,' Joe replied. 'If he and his mates are all carrying knives … do you think … we ought to?'

'He is just showing off, it makes him feel big in front of the others,' replied Josh.

'So, you don't think we should then?' asked Joe.

'Are you mad?' Josh answered. 'Carrying a knife could get you into real trouble, and I mean big trouble. Is that what you want?'

'No, of course I don't! But if Jason and that lot are carrying them, haven't we got a right to protect ourselves?' asked Joe.

They had reached Joe's house and Josh walked on alone. He felt a bit funny about knives. He knew he could never use one on anyone else, but he did find them … just a bit … cool and he suspected Joe did to. He would never have considered carrying one himself, but … if Jason and his mates were carrying … perhaps he ought to … for protection … or was that just an excuse? 'No, it's really stupid,' he said to himself. '… But …'

Focusing

In pairs, ask the students to think about all the possible reasons young people may offer for carrying knives.

● How do you feel about these reasons?
● Do you think they are legitimate reasons or reasons you would support?
● Are they reasons that you would challenge?

Collate feedback from the class.

Look for:

- Reasons from outside – as a deterrent to others, to use in self-defence
- Reasons from inside – to look or feel cool, to reduce feelings of fear or threat.

At the time of writing, carrying knives tends to be a male behaviour. Ask the girls how they feel about this, especially if 'protecting a partner' is offered as a reason for carrying. Does it make them feel protected or uneasy? Would their feelings change if a situation developed where the knife was drawn or used?

Into action

In groups of four, think about the following:

- In the scenario above, what do you feel about Joe's reaction to Jason and his gang allegedly carrying knives?
- How do you feel about Josh's reply? Why may he have more than one feeling about this? Might his feelings be pushing him in different directions?
- What might be the consequences of carrying a weapon such as a knife?

At this point, it is likely that the discussion will focus on the consequences of being caught in possession. Make sure students know it can be illegal.

'Have you heard what happened last night?' Joe was out of breath when he ran up to Josh and Emma who were heading out for school. 'It's Jason!'

'What's he done now?' Emma sighed.

'He's in hospital; his face got slashed open in a fight!' cried Joe.

'And … I would care … why?' Josh replied, trying to appear cool but really wanting to know more.

'Well, turns out on the way home last night he and his mates were mucking about with Danny Brown in Year 9, you know, teasing him. Anyway, Danny must have known about Jason and his mates carrying knives and it turns out he was carrying a small penknife himself, which he got out when he told them to leave him alone. So Jason pulls his knife and starts waving it in Danny's face. His mates said he was just mucking about.'

'Hang on, you do mean THE Danny Brown, the Danny "I am the quietest boy in the entire school, come to think of it, the entire world" Brown?' asked Josh.

'Yep, he's the one,' said Joe. 'Anyway, Danny thought Jason was serious, so he panicked and slashed him across the face. They say it's damaged his eye. Danny ran away but the police arrested him. Jason's mates are all saying they were just mucking about and Danny pulled his knife first.'

In the same groups, think about the following:

- Why was Danny carrying a knife?
- Do you think Danny ever planned or intended to use it on anyone?
- What state of mind was Danny in when he slashed Jason's face? (Who was in charge – his 'feeling' self or 'thinking' self – his 'adult' or 'child'?) What is likely to happen to Danny? How do you feel about this?
- Did the presence of the knives make things worse for everyone?
- How might this incident affect Josh and Joe?
- Who do you think is responsible for everything that has happened?
- Can things happen so quickly that people can't really think about the full consequences for themselves or others? How can you avoid getting in these situations?
- If two people pull knives or weapons, might one back down? What might stop one person backing down? (Look for strong emotions: 'feeling' self taking over from 'thinking' self; 'child' in charge rather than 'adult'; being encouraged by others; presence of someone you want to impress.)

Reflection

On balance, how do you feel about carrying knives? What are the risks of carrying them to us, to others? Do they make us safer or does carrying them make violence more likely? If we are involved in their use, or discovered to be carrying them, what are the real consequences to us and those we care about or who care about us?

This session could lead into further sessions that look at avoiding, defusing (or failing to defuse) confrontation.

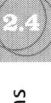
A question of binge drinking

> **D9**
> What do I understand by the term 'binge drinking'?
> Why do I think some people choose to binge drink?
> Do I understand the health and social risks to my personal safety of binge drinking?

To the teacher

'Binge drinking' is an unfortunate and imprecise term because it seems to imply that you need a huge amount of alcohol at one time to 'binge drink'. In fact, relatively small quantities of alcohol can constitute binge drinking as far as our health is concerned. Binge drinking is normally associated with 'drinking alcohol for the purposes of getting intoxicated'. However, medically, over five units of alcohol for a grown man and over four units of alcohol for a grown woman in one session constitutes binge drinking.

A second unfortunate, and rather misleading, term is 'safe drinking limits' for men and women. Young people assume safe drinking limits apply to them and it is vitally important that they understand that they don't. Very low levels of alcohol may protect against coronary heart disease but not until far later in life. There are no *'safe* drinking limits' for young people because they are still growing and developing. Alcohol will have a more harmful effect on young people than a fully developed adult.

A third misunderstanding is that alcohol 'makes you happy'. This drug is not a 'mood giver' but a 'mood amplifier', so, if you are depressed, alcohol may not make you cheerful, it is just as likely to increase the depression. Its effects depend more on how you already feel and where you are, than on how you'd like to feel.

The media may give the impression that most young people binge drink, but this is not the case. It is still a minority activity and our emphasis should be exploring why the majority of young people choose either not to use alcohol at all or use it in a more circumspect way.

Before teaching this session, it might be helpful to have recent figures of young people's alcohol use. These are often available from your local health authority or the internet.

This is potentially quite a long session and you may want to edit it down. A fact sheet for young people to take away may also be useful. In addition, it might be a good opportunity to talk about the need to treat alcohol intoxication as a drug overdose. It is vital to never leave someone who has drunk themselves unconscious alone. If they are on the pavement, place them on a coat or blanket, put them in the 'recovery position' and get medical aid as quickly as possible.

It can be helpful to break the risks of excessive alcohol use into three areas. The effect of alcohol on:

- physical health
- social health
- personal safety.

Although this session focuses on the social and safety risks associated with binge drinking, students should also understand the biological risks. However, take care not to depict binge drinking in a wholly negative light – you may risk alienating the drinkers you seek to engage. Indeed, with older classes it helps to put social drinking into the context of the students' own leisure habits, and their own view of the significance of drinking to those in their close peer group. It is worth bearing in mind that of the young people who *do* drink excessively, not all will necessarily see the 'negative' outcomes of such drinking in the way we do. Professor Chris Hackley, from Royal Holloway, University of London, quotes research that tells us: 'Inebriation within the friendship group is often part of a social bonding ritual that is viewed positively and linked with fun, friendship and good times, although some young people can be the target of humiliating or risky activities.'

The effects of alcohol consumption: information for the teacher

The following is only a rough guide, as each individual's reaction to alcohol is unique to them and is influenced by the context within which it is consumed, as well as by the quantity and the time that has elapsed since drinking it.

For a fully grown man:

1–2 units: increased cheerfulness and increased self-confidence

2 units: increased risk of accident

3 units: usually increased happiness, but significantly impaired judgement

5 units: more severe loss of capacity, greater risk of accidents. This amount of alcohol is likely to impair ability to judge the degree to which alcohol has impaired judgement.

10 units: slurred speech, loss of self-control, may be aggressive

12 units: inability to walk straight, loss of memory

18 units: approaching toxic levels. Continued drinking will lead to unconsciousness.

Note: For women or young people who are physically smaller, the same effects will result from drinking significantly less. Any amount of alcohol may impair driving ability, even when it doesn't put the drinker above the legal limit, leading potentially to loss of driving licence and cause of serious accidents.

To the students

This session explores the risks around the use of alcohol. Most people, young and old, use alcohol safely, drinking only small amounts occasionally. A small number of people drink quite large amounts of alcohol at one time. The media calls this binge drinking.

The purpose of this session is to think about the risks of binge drinking and explore some of the reasons why it might happen.

Focusing

What do you understand by the term 'binge drinking'? How precise is this description? How useful? Who uses it as a term of disapproval? Who might be proud of it?

In pairs, if you had to explain to a Martian what binge drinking is, and why some people do it, what would you say?

Collect some ideas from the class and challenge or unpack anything that is not clear. For example:

- Drinking a lot – what is 'a lot'?
- Drinking a lot of the time – how often is 'a lot of the time'?
- Drinking too much – how much is 'too much'?
- Drinking dangerously – dangerous in what way?
- Drinking for fun – how much of what happens is fun? How necessary is alcohol for fun?

Into action

Part 1

In groups of four, ask the students to read the following statements (you may want to provide fewer statements or give one to each group to focus on).

- Did you see what just happened ... that's really horrible ... (gross/out of order).
- You know who you got off with, don't you? You did ... honest ...
- After what you just said, I'm not surprised they don't want anything to do with you any more!
- Do you think he/she is safe doing that?
- Don't you remember what you did? Do you think you ought to talk to someone?
- Are you going to walk home on your own like that?
- She/he is a right laugh when she/he is drunk!
- She/he is throwing up again!
- We had a wild time last night!

Ask each group to explore:
- What do you feel about those involved?
- What are all the things that could have happened?
- What might happen next?
- How might they be feeling later?

Choose one statement and make three lists of the possible risks the person may be running to their:
- physical health
- social health
- personal safety.

Collect feedback from the class. Ask the wider group to add anything they think is missing.

Extension

Does it make a difference if the person referred to in the statements is a young woman or a young man? Why?

What might the person saying these statements be really thinking or saying inside their heads? For example, 'He/she is a right laugh when she/he is drunk' could really be thinking 'When he/she gets drunk, he/she is embarrassing to be with, does really stupid things that could get him/her and me into trouble, I get really scared and I hate it.'

Now read these two scenarios:

1 *I have woken up in a police cell. I'm feeling terrible. I can't remember anything I did last night. I don't know if I have damaged something or even hurt someone. I am feeling really sick and really scared. I think I must have thrown up because my clothes stink. They have just said they are calling my parents. I think they said something about seeing a duty solicitor after I have been charged.*

2 *I have woken up lying on the pavement. It is really dark and I am hurting all over. I can feel that there is something wet on my face and it really hurts. I can't find my things. I think my clothes are torn. I can't remember anything. I am not sure where I am. I want to get help, but I can't find my phone.*

- What could have led to these scenarios?
- What do you think might happen next?
- Did you assume they were boys or girls? Does it make any difference?

Key issue: List the factors that might mean:

- the enjoyment of drinking *outweighs the risks*
- the risks *outweigh the enjoyment*.

What can be done to ensure the first of these two outcomes actually happens?

Part 2

In groups, explore why you think some people choose to use alcohol like this. How and why do you think it happens?

Collect feedback from the class.

Look for:

- The pressure to conform – if everyone else is binge drinking, it can be hard not to join in
- Curious to know what it's like
- The need some people have to use alcohol to feel confident
- It makes you feel good – *ask specifically how it makes you feel good*
- It helps people have a good time – *ask what is 'a good time' and how alcohol actually helps.*

If these reasons are not given, suggest them yourself.

In groups of four, pick a couple of these reasons. How would you respond to them if someone said these to you?

Collect feedback from the class.

Ask if anyone has experience of being with people who are drunk – how does it feel? Why?

Reinforce that alcohol takes away your ability to make judgements about your own behaviour, and especially your ability to judge your own level of intoxication. (You literally don't know how drunk you are, how dangerous your behaviour might be and the consequences. That part of your brain has been anaesthetised.) Explore students' suggestions about when the risks outweigh the enjoyment, and how hard it may be to be sure it will remain 'worth it'.

Reflection

Working in pairs, discuss the following:

- What are three things that this session has helped you think about?
- Out of everything we have covered in this session, what do you think are the main reasons most young people choose not to use alcohol excessively?
- What can you do that might help keep people you drink with safer?
- As a result of this session, do you feel differently about your own choices and decisions about drinking or not drinking alcohol? Is there anything you feel more strongly about?

A question of coping with stress

S1
Am I aware of what can cause me unwanted stress (stressors) and how this can affect me?
Do I know that stress is something common that affects everybody in some way, and can have both positive and negative effects?

S2
Am I aware of how this affects me personally? How good am I at recognising unwanted stress in myself (and others)?

S4
Do I know how simple changes in my breathing and body posture can actually change the way my brain and body respond to stressors, and help me feel less stressed?

To the teacher

This session helps students to understand the reality of stress – that the stress response is something normal and common to everyone – and to be aware of causes and effects of stress. Through the experience of the 'soap' characters and a group activity that takes a light-hearted approach, the session also facilitates some reflection on students' own stressors – initially, in a safe and dissociated way – and then introduces a rapid stress relief technique as 'first aid' to use if feeling the effects of 'destructive' stress. Some notes on stress have been provided to assist you on page **266**.

The session links the content boxes above and also touches upon box Year 10, S8.

Note: A photocopiable sheet of the script below can be found on page 187.

To the students

This session is about stress, people's attitudes to it and coping with it. You hear people talk about 'stressing', but most people don't know that it's a real reaction that happens in your brain and body, that it happens to everybody and it's not always a bad thing. It can be stimulating, motivating and really **constructive**. Of course it can also be negative or **destructive** – that's when people say they're getting 'stressed'.

Josh was sitting struggling with his maths revision, scratching his head, wishing he was playing football and wondering whether it was time to take a break for a small snack (which would only be his third since he got home). His concentration (which wasn't that great anyway) was suddenly broken by a crash in the kitchen, followed by swearing, followed by the unmistakable sound of his sister, Emma, crying. Josh was in the kitchen faster than a penalty shot.

Emma was sitting on the kitchen floor sobbing, surrounded by a broken mug and a pool of coffee. She was attempting to pick up sticky wet pieces of mug. Josh breathed a sigh of relief.

'I thought you'd really hurt yourself,' he said. Then he looked at her with a puzzled expression. 'Whatever's the matter, Emma? It's only a mug and a drop of coffee. Why are you crying? Is it, you know, that time of the month?' he asked, helpfully or so he thought. Emma's expression suddenly made maths seem like a really good option.

'No, it's not!' Emma shouted at him. 'Why do boys always think girls aren't allowed just to be really upset and angry – just because they are!!' Then she started crying again. 'I thought twins were supposed to understand each other.'

Josh thought it would be a good idea not to say anything else; he just put his arm round his sister.

'Oh, I'm sorry, Josh,' she said, after a moment or two. 'I've had such a rotten day. I was late for the bus, I forgot to take my books for the library and now they're overdue, Miss Beale was in a funny mood and I had a row with Sara about our project. Now we'll probably make a mess of that … I just want to run away … the coffee was just the final disaster!'

Josh didn't think any of it sounded like a disaster to him, but wisely didn't say so! 'It's OK, Emma,' he said. 'You take a deep breath and sit down. I'll do this, and then we can think about the other stuff together …' He bent down and starting picking up bits of broken mug.

*Josh was still feeling puzzled though. His sister usually coped with much bigger stuff – she seemed to thrive under pressure. Like when she helped organise the school play **and** acted in it – there was so much involved and a deadline to meet **and** being on stage. It would have got **him** stressing like mad, but she was just buzzing.*

Focusing

- What do you think about Emma's explanation for getting so upset about smashing the mug of coffee?
- Did Josh do anything that was helpful?
- Why do you think she had responded so differently to the other stuff Josh was recalling – such as the pressure of the school play?
- How do you think Josh responds to stress?

Students could raise a variety of ideas including: lots of little things can add up; Josh offered to talk it through; she enjoyed/was good at the other stuff; people can snack a lot when they're stressed, etc.

Divide the class groups and give each group a sheet of flip-chart paper and some marker pens. Explain that their group task is to draw a stressed person. They can be as creative as they like and add pictures and words to illustrate all the things the person is stressed about. The group can include anything that comes to mind when they think about stress.

Note: *Emphasise that the drawing doesn't necessarily have to be brilliant (although of course it might be). It can look however they choose. Even if one person does the drawing, everyone should make suggestions.*

While the groups are working, circulate and encourage the students, without editing or suggesting anything yourself. When all the groups have created their picture of a stressed person (which could be a young person or an adult) with plenty of images and words, ask one person from each group to hold up their sheet so that everyone can see. Ask each group in turn to explain what they've drawn and written.

Look for:

- Frowns, worried faces, lines, tears, sweat
- 'Bad hair' and spots (quite logical, stress affects blood flow, including to the skin and scalp)
- A clock (time pressure), big weights (for example on shoulders)
- Piles of paper and books (homework, exams or, if they have depicted an adult, work-related things, bills, etc.)
- Jobs they have to do at home
- Long lists of things that have to be done
- Lots of arms juggling stuff, legs running to keep up
- People surrounding them, tugging at them, nagging at them (family, toddlers, teachers, other students, bosses, etc.)
- Bars of chocolate, bottles of alcohol, fat stomachs (resulting from these) or thin (not eating)
- Cigarettes, sleeping pills, other drugs
- Sometimes toilets are featured
- More unusual things – whatever comes up reflects students' perception and it's useful and usable.

Praise what students have come up with and show appreciation for any humour, their observation, perceptiveness, etc. Draw out from the discussion how some of the things they have depicted relate to **causes** *of stress and how some identify* **effects** *of stress.*

Bring out from the discussion how effects can be physical, behavioural or psychological – but emphasise that stress is **not** *something 'imaginary', even when the results are psychological. Tell the class very simply that stress is a* **real** *response by the brain and body to demands that are made on us, and that this response was designed to ensure our survival – to get human beings ready to 'fight' or 'run away' if threatened; emphasise that it happens to everyone automatically. Unfortunately, it's not so easy to fight or run with present-day demands like exams, so that brain-body reaction can make us feel bad or even unwell.*

Use the discussion to explore in a dissociated way, young people's awareness of their own stressors (and perhaps how they deal with them). You could signpost sources of support. Link back to the scenario with Emma and Josh and point out that self-awareness does make a difference and influences whether we see the demands on us as 'low' or 'high' level, along with our ability to cope. Like Emma's coffee cup and chain of 'disasters', something doesn't have to be a major life event to be experienced as a major demand if we're already stretched to our limit. Refer back to Emma and the school play to point out how, even if something is a major demand, that same brain-body response can lead to it being experienced as challenging, motivating and stimulating because we see ourselves as well able to cope. Remember, too, that Josh would have reacted to the stress differently. Perhaps he wouldn't have cried, but he might have eaten lots of snacks.

Into action

Inform the class of the good news that there are lots of things you can do to deal with negative or destructive stress:

- change how we see the demand
- strengthen our abilities to cope
- deal with the brain-body effects.

*Tell students that you're going to teach them one simple stress-busting technique now – the **quick stress release**.*

Quick stress release

Point out that Josh's suggestion to Emma to 'take a deep breath' was really quite clever, because how we're breathing is usually the first signal to the brain that we're facing a stressor. Often our first reaction to a threat is a sharp 'in' breath that we don't even realise we're doing. That acts like a text to our brain and instantly triggers the brain-body reaction – lots of stress chemicals are pumped around our body and our nervous system is put on full alert.

So, when you're in a situation that stresses you, try this:

1   Take an easy deep breath and let it out S-L-O-W-L-Y and gently.

2   As you do so, **think** about your shoulders – they will probably be tense and raised – and deliberately R-E-L-A-X and LOWER them.

Invite the class to practise this technique.

This technique can be performed very quickly without anyone noticing. It changes our breathing INSTANTLY and lets go of some muscle tension. It's like sending our brain a quick text message: 'It's OK.'

The technique can be done so quickly that you can do it:

- as you walk into a room
- as you go to take a penalty kick
- when you walk out on to a stage
- when you're revising or doing coursework
- as you go into/start an exam.

The results can be instant – hands that were shaking stop shaking, the mind can think straight, you feel more CALM … so perform better …

Reflection

Privately, ask yourself: When are the times I might want to use this method?

In the scenario with Emma and Josh, it was a good thing that Emma had Josh to talk to and he offered to talk it through with her. It's important to have somebody to talk to. If you felt you had demands you were struggling to cope with and were feeling unpleasant effects of stress, who could you talk to?

This session is adapted from 'Stop Stressing' and various stress training materials by Alan Van Loen, Aware Consultancy.

2.5 Year 11 themes and pathways

The content boxes shown in bold have been expanded into suggested sessions.

Theme 1 – Focus on relationships

Pathway		Content boxes					
1	Taking stock of 'me'	G1	**G4**	G7	G8	G9	**G11**
2	Managing 'parent', 'adult' and 'child'	G2	G3	G10			
3	Is help there …?	G5	G6	G12			

Theme 2 – Focus on me as a learner

Pathway		Content boxes					
1	Me as a learner	L1	L3	L8	L12	L11	L14
2	How is my learning going?	L2	L4	L5	L10	L9	L16
3	Ready for exams?	L6	L7	L13	L15		

Theme 3 – Focus on economic wellbeing and the world of work

Pathway		Content boxes					
1	What shall I do?	W1	W2	W4	W15	W16	W17
2	I may need guidance	W3	W12	W18			
3	Starting out	W5	W8	W14	W19		
4	Knowing the terms	W6	W7	W9	W10	W11	W13

Theme 4 – Focus on work experience

Pathway		Content boxes					
1	And this is how I feel …	E1	E4	E13	E14	E15	**E19**
2	Understanding what I need to …	E2	E11	E12	E17	**E18**	
3	Let's get practical!	E3	E5	E6	E10	E16	
4	It's over! Looking back …	E7	E8	E9			

Theme 5 – Focus on health and healthy futures

Pathway		Content boxes				
1	It's my responsibility!	H1	H2	H3	H6	H8	
2	I should know this …	H4	H5	H7			

Theme 6 – Focus on managing my health, risk and keeping myself safe

Pathway		Content boxes					
1	Personal safety: reflection time	K1	K5				
2	Personal safety: decision time	**K6**	K7				
3	Keeping my money safe	**K2**	K3	K4			

Theme 7 – Focus on drugs

Pathway		Content boxes					
1	Taking stock	D1	D6	D7	D14		
2	From my point of view	D2	**D4**	**D11**			
3	It's what I know	D5	D9	D10			
4	Can I foresee …?	D3	D8	D15	D16		
5	Help and safety	D12	D13	D17			

Theme 8 – Focus on relationships and sex education

Pathway		Content boxes					
1	Friends and relations	R2	R5	**R17**	**R18**		
2	Very close friends	R1	R4	R16	**R19**		
3	Powerful feelings	**R3**	**R8**	**R9**			
4	Me and my needs	**R6**	R14	R15	R20	R21	
5	Questions of contraception, mostly	R10	R11	R12	R13	**R22**	R7

Theme 9 – Focus on managing stress

Pathway		Content boxes					
1	Putting myself first	S1	S3	S7	S6		
2	Managing my stress	S2	S4	**S5**	S8		

Theme 10 – Focus on being a parent

Pathway		Content boxes					
1	A parent? Me?!	P1	P2	**P3**	P4	P5	P12
2	If and when	P6	P7	P8	**P9**		
3	The meanings of 'parent'	P10	P11	P13	P14		

Theme 11 – Focus on 'moving on'

Pathway		Content boxes					
1	How am I?	M1	M2	M4	**M6**		
2	Looking ahead	**M7**	M3	M10	M5		
3	Moving forwards	M12	M8	M9	M11		

Becoming everything I can be	Taking charge of my healthy and safe lifestyle	Managing my changing relationships
Focus on relationships		

Becoming everything I can be

Focus on relationships

G1 Do I like myself? Do I like who I am becoming? Would I choose myself as my own best friend? Am I proud of me? Would I swap places with myself, if I were someone else?

G2 How good am I at managing my inner 'child' and inner 'parent'? Is my inner 'adult' able to judge whether to be influenced by my inner 'child' or inner 'parent', either of which may be appropriately or inappropriately encouraging me to do something? Can I ignore them if I need to?

G3 How well do I understand my inner 'parent' voice and my inner 'child' voice? How good am I at judging when to be guided by them, and when to trust my own 'adult' judgement? How confident do I feel about dismissing these inner voices when I need to?

G4 What do I understand by 'self-talk'? When I talk to myself inside my head, do I usually build myself up or usually knock myself down? Do I give myself encouragement? Do I congratulate myself or praise myself when I am successful? Can I balance appropriate critical self-reflection with positive self-praise?

G5 Do I have a strong network of people who can help me? Do I need to expand this network to include new people?

G6 Do I have someone who I know I can talk to, and who will be able and willing to help me no matter how bad things might become or what I might have done?

G7 Am I a role model? How can I tell? To whom? In school? Out of school? At home? How do I feel about this? Would I consider myself a 'good' role or a 'bad' role model?

Taking charge of my healthy and safe lifestyle

G8 Has my view of a healthy lifestyle changed? How would I describe a healthy lifestyle? How does my lifestyle rate?

Managing my changing relationships

G9 As I become more independent, what new responsibilities do I have towards myself? How do I feel about being fully responsible for looking after myself?

G10 Am I becoming more skilled at recognising when others' inner 'parent' or inner 'child' have taken over from their own inner 'adult'? Am I getting better at managing others' inner 'child' or inner 'parent' if I feel this is appropriate?

G11 How good am I at balancing being sociable or popular, whilst maintaining my own independence and principles? What do I understand by the term 'exploitation'? Can I recognise when I'm being used?

G12 Are my responsibilities towards others who may be being treated unfairly, threatened or in need of help changing as I get older? How is my understanding of prejudice, discrimination, racism or stereotyping changing? If I believe any of these behaviours are happening to me or someone else, do I feel able to challenge it or talk to someone who can?

Becoming everything I can be	Taking charge of my healthy and safe lifestyle	Managing my changing relationships

Focus on me as a learner

L1 How am I doing? Am I still on track to meet my dreams? Are my dreams realistic? Are they limiting me? If I achieve my dreams, what will this give me? Are my current dreams the only way of getting what I want? Are my dreams changing? Do I need to do anything differently if I am to achieve my dreams?

L2 Am I still learning as well as I can? What do I understand by 'a good learner'? Do I need to change anything in the way I learn? How important is speed? How is my organisation? Am I still motivated or are other things distracting me? Can I make compromises between my leisure interests and my school work? Do I see what I am doing at school as relevant to my future?

L3 What am I trying to achieve? What am I really good at? What choices will I have this year? What choices do I think I will make and why? If I make those choices, what might be the long-term consequences or benefits?

L4 How do I organise my approach to any coursework or modular tests? How do I plan my time? How good am I at keeping to my time plan?

L5 How is my expertise in studying and revising effectively continuing to develop? Am I able to motivate myself to study and revise? How good am I at recording, recalling and applying what I have learned?

L6 What have I learned from 'mock' or 'practice' examinations? How do I feel about my performance in these examinations? Have they increased or decreased my confidence in myself and my abilities? Am I more or less motivated?

L7 Do I need to make changes in my approach to learning or revising as a result of mock or practice examinations? Do I need to change my focus; do I need to alter my priorities?

L10 Is my style of learning changing? How am I evaluating and using new sources of information? How do I organise my time, especially on coursework?

L11 How much do I know about the world of work? Am I feeling attracted to some areas of work? Are there areas of work I want to know more about? Have I rejected some areas of work already? Is this the right time to do this?

L12 Do I know who I need to talk to if I am not sure what to do next year, or what options are available to me?

L13 How do I feel about examinations? Am I able to manage my emotional state to make sure I can perform to my full potential in examinations?

L14 Do I know who I can talk to, when, where and what to say if I feel stressed about my work or anything else that might be worrying me? Do I understand what I can expect to be kept secret and what may have to be passed on?

L15 How good am I at managing my work/life balance, especially in the lead up to examinations? How good am I at knowing when I need to adjust the balance, for example in the run up to examinations or important coursework?

L16 How good am I at managing others who try to disrupt my learning, either individually or as part of a group?

Becoming everything I can be	Taking charge of my healthy and safe lifestyle	Managing my changing relationships
L8 What choices can I make for next year? How will those choices affect my future plans? Who can I ask if I need advice? L9 What choices have I made in the past that I would make differently next time? What have I learned? What do I believe I am 'bad' at? Why do I believe this? When did I learn I was bad at …? Can I unlearn this conclusion? What can I do differently? What would make me a good learner at this subject?		

Focus on economic wellbeing and the world of work

W1 Have my thoughts about a future career changed? Do I know generally or specifically the type of career I want? What research am I doing to pin down exactly what qualifications and/or experiences I need to have in order to be able to apply for my chosen career? W2 What am I prepared to do to get the type of future employment I want and/or the rewards it brings? W3 Is it OK if I don't yet know what I want to do when I leave school? Do I know what the best strategy is to keep my options open? W4 What experiences and skills do I have, what responsibilities have I held that might give me a competitive advantage over others applying for a similar position in employment or further education? What could I do to increase these? In school? Out of school?	W5 Do I know how to set a personal budget? Do I understand the difference between 'gross' and 'net' pay? Do I understand the term 'stoppages'? Do I understand 'income tax' and 'national insurance'? How do I feel about budgeting? Do I know who can help me if I need accurate, trustworthy support and advice with managing my finances? W6 Do I understand the term 'credit rating'? Do I understand how my credit rating can affect my life? W7 Do I understand the full range of risks of getting into debt? Do I know how to evaluate a potential source of a future loan? Do I understand the range of consequences that can happen when people cannot repay their loans? W8 Do I understand the difference between 'credit cards' and 'debit cards'? Do I understand how to protect myself from other people using my credit or debit card details? W9 Do I understand how apparently small differences in interest rates can have huge implications on the cost of borrowing money and the time it will take me to repay a debt? W10 Do I understand the terms and full implications of 'paying the minimum amount' on a credit card, 'interest rates', 'debt management' and 'bankruptcy'?	W15 How do I feel about possibly competing and having a career or job in a 'global market'? W16 Do I understand that in a competitive global market having the minimum entry requirements may not be enough to secure me my chosen job or career? W17 How do I feel about having a part-time job? Do I know what I can legally undertake? How would I balance school work, a part-time job and leisure? What do I understand by the term 'work/life balance'? W18 If I need help with exploring future career choices, do I know who can offer information and guidance? W19 Do I know what an enhanced police check is? Do I know what it contains and which employers may request one or be required by law to request one?

Becoming everything I can be	Taking charge of my healthy and safe lifestyle	Managing my changing relationships
	W11 What does 'the rate of inflation' mean? How does this affect me? How does this affect the interest on people's savings or debt? W12 If I need unbiased, professional help with my finances, do I know which organisations I can trust to give me free, honest and impartial financial advice? W13 What does the term 'insurance' mean? What insurance should I have? If I want to take out insurance, how do I select a provider? W14 What do I understand by the term 'pension'? How do I feel about saving for my old age?	

Focus on work experience

E1 How do I feel about possible future work experience opportunities? Am I nervous or excited? How do I feel about meeting new people and doing new things? Am I nervous or excited? What expectations do I have? Are they realistic? What am I looking forward to? Do I have any concerns or fears? E2 Do I understand the difference between 'work experience' and 'career tasting'? E3 How will I choose my work experience placement? What will influence my choice? Can I find opportunities for myself? Why am I choosing this opportunity? What do I think it will offer me? Am I avoiding a placement I should consider more carefully? E4 Will it challenge me or am I taking an easy option? Am I choosing a placement that will really stretch me or am I limiting myself? E5 What will help me to say work experience was 'time well spent'? What could be all the possible benefits to me of having a good work experience placement? What do I hope to get out of it? What do I need to do to play my part in achieving my outcomes?	E10 In what ways will I need to change my personal organisation in order to attend work experience? How will I travel to my work experience placement? E11 What risks might there be to my health and safety at my work placement? What health and safety regulations do I need to be aware of? E12 Am I clear what I have to do if I am ill or going to be late to my work experience placement? E13 How do I feel about being asked to do tasks that are well below what I think is my potential? Do I understand why this might be? How do I feel about being asked to do repetitive tasks that might be boring? E14 If I am unhappy during my work placement, what should I do? Who should I contact? When and how should I contact them?	E15 How am I getting on when working with other people? Am I a good listener? Do I get on well with others? Can I work to others' instructions? How do I feel about working with others who I may not have met before? Can I say 'I don't understand'? E16 If I need help, who will I ask? How will I find out what I can do without direction; what I need to take advice about and what I need to do only as instructed? Do I know what to do if I make a mistake? E17 Who do I expect I will be working with or for? Is there a difference between working with a member of an organisation and working with a client or member of the public on behalf of that organisation? What expectations might my work experience placement have of me? E18 Do I know what factors might lead to my making a good impression? Do I know how enthusiasm or exuberance could lead to taking risks or even real danger at work? Do I understand the importance of following instructions?

Becoming everything I can be	Taking charge of my healthy and safe lifestyle	Managing my changing relationships
E6 How will I record my experiences and the learning I gain through my work experience placement? E7 Once my work experience is over, what have I learned about this type of work? What have I learned about other people/about myself? How did it feel to work with people I hadn't met before? Was I able to work well in a new team? E8 Did I behave differently or in new ways during my placement? Was I a different person? Do I want to keep parts of that new person? Which parts, and why? E9 What parts of my school curriculum did I make use of? Has it influenced my ambitions or approach to learning? Will I make any new choices as a result of this experience?		E19 How do I feel about being interviewed as part of my work experience? How can I really demonstrate my skills and personal qualities to people who do not know me at an interview? What do I know or do, what special skills or experiences do I have that make me really employable?

Focus on health and healthy futures

H1 How do I feel about booking an appointment and attending a doctor or clinic on my own? How do I feel about talking with a doctor, nurse or other health professional on my own? Do I know what they will keep confidential? H2 How good am I at recognising stress in myself? What do I understand by the terms 'anxious' and 'depressed'? If I felt I was having difficulties with my mental health, how would I feel about seeking support from others? Who would I talk to? What would I say?	H3 How are my community's, family's and society's expectations of me changing? How could these expectations affect me and my lifestyle? H4 What do I think are the latest healthy lifestyles? What do I feel about them? H5 Do I understand the difference between a 'balanced diet' and 'dieting'? H6 How do I feel about exercise now? To stay healthy, do I understand how much exercise I need to take and how often? In what ways do I enjoy taking exercise? Are they changing? Do I know that exercise can help me feel better? Do I know that any initial feelings of discomfort, of being out of breath lessen as I get more used to exercise? H7 Do I understand what it means when the media reports a health risk has 'increased by' or 'decreased by' a particular percentage?	H8 What new responsibilities do I have towards others? Are they responsibilities that others *require* me to fulfil? Are there some I believe I *should* fulfil?

Becoming everything I can be	Taking charge of my healthy and safe lifestyle	Managing my changing relationships

Focus on managing my health, risk and keeping myself safe

K1 Am I taking more risks in my life? Am I generally impulsive, or do I spend time thinking things through before making a decision? Are there times when it is OK to be impulsive? Are there times when it is really important to stop and think? Are some risks worth taking? Do I think about the minor and severe, short and longer-term consequences of something going wrong? How likely is it that something could go wrong and in what ways? How do I assess my decision as being worth the risk?	K5 Do I realise that some companies will perform an internet search on my name to provide an initial first impression of me? How do I feel about this? How can I protect my reputation?	K6 Could I manage a situation where I am offered a lift in a car where I suspect the driver may have been drinking alcohol (using cannabis or other drugs that might impair competence)?
K2 How do I feel about gambling? What are the alternatives to gambling? What are the risks of gambling for me? Why do I think people gamble? If I or someone I knew had a problem with gambling, would I know where to get help?		K7 How do I feel about someone paying me unwanted attention? Do I know what to say and do if someone's attention towards me is making me feel uncomfortable? Do I understand what harassment is? Would I know what to do if I feel someone is harassing me?
K3 What do I feel about saving? What do I feel about getting into debt? Do I understand compound interest and the true cost of borrowing? Do I understand what is meant by the term a 'secured' loan?		
K4 If I have to have a loan in the future, how do I choose who to borrow money from? What questions do I need to ask? What are the consequences to me if I cannot make the repayments?		

Focus on drugs

D1 What do I remember from previous education or learning about drug use? How do I feel now about the use of drugs, especially when tobacco, alcohol and illegal substances are the cause of so many health and social problems?	D5 What new questions do I have about alcohol and drug use? What do I remember about the most commonly available drugs, their effects on people's physical systems and the social and legal consequences of their possession, dealing and use?	D11 Do I think the opinions of others around me are changing about alcohol or drug use? Why do I think this? Do I think people of my age are using alcohol or tobacco more regularly? What do I feel about this? Are my feelings about the consequences changing? Do I know for sure whether those (my age) around me are, or are not, using drugs? What do I feel about those making the same choices as me? What do I feel about those making different choices from me?
D2 Are my views changing? As I get older, am I revising my view of new risks and consequences for my own drug use? Am I confident that I know enough to be able to manage invitations to go out with others to places where drinking alcohol and other drug use might be involved?	D6 What do I know, or remember from previous learning, about the possible short and long-term consequences of alcohol use?	
	D7 How do I feel now about binge drinking? Do I remember the health and social risks to my personal safety of binge drinking?	

Becoming everything I can be	Taking charge of my healthy and safe lifestyle	Managing my changing relationships
D3 Could I find myself in situations where alcohol or drug use is 'acceptable' or even 'expected' by others? Might I feel a pressure to conform to the expectations of others? How do I feel about this? How might I manage my feelings in a situation like this? What strategies could I use to stay safe?	D8 Am I becoming more at risk of drink spiking? Do I know how to guard myself against someone who might spike my drink?	D12 Do I know how the use of alcohol can change a drinker's behaviour? Do I know how this could affect or be a risk to them and their relationships with others, including friends, family and school?
D4 Why do I think we hear so much about *illegal* drugs in the media, on the news and in films? If I read, watch, listen carefully to the media, can I find examples of local and national concern about legal drugs, too? Do some of these concerns relate to the health of users of these legal drugs?	D9 Do I know that mixing some drugs, including using drugs with alcohol, can be a potentially lethal combination? Do I know which combinations may be lethal?	D13 Do I understand how my own and others' use of alcohol, cannabis and other drugs can seriously affect my ability to keep myself and others safe?
	D10 Do I understand that future employers may have strong policies on employees' recreational drug use, both in the workplace and outside the workplace, and that even recreational drug use can have a serious effect on my future career prospects? Do I know that a prosecution involving illegal drugs can stop me ever visiting some countries?	D14 Am I becoming more or less at risk from others' alcohol or drug use? In what ways? How good do I think I am or will be at managing these risks?
		D15 How will I manage if I am offered a lift in a car or on a bike being driven by someone who I believe might have consumed alcohol or drugs?
		D16 Are my feelings about how I will manage, and what I will say and do if I am in a situation where I am offered something suspicious or something I don't want to consume still the same? What if it is offered by a friend or someone I really like, or someone who is in a position of authority over me? For example, an employer. Can I express my feelings and intentions firmly and assertively in such a situation?
		D17 Do I recall how to get immediate medical help and longer term support for someone who is having difficulties with drug or alcohol use? Do I know the consequences for them of getting such help?

Focus on relationships and sex education

R1 How are my feelings about being a boyfriend or girlfriend changing? What do I expect having a boyfriend or girlfriend will involve? How do I feel about this? Do I feel anxious that I won't be liked? Do I feel anxious that I will be left on my own?	R10 Do I still have questions about different types of contraception, their pros and cons, use and availability?	R16 How do I or others feel when friends are making new relationships? How does it feel to be the odd one out?
R2 How do I feel about being rejected? How do I deal with embarrassment? How does it feel when others know I really like someone? How does it (or would it) feel when others know I have been rejected?	R11 Do I remember how to use a condom to ensure I don't put myself or someone else at risk? Will I remember what to do if I fear that a condom hasn't worked, and that I or someone else might be at risk?*	R17 How does my family feel about me becoming an adult and forming new types of relationships? What do they expect from me? Do other people or groups have expectations about how I should behave? How do I feel about that? Do I agree?

* **Note to teacher**: Condoms are normally an excellent barrier to pregnancy and STIs. However, the method can fail if condoms are not used properly, or are (rarely) faulty.

Becoming everything I can be	Taking charge of my healthy and safe lifestyle	Managing my changing relationships
R3 How might relationships help or hinder my learning? How might they affect my plans for the future? R4 How are my feelings about having a sexual relationship changing? Are they getting stronger? What do I feel about that? How might my feelings affect what I do? What else could influence me? R5 Do I understand that, although it may seem like everyone else is having sex (or saying they are), in fact they are still not? Do I understand that the number of young people of my age who have experienced sexual intercourse is still a minority and that, if I haven't, I am normal? **R6** Do I know that I have a right to only do what I feel comfortable with? Do I know that I have a responsibility to protect others' rights to be safe and feel comfortable? R7 What questions do I still have about sexual behaviour? Are there some things I am not clear about? Do I feel able to ask about what I don't yet know? **R8** Am I aware that people's feelings of sexual attraction, their sexual behaviours and their sexual identity are not necessarily 'fixed' throughout their life? Do I understand that, for a variety of reasons, these three things might not always coincide and that trying to fit people to stereotypes and labels is not helpful? How do I feel about this in relation to me and other people I know, or groups of people? Do I feel comfortable with my own sexuality and other people's? **R9** Are any of my views and feelings about relationships and sexual issues changing as I get older? Am I able to help others explore and discuss their views and feelings?	R12 Do I remember where to obtain emergency contraception? How would I feel now about approaching someone to ask for emergency contraception? Do I understand issues of confidentiality? Do I remember how quickly emergency contraception has to be used in order for it to be effective? Do I have up-to-date knowledge on who to get support and advice from if it has been left too late? R13 What questions do I still have about sexually transmitted infections? R14 Do I know who I can go to in order to get reliable help and advice? How do I know I can feel confident in the advice they offer me? How do I feel about approaching someone to ask for help or advice, especially if they are a professional I have not met before? Do I understand that counsellors will not advise, but will help me find my own way forward? R15 What do I know about how the use of alcohol and other drugs might make me vulnerable to others, or change my own ability to make decisions and keep myself safe?	**R18** What different pressures could be involved in my relationships as I am getting older – now or in the near future? How will I handle these? **R19** Do I expect relationships to go on, to change or to stop? How do I feel about breaking up with someone I care(d) about? How would I feel if someone I cared about or still care about now wants to be close to someone else? R20 How do I negotiate the use of contraception with someone else? R21 How would I feel if I felt I should use emergency contraception but my boyfriend doesn't feel it is necessary? How would I feel if I felt my girlfriend should use emergency contraception but she doesn't want to or feel it is necessary? **R22** What are my views on termination of pregnancy? How do I respond to people whose views might be different from my own on this and other controversial issues? How would I handle differences like this with a boyfriend or girlfriend?

Becoming everything I can be	Taking charge of my healthy and safe lifestyle	Managing my changing relationships

Focus on managing stress

S1 As I get older, are the sources of my stress changing? Am I developing my ability to recognise unwanted stress in myself?	S4 Do I know that I can experience unwanted stress from self-imposed demands and that I can often remove or reduce these?	S7 How good am I at managing my work/life balance? How good am I at knowing when I need to adjust the balance, for example in the run up to examinations or important coursework?
S2 How effective am I at managing unwanted stress?	**S5** Am I aware that stress can result from what we believe about a situation and that changing my thoughts about something can change my feelings?	S8 How good am I at being assertive in order to remove or reduce demands that cause unwanted stress for me?
S3 How do I feel about examinations? Am I able to manage my emotional state to make sure I can perform to my full potential in examinations?	S6 Do I know who I can talk to, when, where and what to say if I feel stressed about my work or anything else that might be worrying me? Do I understand what I can expect to be kept secret and what may have to be passed on?	

Focus on being a parent

P1 How do I feel about one day being a parent?	P6 Do I believe there are some things only mothers should do and some things only fathers should do, or should everything be a shared responsibility?	P10 How would becoming a parent affect my relationships and lifestyle, now and in the future?
P2 What would becoming a parent give me? What would I *have* to give up? What might I *choose* to give up?	P7 Do I understand that not everyone can become a parent? Do I understand that not everyone will want to become a parent? If someone cannot become a 'biological parent' what options are open to them to still be a parent?	P11 What do I feel makes a good parent? What do good parents say and do, what don't they say and do?
P3 How will I know I am ready to become a parent? Are there experiences I want to have first? Are there things (for example, knowledge, skills, attitudes of mind) I would need to bring a child up safely and healthily that I don't yet have? How can I make sure I have these when I need them?	P8 Do I understand that there are biologically better times for both men and women to become a parent?	P12 Is choosing to have sexual intercourse with someone different to choosing to have a child with someone? In what ways?
P4 Would I have to give up more or less than my partner? Might I become financially dependent on someone else? How do I feel about this?	**P9** Do I understand that biologically ideal times and socially ideal times can be different? Do I understand the risks of having children very early in life and the risks of leaving it too late to try to become a parent? Do I know that the biological risks are different for men and women?	P13 What qualities would I look for in someone I would want to have a child with? Why would I choose these qualities? Are they different from the qualities I would look for in a boyfriend or girlfriend?
P5 What qualities do I have that I feel would make me a good parent? What might I need to change or work on changing?		P14 What do I feel about marriage? Do I think marriage is important before becoming a parent with someone? Why? What if my partner feels differently – will I be ready to explain/compromise/alter?

Becoming everything I can be	Taking charge of my healthy and safe lifestyle	Managing my changing relationships

Focus on 'moving on'

M1 Thinking back over the last five years, how have I changed in my attitudes, my skills and my relationships?	M8 What are my options? What opportunities do I have? What are the pros and cons of each option?	M11 Who are all the people who can support me in deciding what to do next? Why do I think they are the right people? Are there other sources of support that I don't know about? How can I find them?
M2 Am I proud of what I have achieved? Do I like what I have become? As I approach the end of this year, where do I want to go next?	M9 Are there any practical issues I need to take into account or overcome? Am I mentally closing off options I could consider more carefully?	M12 What opportunities are there for me to get new training or learning experiences?
M3 Are my ambitions changing? Am I still on track to achieve my ambitions or dreams? If not, are there aspects of my dreams or aspirations that I can still achieve but in different ways?	M10 Is there extra learning or experiences inside or outside school that will help me achieve my ambitions or dreams? What skills or experiences do I have or could I get that 'mark me out' as special? How can I go about getting them? (For example voluntary work, outdoor activities, personal challenges, etc.)	
M4 What are all the things about me, in school and outside of school that I am particularly proud of? What do I think I am really good at? What am I OK at? What am I fantastic at? What would I like to do more of? What am I looking forward to? What do I want to learn more about?		
M5 Can I keep doing things I want to in my further education? Can I eventually make use of them in a future career or job?		
M6 Do I like myself? Do I like who I am becoming? Would I choose myself as my own best friend? Am I proud of me? Would I swap places with myself? How do I hope people think of me? How do I hope they will remember me?		
M7 Is there anything about me I want to leave behind when I move on? Are there changes I want to make in me, things I want to do differently, especially if I am moving on to a new place with new people?		

Becoming everything I can be	Taking charge of my healthy and safe lifestyle	Managing my changing relationships

A question of self-talk

> **G4**
> What do I understand by 'self-talk'?
> When I talk to myself inside my head, do I usually build myself up or usually knock myself down?
> Do I give myself encouragement?
> Do I congratulate myself or praise myself when I am successful?
> Can I balance appropriate critical self-reflection with positive self-praise?

To the teacher

This session focuses on self-talk – the voice inside our heads that comments on what we think, believe and do. The nature of this inner voice can indicate, and influence, our attitude towards ourselves and others and it is powerful. It can affect how we perform in our daily lives. Our self-talk relates closely to how OK we feel, and how OK we feel others are, and our general readiness to be passive, assertive or aggressive in our interactions with others. A person who is inclined to be passive, may be more inclined to negative self-talk: 'I can't cope!'; 'I'm not worth the effort!'; 'It'll all go wrong!'; 'I'm so stupid!' More positive self-talk often accompanies more assertive actions: 'I can do this if I try!'; 'I'm worth the time it'll take to get this right!'; 'I'll do my best, it's the least I can do in return!' Negative self-talk may be more likely for someone who is more inclined to be aggressive: 'Everyone's so stupid!'; 'They're just behaving like this to spite me!'; 'I'll show them – I'll spoil their fun!'

The session provides an opportunity to think about self-talk, the forms it usually takes, and how to challenge and change negative self-talk – encouraging more assertive and pleasant behaviour.

In addition, the unconscious mind seems to 'listen' to the conscious mind and tries to help. Self-talk such as 'I know I can do this' brings on-line our inner resources, whilst 'I can never do this' has the reverse effect. The self-talk is more than just a coach; it can actually impact on neurological activity. Whether you think you can or whether you think you can't you are probably right!

To the students

In this session we are going to explore and begin to take control of 'self-talk', the quiet voice, or sometimes loud voice, that we hear inside our heads. Sometimes it is really helpful or supportive, and sometimes it is really critical or even nasty. Sometimes we can literally be our own worst enemy, sometimes we can be our own best friend.

Have you noticed the comments you make to yourself – inside your head – when things go well? Or when things go badly wrong? Or when you're scared how they might turn out? Or when you know exactly what you should have said, but it's too late now? Or when you'd like to say something to someone, but you don't dare? The little voice inside our head can appear at any time, talking to us – we call it self-talk – telling us what we should or shouldn't have done, what might happen, and how.

Becky had bought a nice top. It was quite expensive, but was from a good shop so it should last a while. It was quite sexy, too! She hoped that Nathan would like her in it when they went out on Friday night. She hoped her mum wouldn't complain about the cost, or that it was cut quite low … She thought to herself, 'Mum'll hit the roof! She'll say it cost too much and that I look like a slut wearing it – I'd better not show her.'

Becky: *(Steeling herself for criticism)* 'Hi, Mum.'
Mum: 'Hallo, Becky! You're back sooner than I expected. How did you get on?'
Becky: 'I found a top I liked.'
Mum: 'Oh, that's great! Did you get it in PriceCut? Oh, don't go upstairs – I'd love to see it. Will you try it on for me?'

Becky comes slowly down the few steps she'd run up.

Becky: 'You wouldn't like it. What's for tea?'
Mum: *(Ignoring the tea question)* 'How much was it? Where did you find it?'

Becky sighed. Now for the row. 'It was in "Janice Proud". It's really good quality – it'll last ages.'

Mum: 'Janice Proud?! You always said their stuff was too expensive! Let's have a look …'
Becky: 'You're always criticising my choices! I'm NOT taking it back!'
Mum: 'Hang about, I haven't seen it yet! Hey, that's really nice. Wouldn't mind it myself. I bet it'll give Nathan ideas! How much was it?'
Becky: 'It was … well … £22! I **knew** you'd have a go at me!'
Mum: 'No, it looks good quality to me. You've done well! Wait a minute – what's this? It looks like a stain …'
Becky: 'Where? Oh – wow that's awful! Why didn't I notice? Just my luck. Now I s'pose I WILL have to take it back!'

She snatches the top back and rushes upstairs. She thinks to herself, 'I won't know what to say – I'll mumble and look silly! They'll say it's non-returnable and then I'll feel terrible! They'll just think I'm making a fuss! They'll hate me for bringing it back!' She puts her head in her hands.

Focusing

This is an opportunity for self-reflection and to work in pairs. Reassure the class that they need only share what they are comfortable with.

Many of us think with a voice in our heads, sometimes there is more than one voice and perhaps you even find yourself arguing with yourself! Some people find their self-talk is really cruel, they are more spiteful to themselves than they would ever accept from anyone else.

Think about the way you talk to yourself. Do you tend to encourage yourself? Do you generally praise yourself? When things go a bit wrong, do you tell yourself off or do you encourage yourself to try again, or do better? Are you a friend to yourself or a critic?

What is the voice in your head usually like?

Into action

In pairs, talk about Becky's self-talk:

- What does it say about Becky, and her level of self-confidence?
- Was Becky right about how her mum was going to react?
- Might there have been a row if Becky's mum had risen to the bait? How influential would that have made Becky's self-talk?

Now think about the trip to return the top:

- What are the chances of Becky returning the item?
- If she does return it, how might the conversation go?
- What could she say to herself that might change her attitude, and make a polite, assertive conversation more likely?

It's time for a mini-lecture about self-talk …

Sometimes our self-talk doesn't sound like our own voice, it copies a parent's, a teacher's or a friend's. Sometimes these imported thoughts can be helpful, but not always.

Remember self-talk is *self*-talk. No one can hear it except you – so why not praise yourself, why not thank yourself for doing something for you or encourage yourself – who is going to know? If you don't like the voice in your head, change it, it's your voice.

Since it is in your head and no one else can hear you, how about imagining someone else's voice, for example someone you know who cares for you, or your favourite movie or music star. Try experimenting with different voices. You can tell yourself whatever you choose to say.

There is a difference between the sensible voice in your head that is warning you about something, and the voice that is simply putting you down. The sensible voice may be telling you helpful thoughts to protect you from possible harm that your brain has identified. The trick is to stop and think, and perhaps even think again. Is this voice trying to help me or just limit or criticise me? Whatever the *source* of these two kinds of self-talk, it may help to distinguish between them like this: does the voice sound like a *caring* parent, trying to look after me, or maybe even an *experienced adult* warning me about a danger I recognise? Or does it sound like a more negative and critical parent-voice, trying to discourage or limit me? If you *have* been put down, you may even learn to keep the criticisms inside you, ready to limit you even when there's nobody there to criticise you – except yourself. These limiting commands or 'injunctions' can be learned and stored inside our heads. *Be perfect! Hurry up! You'll never amount to anything! Please me!* They stay there, ready to be trotted out whenever we might do something that someone might disapprove of for a reason that is NOT in our best interests.

If we choose to, we can listen only to the helpful caring voice, or replace it, if it seems to have a mind of its own, with our own chosen voice, telling us only helpful, sensible and encouraging things. This can be *very* powerful.

… and now, back to the session …

What might someone say to themselves in the following situations using positive self-talk?

- You have been given a really challenging piece of home learning to complete by tomorrow.
- You have just been told there is a test tomorrow in a subject you find challenging.
- You have been invited to a party and you won't know many people there.
- You want to be asked out by someone you find really attractive, or you want to ask someone out who you find really attractive.

Into action

Imagine someone of your age telling you their voice kept saying to them:

- 'You can't do that.'
- 'You are so stupid you are *always* going to fail.'
- 'You're no good at learning new things.'
- 'You could never be good at this.'
- 'You will end up on your own.'

Perhaps you can think of some more. The problem is that this person might believe these statements, and it may turn into a self-fulfilling prophecy. By listening to our own negative self-talk, we actually create the conditions where it's more likely our negative thoughts will come true.

Working in pairs, discuss how you would advise them to change their self-talk into something more helpful.

For example, turn the internal voice that says, 'You can't do that!' into self-talk that says, 'I CAN do it! I'm *going* to do it! I'm going to try my best and then *see* what I can do!' In pairs, try to turn the other statements around.

Although it sounds daft, the voice in our heads can cheer us on or really limit us. People who are capable of extraordinary feats are actually not much different from everyone else; they do, however, make sure the voice in their heads is totally on their side. This can help them use all of their skills, talents and physical abilities – and learn new ones.

If it is not helping, then the trick is to literally tell it to 'shut up'! Then, if you replace it by positive self-talk, it can help you gather your resources and do better than you ever thought possible. It can't work miracles, but telling yourself you can succeed can genuinely make success more likely, and help you achieve the maximum of which you are capable.

Reflection

Over the rest of today, listen to the voice or voices in your head. If the voice isn't helpful, tell it to 'shut up'. Instead, take control and tell yourself what you would prefer to hear. It can make a real difference.

A question of balancing popularity and independence

> **G11**
> How good am I at balancing being sociable or popular, whilst maintaining my own independence and principles?
> What do I understand by the term 'exploitation'?
> Can I recognise when I'm being used?

To the teacher

We come from strongly tribal creatures and for many adolescents the drive to be accepted by, or be popular with, their peers can be very strong. Therefore, young people may naturally want to be like their peers, talk like them, walk like them, and be liked by them. However, they may also want to be individuals with minds, personalities, beliefs, values, priorities and plans of their own. This may cause tension and, on occasions, uncertainty about what to do. Relationships in the peer group or circle of close friends can suffer when not everyone is in accord, but may also be where ideas are tried out, confidences and discomforts shared, lessons learned and significant choices made. Sometimes, conflict may lead to changes of friends, even change of friendship group. Sometimes, particularly where close friends unite against a common idea or adversary ('unfair parents' for example – aren't *all* parents of 16 year olds unfair?), friendships may be strengthened.

Indeed, the tensions may be worse when family values, expectations and pressures conflict either with local young people's perceived 'norms' or with a particular offspring's wishes. Such is life when growing up in families, schools and society.

There is a phenomenon known as 'groupthink'. The term was coined in 1952 by William H. Whyte in *Fortune*:

Groupthink is a type of thought exhibited by group members who try to minimize conflict and reach consensus without critically testing, analyzing and evaluating ideas. During groupthink, members of the group avoid promoting viewpoints outside the comfort zone of consensus thinking. A variety of motives for this may exist such as a desire to avoid being seen as foolish, or a desire to avoid embarrassing or angering other members of the group. Groupthink may cause groups to make hasty, irrational decisions, where individual doubts are set aside, for fear of upsetting the group's balance. The term is frequently used pejoratively, (and) with hindsight.

It can happen that the peer group itself is the cause of tension, by suggesting, assuming, pressurising or commenting in such a way as to throw into sharp relief the very principles of one (or more) peer group members. This can happen where proposed action or inaction are at variance with what one (or more) of the group feel is appropriate. It may be that the majority are doing the proposing, or a strong member with a leadership role, or it's perhaps even *assumed* that something will be done which demands either complicity, often silent complicity, or else an explicit stand.

This session expands on the first question in content box G11, and aims to encourage exploration of what is good about peer groups and friendships, and what may make it hard for tensions, when they occur, to be resolved one way or another so that everyone's independence and integrity can remain intact.

To the students

The purpose of this session is to explore something called 'groupthink', to help increase your awareness of when 'groupthink' is happening, and how to challenge it when it does.

How often have you done 'what everyone else does' in your group of friends? How often, when you think about it, has this meant doing something you might not (or definitely would not) have done if you were on your own?

It's true that groups sometimes seem to act as though the group has its own brain and decision-making skills quite independent of the group members. Of course, it's quite possible for a group to make a group decision, perhaps by discussing it, perhaps even by voting – but what about the times when decisions are unspoken? Is everyone in the group sure that everyone else agrees with what is done, or said, or ignored or responded to? What if they aren't, does it matter? When it *does* matter, what makes it matter?

Focusing

In pairs, can you think of any times when what you really wanted to do, or thought was right, was put to one side because you were in a group? List some examples. Were they mostly minor things, like being a bit noisy in the street, or not moving over to let a pedestrian pass the group without having to step off the pavement? Or were there some more serious ones?

Into action

It's well known that when people are in groups, they sometimes behave in ways that invite the terms 'herd' or 'sheep'. It may sometimes just be an outsider's perception that everyone is thinking and acting in the same way, but it may mask a real issue: when do I do what the group does, or what my friends do, or what 'everyone expects' me to do, and when do I stand up and assert my own, rather different views?

In groups of at least four, discuss:

- What are the good things that you get from feeling part of a group of people your own age? Are there other ways of getting these?

There possibly are, but there's nothing like the feeling that you are 'in' – accepted, valued and counted as one of the group. Groups are very valuable to us. That's why it can feel so painful to feel rejected or discounted by a group of people whom you admire and value, and who are your friends.

- Is it sometimes easier just to 'go along with the others'? What is it that makes it easier?
- What can make it hard to stand up to a group (or its leader) and disagree with a popular decision, or refuse to 'go with the flow'? What are the risks? What do you stand to lose?
- How real are these risks? What do people your age think of someone who gently and firmly stands up for their own (possibly minority) view?
- What skills does it take to do this, and how much self-confidence?

In your groups, explore the ways in which you might express a minority view, challenging ideas and actions, rather than the people who hold them. What personal qualities does it take to do this? Are these qualities that the group might respect and admire? Discuss this as a class. Perhaps challenging ideas may not be such a risky thing.

Think about the group discussions you have just had in this session:

- Were there any minority views?
- Were these minority views expressed in an assertive and constructive way?
- Did some people feel unable to speak? You may need to check …
- If there were, why was this?
- Was there anything the group could have done to ensure everyone felt able to speak openly?
- What can friendship groups do to try to ensure everyone is respected as a person and has their views listened to?

Reflection

Although standing up for your views can feel risky, in reality it may not be if you are both respected and take care to be polite. It works both ways, though, and each person in the group shares responsibility to listen to others and *their* views, too. It is a strong group that respects and gathers the opinions of all its members, rather than assuming or imposing 'support' for a single view.

Critical reflection can work *for* groups, as well as *in* groups.

Session extension: 'groupthink'

To the teacher

Irving Janis, who has done extensive work on the subject of groupthink, suggests that it is:

A mode of thinking that people engage in when they are deeply involved in a cohesive in-group, when the members' strivings for unanimity override their motivation to realistically appraise alternative courses of action.

The warning symptoms of groupthink are:

1 *illusions of invulnerability* – creating excessive optimism and encouraging risk taking
2 *rationalising warnings* that might challenge the group's assumptions
3 *unquestioned belief* in the morality of the group, causing members to ignore the consequences of their actions
4 *stereotyping* those who are opposed to the group as weak, evil, disfigured, impotent, or stupid
5 *direct pressure* to conform placed on any member who questions the group, couched in terms of 'disloyalty'
6 *self-censorship* of ideas that deviate from the apparent group consensus
7 *illusions of unanimity* among group members, silence is viewed as agreement
8 *mindguards* – self-appointed members who shield the group from dissenting information.

This can lead to a pressure to conform to group norms, even if the individual realises this might not be in their best interests in other areas of their lives. Yet, this is not always the case, some young people can go completely the other way, celebrating their individuality and deliberately refusing to conform and creating their own unique and often idiosyncratic style.

The group or individuals in the group can feel their own decisions are validated by others' willingness to join in. If we want to do something that we perhaps know is unwise or harmful, it can sometimes feel better if others agree to make the same choice. Young people often feel that failure to join in everything their peer group does will lead to being isolated. This may or may not be true.

This session extension is intended to help students identify when groupthink is happening, get in touch with whatever feelings they have inside themselves and consider how these feelings might influence their decision making.

To the students

In this session we are going to look at how we balance joining in activities with our friends while remaining true to our own principles and beliefs. Have you ever been in a situation where you are with a group of people who you like and who all want to do something you are not sure about? How does that moment feel? Is it one feeling or lots, perhaps, conflicting or pushing in different directions?

Think about these:
So, we are all going. Are you coming?
We're all going to try it. OK?
Right! Let's all do this! Come on!

Focusing

In pairs, or small groups, quickly think about young people of your age in your community. What sort of situations or activities might be happening that has prompted someone to say these three statements above to someone else? List as many as you can.

Collect feedback from the class.

Into action

For each of the situations you have suggested, first imagine an unexceptional member of the group who does not want to act as the group is choosing to do, and who would behave differently if he or she was on their own. When a group all appears to want to do something that one person might think is not such a great idea, one or more different things can be happening.

Discuss, and write down in your pairs or groups, what you think is the self-talk of your imagined group member. Perhaps it is a justification of the action or inaction; or maybe it is anxieties that are *thought* but not *expressed*.

Compare some examples.

Look for:

● Justifications – 'It's bound to be OK! If everyone else thinks it's all right, it must be! The chances of it going wrong are tiny! They must've done it loads of times before.'

● Unexpressed worries – 'I hope we aren't seen! They'll think it was someone else! I can't be held personally responsible! I don't have a choice, everyone else is doing it! I'm the only one who's worried.'

● Indecision – 'What could I say to get out of it? If I say anything, they'll think I'm mad! They may throw me out of the group. What if it all goes pear-shaped? I don't know what to do!'

Might this imaginary, but typical, group member even go along with the proposal without thinking *anything*, perhaps only 'waking up' later when it's too late?

In fact, almost everyone else in the group may actually be equally worried but *everyone* goes along with what they feel everyone else wants to do. Sometimes something called 'groupthink' happens. This is when a group all appear to think something is a really good idea and, because they know each other well, no one wants to upset the consensus, or what appears to be a shared agreement. Nobody checks what others are feeling.

A man called Irving Janis in 1977 said groups are really susceptible to groupthink if the following symptoms are present:

1 *Illusions of invulnerability* – the belief that if the group sticks together it can do anything (and get away with it).

2 *Rationalising warnings* – anyone warning against what the group believes or wants to do is stupid.

3 *Unquestioned belief* – what the group believes is always right. Everyone else is wrong, no matter what happens.

4 *Stereotyping* anyone who disagrees with the group as weak, evil or stupid.

5 *Direct pressure* – any member who questions the group is challenged, ridiculed or called disloyal.

6 *Self-censorship* – any ideas that go against the group's beliefs are ignored.

7 *Illusions of unanimity* among group members, silence means you agree!

8 *Mindguards* – there are self-appointed members who stop the rest of the group seeing or hearing any conflicting information. Anyone presenting conflicting views is silenced, or maybe challenged or ridiculed.

In groups, think about these symptoms. Can you recall situations where your group experienced groupthink? How many of Irving Janis' points were working in those situations?

Think about the statement: 'Critical reflection can work *for* groups, as well as *in* groups.' What can a group and its members do to make groupthink less likely? How can it encourage critical reflection before making decisions? List some realistic suggestions.

Reflection

Think of your own groups of friends, and how decisions are made in these groups. Think about times when you have felt worried, powerless, undecided or pressured, and have gone along with a decision you didn't like. Ask yourself: what can *you* do to strengthen your group's reliance on the good sense of its members? How can *you* help make it OK for everyone's views to be expressed and listened to?

A question of making a good impression

E18
Do I know what factors might lead to my making a good impression?
Do I know how enthusiasm or exuberance could lead to taking risks or even real danger at work?
Do I understand the importance of following instructions?

To the teacher

For many students, going to their first day of work experience can be both scary and exciting. This session explores some of the mixed feelings we might have and, in particular, considers how it feels to be asked to do tasks that are possibly well below our potential. A further surprise for students is that, after the pace of a secondary school, many workplaces are actually quite slow.

Young people are the highest risk group for accidents in the workplace. These accidents are often triggered by them overreaching themselves in a desire to make a good impression before they have appropriate training or experience. For many students, work experience is a rich and rewarding period in their education. For others, it is dull, repetitive and often boring.

To the students

The purpose of this session is to explore 'first impressions' and consider ways we can positively influence people's first impression of us.

Work experience is just that – a chance for you to experience going to work on a regular basis for a few weeks. First impressions are really important. Have you ever met someone who you thought was one type of person, but actually were quite different once you got to know them? When we meet someone for the first time we know nothing about them so, rightly or wrongly, we quickly try to work out what they are like based on what we see and hear. Once we have made that judgement, it can lead us to make all sorts of fair or unfair judgements about that person. We can turn this to our advantage by making a good first impression.

'You nervous?'

'What about?'

'Starting work experience.'

'Not really.'

Actually, that wasn't true. Both Josh and Emma needed to have an interview before their placement and, whilst Josh thought it would be OK, he was a bit anxious. He didn't really enjoy meeting new people, especially when he wasn't sure what they would ask him. He was also a bit worried they might give him some sort of test. Emma was feeling the same way.

'Look,' Hannah said. 'It will be fine. All the people who offer placements want to help young people, they don't have to offer work experience placements. No one is trying to catch you out; they just want to help you.'

Focusing

In pairs, think about your work experience. What are you looking forward to and what would you rather avoid? What, if anything, are you nervous about?

Into action

In groups of four, think about either your interview or your first day on your placement.

Either:

● What impression do you want people to have of you? What do you want people who have never met you to think you are like?

Or:

● Imagine you are an employer who is expecting a student to join your organisation for a work experience placement today.

● What type of person are you hoping for? What characteristics do you hope they will have?

● Why is this important?

Collect some feedback from the class.

Look for:

● Appearance (appropriate to the work – unless it is an interview)

● Punctuality (not too early but not late)

● Confident (unpack this one – how confident?)

● Enthusiasm

● Interest in the work

● Some prior knowledge of the company (someone who has done some research)

● A good listener, someone who pays attention

● Good communicator (someone who can talk to people)

● Smiles (we are going to have to work together).

In groups, students pick one or two qualities from the list above (make sure all are being considered by at least one group).

Either:

● How might an employer judge whether you have the qualities they are looking for?

Or:

- What are all the things you can do to make sure they have a good impression of you?

Collect some feedback from the class and discuss.

Look for:

- Dress appropriately – if in doubt, telephone and ask.
- Check out the route, bus times, etc. prior to the interview or first day.
- Check out where the entrance is if the company is large.
- Know the company's telephone number.
- Arrive not more than ten minutes early and not less than five minutes early. (If you are going to be late, make sure you telephone and let them know as soon as you can.)
- Check out if the company has a website and learn about them.
- If possible, know who to ask for when you arrive for your interview or first day.
- Take a note pad and pen, so that you can write notes if you need to. (Remind them that virtually all of us find it hard to remember what we are being told if we feel nervous – it's OK to take notes.)

A word of warning ...

Is it possible to be too enthusiastic?

Imagine you are in your placement and you want to make a good impression. You see something that could be done quicker, or could be done better.

In pairs, discuss the risks of doing something or changing something without asking.

Explain that:

- there may be very good reasons why things are done as they are, even if they seem strange or stupid to you.
- some things that look really easy may not be. They might involve a risk to you or cause a risk to others of which you are not aware.
- companies do not want their computer systems improved. (Many companies rent their ICT systems and 'improvements', even if they work, can be serious breaches of contract.)

It is essential that you ask before doing anything that you are unsure about, or which you have not been asked to do or had explained to you.

Reflection

Think about making a good first impression. Of all the things we have discussed in this session, which are you confident you have got sorted out and which might you need to work on?

If students say they still lack confidence, this is an opportunity to use a 'future pacing' exercise (see page 250).

A question of 'brand you'

> **E19**
> How do I feel about being interviewed as part of my work experience?
> How can I really demonstrate my skills and personal qualities to people who do not know me at an interview?
> What do I know or do, what special skills or experiences do I have that make me really employable?

To the teacher

Achieving success in examinations and accumulating relevant life experiences are obviously vital parts of securing employment or access to further education. However, there is another hurdle – the interview. Many students do not understand the processes that companies use, for example a job description and a person specification. Because of equal opportunity policies, many companies are quite mechanical in their shortlisting, comparing the application with the person specification. Many students do not know how to put together an application or curriculum vitae that gives them the best chance of being shortlisted for interview.

This session focuses on helping students pull together a 'rich picture' of what they have to offer. In reality, this session should be part of a wider programme and may need to be adjusted to fit the skill level of your students. It could also be broken up into two or more sessions.

To the students

Many of us will need to be interviewed as part of our work experience and the purpose of this session is to help you prepare for it. The truth is, most people don't like being interviewed and feel a bit nervous before and during the event. The more relaxed you are, the easier it is to be you, answer questions and effectively sell yourself. Having the opportunity to really think about what you can offer can help. Many people are surprised that the people conducting the interview are often equally as nervous. You will almost certainly tell your friends how they behaved towards you, so they also have to protect their reputation and, perhaps, company image.

A work experience interview is good practice for interviews you might have in years to come, so take it seriously. Many people find that the more interviews they do, the easier it becomes. When you go for interviews in the future, you will almost certainly be competing with other people for the college place or job position. Remember, if you get invited for an interview, you know you have already done well, the chances are that the majority of applicants will already have been rejected.

'When is your interview?' Emma asked.

'Wednesday,' Sara replied.

'Mine's tomorrow,' Emma said.

'You'll be fine. You don't have anything to worry about,' reassured Sara.

Emma felt anything but calm. She knew she was pretty good at school work, but when it came to meeting new people and talking about herself she never knew what to say and ended up coming across as really quiet. When people asked her things, her mind seemed to switch off! She always knew what she should have said afterwards, just never when it mattered. Not like Sara, she never worried about anything.

Actually, Sara felt really nervous. She knew that when she was nervous she talked far too much. She was really worried about being asked questions she couldn't answer and coming across as a complete idiot.

Focusing

Imagine you are in advertising. Think of some different products that you know are being advertised right now on the television or radio. List these and talk about how the advertisers promote their brands. What do the adverts tell people their lives will be like if they buy them? Have you ever thought that you might be a 'brand'? Your qualifications will be vitally important. These are what get you and the others you are competing against into the interviews. Now you simply have to convince them that you are the person they want.

Into action

Imagine you have been given the job of advertising the brand 'you'. This can be a good pairs activity – one person recording and coaching the other. Today, you have permission to really show off.

First, think about 'you' from your own point of view. What skills do you have – things you can do, things you are brilliant at, good at, or just OK (competent) at. You don't have to be brilliant at something to have a skill. Being competent or OK at something is often fine.

Think about your:

- technical skills – what can you do really well? For example, 'I am really good at ICT or art and design.'
- people skills – how do you work with others? For example, 'I can handle difficult people well.'
- personal skills – what sort of a person are you? For example, 'Once I start something, I always try to finish it.'

Write down your responses as quickly as you can. Think really widely. Even if you are not quite sure of the level of a skill, still put it down for now. What experiences have you had in school, outside of school? What skills have these given you? If you are doing this in pairs, help your partner challenge themselves to identify as many skills as they can – don't let them be modest.

Then, try to think of an example of when you have used or demonstrated each skill. The example can be quite small, such as 'I helped my mum get online'. It's demonstrating that you have the skill that matters, not where you used it. If you wrote down skills you were not confident you really had, really search through your memories and see if you have ever had to use this skill.

Now the tricky bit …

We need to turn it around and try to see 'you' from an employer's point of view. *This could be a private reflection, but is best done as a pairs activity, with one person listening to what the other feels they have to offer and prompting them using their own knowledge of their partner.* What sort of person will a possible employer see? What personal characteristics do you have in addition to your skills? Consider:

- are you friendly?
- are you an attentive listener?
- are you careful to follow instructions?
- are you ready to work hard?
- are you ready to learn new skills?
- do you make eye contact easily?
- do you smile lots?
- do you speak clearly?
- do you appear self-confident?

Be ready to prompt your partner if you think they are missing important attributes they have (or need to note down some they haven't). Along with your skills list, write down all the characteristics you have identified. This is your 'brand'. Brand 'you'.

Now, imagine that during the interview the employer is thinking, 'How will employing you benefit me?' During the interview, the interviewer's task is to try to answer this question by taking account of what you say, how you respond, how you look and how you behave. You need to try to show your 'brand' as clearly as you can.

Try to complete the following statement (about you) honestly, from the employer's point of view:

'If I employ this person, I and my company will benefit because …'

Still from the employer's perspective:

- What are you convinced about?
- What more would you like to know about this interviewee?
- What are you still wondering and uncertain about?

Switch back to being you. You now know what the employer is convinced about and what they are not. How will you convince them? How will you 'win them over'? If you need to strengthen your list of skills (your 'skill set'), do you need to acquire more skills? Do you need to develop those you have? Perhaps you need to do both. What about the way you are seen by others – has your partner helped you identify characteristics to think about or work on that will strengthen the brand 'you'?

Reflection

This session has been about putting your whole brand together. When you apply for any career or college course, you obviously need to pick out which bits of your brand 'you' to really emphasise.

Visualise your future employer. Imagine they are in a 30-second advert being an amazing employer. They are explaining why they are an amazing employer by talking about a fantastic appointment they made. They are talking about you. They begin by saying, 'I employed … and this is what they did for me and my company.' What are they saying?

A question of gambling

K2
How do I feel about gambling?
What are the alternatives to gambling?
What are the risks of gambling for me?
Why do I think people gamble?
If I or someone I knew had a problem with gambling, would I know where to get help?

To the teacher

Gambling is mostly not a horror story. It could be considered to be a long and well-established activity in our society, though in some cultures and religions in the UK gambling may be frowned upon, or even considered a sin. Gambling takes many forms – the large-scale activities such as the national lottery, bingo halls and casinos, horse and greyhound racing, through to smaller, local-scale ventures such as office sweepstakes, raffles and the tombola at the school fête. It is often an occasional and enjoyable activity where the gambler risks relatively little and where wins are a nice surprise. Few who risk a small gamble expect to win anything, and even those who gamble in 'the lotto' recognise that the chance of a sizeable win is small at best. For most, the excitement is in the element of chance and the outside possibility of being a significant winner. For many, it is indulged in openly and socially.

However, the subject needs to be looked at because problem gambling is a reality for some, and a small percentage of adolescents could even be described as pathological gamblers with severe gambling-related difficulties. Common amongst them are those who gamble alone, and even on the internet, often 'chasing' losses, and always encouraged by what they perceive as 'near misses'.

- Reasons young people give for gambling include: fun; enjoyment; excitement; buzz; adrenaline rush and to win money.
- Explanations for not gambling include: to avoid debt; fear of becoming addicted; too risky; a sin; unlikely to win.
- Gambling among young people is a growing problem in society.
- Young people are more vulnerable to the negative effects of gambling than adults.
- Male gamblers outnumber females in the 16–25 age range.
- Gambling is often referred to as the 'hidden addiction' because, unlike other dependencies, it is much more difficult to identify when someone's gambling is out of control.
- **One of the most problematic types of gambling to date appears to have been fruit machine gambling.**
- 78 per cent of 15 year olds say they have gambled and (according to MORI and the International Gaming Research Unit) one-third of adolescents will have played fruit machines in the last month.
- Problem gamblers are more likely to be in the 16–25 age range, to have begun gambling at an early age (as young as eight) and to have been bolstered by a big, early win.
- It may be that the 'new' forms of gambling, such as the machines inside bookmakers' premises, and online poker and bingo (both of which are growing in popularity), will be the future focus of problem gambling.

The purpose of this session is not to frighten or forbid, but to look at gambling from all angles in order to recognise that it is sensible to treat it cautiously and rationally. The session involves exploring gamblers and non-gamblers *as groups* with a particular focus on fictitious characters. Judge whether to encourage – or even allow – personal disclosures that could be sensitive, or allow any focus on a real individual in the class. You may need to re-visit the class ground rules to ensure clarity.

To the students

Ever bought a raffle ticket? Did you win? (Probably you didn't but you *might* have done.) Gambling is very common. Many, perhaps most, of us have gambled at some time or another. When did you last have a bet? Was it just a verbal one? ('I bet you won't dare ask Emma out!' said Josh to Joe over lunch.) Or did it involve money? ('I bet you a quid Arsenal beat Chelsea next Saturday!' Nathan challenged Jack.)

The purpose of this session is to explore gambling – what it is and the forms that it takes – and why it is so popular. It's also intended to look at when (and why) it can get out of hand for some people, what happens to problem gamblers and where help and support can be found for anyone needing it for themselves or others.

Focusing

What is gambling? Can you describe it and create a definition? Talk in pairs for a minute or two and then write down some ideas.

How many of the ideas had the words 'luck', 'chance', 'risk' or 'stake' in them?

Clarify the essence of gambling, if necessary.

However you choose to define it, there is a *stake*, a *risk* that you will *lose* that stake, and a *chance* (even when there's some skill) that you may *win* back more than you risked. If so, luck will be involved, even if the gambler adds in as much experience, skill and judgement as he or she can. Most gambling is based on the chances of winning being smaller than the chances of losing. That way, the person (or organisation) taking the bet is more likely to win. In the long term, it's the takers, not the punters, who become rich. That's why people are keen to open casinos, the owners of betting shops are all rich, and the national lottery has raised £17 billion for 'good causes' of one kind or another. The rest of us have good fun, but pay for the privilege, just as we generally have to pay for any commercially provided entertainment.

Into action

What counts as gambling? Bets between friends? Buying a raffle ticket? As a class, generate a list of as many varieties of gambling as you can.

Write class feedback on the board or a flip chart.

Then ask how many of the class have ever gambled using any of these forms. It may be interesting to see the spread of gambling activities represented in the class, without putting undue focus on anyone. Tell the class you want to explore why people do it, and what feelings they get from it. Judge whether it is appropriate to probe a little (how often, how much do you spend, what's it like when you win/lose, etc.)

Ask the class what they think of gambling – do they have views and feelings to share?

Suggest that the class plays 'Inside, outside, upside down'. You need six groups. Two will focus on occasional gamblers, two on non-gamblers, and the remaining two on gamblers having trouble controlling their gambling. Both gamblers in the latter category play fruit machines in the local arcade. Explain that there are upsides to gambling whether or not you can control it (entertainment value, anticipation, the thrills of playing, the 'rush' from the 'near miss', the excitement of winning, etc.) Equally, there are downsides for all gamblers (disappointment of losing the bet/game/spin, feeling time has been wasted, going home empty-handed, etc.)

Assign each group a category, or allow them to choose. Ideally, you need all three categories to be represented twice. A crib-sheet is provided below for each category. Make it available to groups wanting to see it. Not every character will fit everything on the crib-sheet.

The activity involves each group choosing a person to play the role of gambler (or non-gambler). The group's task is to prime the chosen person with as much detail as possible about what they think, how they feel, what they believe, how they 'see' gambling, so that when they are questioned in role, they can paint a full, credible and accurate picture of such a person. They should try to create a realistic picture of the person in relation to the issue of gambling, but can add any personal details they like, as long as they fit the gambling behaviour. When the groups are ready, put each character in role into the spotlight in turn. Encourage questions from the whole class that will probe this fictitious person's views, experiences and feelings, and attempt to discover why this person acts the way they do and how they feel about themselves. Try to discover how they feel at various points: when they are gambling; when they're not gambling; when they win; when there's a near miss; and when they lose. Allow them to consult with their group if they aren't sure about how to answer questions they hadn't planned for. **Be sure to de-role each role-playing student before the session ends***.*

Note*: It is vital that each category be given equal status – it is quite possible that, in reality, all three categories are actually represented in the class.*

Crib-sheet for unrestrained gambler

- Loves the thrill of playing – can't get enough of it; sees gambling as an important part of their lives.
- Experiences adrenalin rush at start of session, and at near misses as well as wins.
- When playing, often has a dry mouth, sees and thinks of nothing else.
- When not playing, often thinks of (or 'lives for') the next time they can gamble.
- Usually plays alone.
- Has a favourite machine; if someone else is on 'their' machine, the gambler feels jealous and possessive.
- May start to sweat as losses mount.
- Is excited by near misses – each feels like a success and spurs the gambler on to try again. (Near misses, for example two treasure chests followed by a third treasure chest just above, or just below, the win-line are programmed into the machines by the manufacturers to encourage the user to continue. In reality, there is nothing 'near' about the miss. Gamblers usually either don't know or don't take account of this.)
- May feel the need to 'chase' losses (continue gambling to try to win back lost money).
- Each win *justifies* continuing – each loss *demands* that the gambler continue.
- If there is time, spends every penny they have before leaving – including winnings.
- Frequently late for next activity/event/appointment.
- Often has trouble getting enough money for the habit – may sell, lie or even steal to get more money.
- May have low self-esteem.
- May have started gambling *very* young.
- May have had a 'big' win (or one that seemed big) early in their gambling career.
- May have parents who gamble.
- May be, or feel, awkward when socialising with others.
- Wants that really big win that will wipe out all the losses, lost time and personal clouds.

Crib-sheet for non-gambler

- May not approve of gambling.
- May not approve of gamblers.
- Is fearful of becoming addicted.
- Is keen to avoid debt.
- Feels most gambles are too risky, and you're unlikely to win.
- May feel it is a sin.
- May feel compelled to follow parents' instructions (not to gamble).
- Doesn't enjoy anything about gambling.
- Is naturally not a risk taker.
- May be a bit shy.
- Likes to feel safe.
- Doesn't get a lot of pocket money.
- May view gambling as a waste of time that could be spent doing better things.

Crib-sheet for restrained gambler

- Says gambling is a bit of a laugh, and actually rather enjoys it.
- Sometimes plays cards for money when bored.
- Won a bottle of wine in a tombola once and gave it to Dad.
- Doesn't have much money, and would usually rather do other things with it.
- Doesn't think about gambling when not gambling.
- Gets a 'rush' when winning, but hates losing and can 'quit while ahead'.
- Views gambling primarily as a form of entertainment.
- Understand that, mostly, the odds are stacked against gamblers winning.
- Realises that a big win is unlikely and feels it's not worth chasing.
- Understands the wisdom of the saying 'avoid throwing good money after bad'.
- Has plenty of other things to do with friends, with time and with money.

When all characters have been grilled, encourage discussion allowing anyone – characters and questioners – to say what they have learned and whether their views or feelings about gambling have been reinforced or changed in any way. Encourage the class to try to put themselves in the shoes of people with a different attitude to gambling from their own. Ask them to say what they think leads to them feeling and behaving as they do.

Ask the class the following:

- Can you suggest what makes gambling popular?
- Why do so many people do it? Is it *just* the lure of the money they might win, or is it more than that?
- Will lots of money actually make the gambler happy?
- Are the reasons why a person finds it hard to control gambling to be found by studying gambling, or should we look elsewhere? Where?
- The same choices face everyone who loses, so what determines whether a gambler stops or continues?

Ensure that the contact details for the national helplines for gamblers are available, if necessary.

Reflection

Do you know which category you're in (non-gambler, occasional gambler, gambler who finds it hard to stop)? Are you in the category you *want* to be in? Are you able to change category? If you can't, do you know who to turn to? If you, or someone you know, needed help to look at the issues, do you feel able to seek it?

GamCare
National telephone helpline: 0845 6000 133
http://www.gamcare.org.uk

Gamblers Anonymous (UK)
Helpline: 020 7384 3040
http://www.gamblersanonymous.org.uk

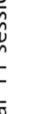
A question of taking a lift with an unsafe driver

> **K6**
> Could I manage a situation where I am offered a lift in a car where I suspect the driver may have been drinking alcohol (using cannabis or other drugs that might impair competence)?

To the teacher

Young people can find it difficult to manage situations where their peer group members are all choosing to behave in a certain way. There may be a tendency to 'hope for the best' or deny the possibility of something that is known to be risky actually happening. This session offers a number of possibilities, including managing the immediate situation, exploring the effect even small amounts of some drugs can have on our ability to make choices and manage situations, and also the full implications of an incident such as a road accident. The session offers an opportunity to explore the timeline, looking for critical moments and exploring why people might make the choices they did, and what choices they might wish they had made after the event.

The critical issue to explore is why, if the risks are apparent, do we sometimes pretend they aren't real or won't really happen and hope for the best? Do we ever let a desire 'not to make a fuss' or conform to the group put us in real jeopardy? If people were with a group of strangers rather than friends, would they make different choices? If you are with your friends, do you feel pressures to follow 'unwritten rules' or not to 'inconvenience' them by appearing awkward or uncool? If the worst did happen and you could look back and give yourself advice, would you suggest a different choice?

This same session would work for using illegal drugs such as cannabis. The session also links well with Year 11, G11 on page **134**. Nathan and Becky act as the bystanders in this scenario. You might use different names in order to change the genders of the bystanders. It can be interesting to explore whether or not students have different expectations for young men and women in this situation.

To the students

Have you ever been in a position where everyone around you is doing something that you feel might be risky or even dangerous, but they all seem to be ignoring the risks or danger and tell you it will be OK? How does this make you feel? How easy is it to be the odd one out, especially if you feel it might inconvenience everyone else?

In this session, we are going to look at a situation where a small amount of alcohol may have caused a serious crash. What we are going to explore is why everyone told each other it would be all right, when really they all knew there were real risks.

It was after the party and Julie was being encouraged by her friend Sue to have a lift with her and Matt. 'Come on, Julie, he is fine. We all want to get going. Are you getting in or are you just going to stand there in the rain?'

Becky was leaving with Nathan. 'I can't believe it, they are going with him!'

'What's the matter with that? Matt is fine. He didn't drink/use any more than he normally does. What do you expect them to do? It's raining like mad outside and they aren't going to pay for a taxi! He's not drunk, and he is not likely to risk that car of his.'

'Well, I know Julie didn't want go with him; she only went because Sue insisted it would be OK,' Becky replied.

'Yeah, well, you know what Julie's like. She's scared of everything!'

They watch the car speed away from them. After a few seconds of erratic driving, the young people see it cross the road and crash head on into another approaching vehicle. After the initial noise of the crash, there is silence. No one is getting out of either car.

'What are we going to do?'

Focusing

Questions to explore the present:

- What are Becky and Nathan feeling right now?
- What will they do next? What *should* they do?
- Do you think the drivers and passengers will walk away?

Into action

When the vehicle is being towed away, Julie's body is found inside. A post mortem reveals she has no alcohol in her system. In groups of four, discuss:

- Do you think Julie knew it was dangerous to get in the car?
- Why do you think she got in the car with this driver?
- What pressures might have influenced her decision? Where might these pressures have been coming from? For example, outside or from feelings within her.

Look for:

- Not wanting to appear awkward
- Not wanting to appear stupid or childish
- Not wanting to be left behind

- Fear they would all laugh at her after they had gone
- Wanting to be like them and liked by them.

- Is it possible to put pressure on someone so they actually make your decision rather than their own? If this happens, who is responsible for what happens next?
- Does that pressure have to be really strong persuasion, or can it be quite subtle?

Look for:

- The 'look', or the expectant 'wait' – in this case perhaps holding the door open
- The comment about the rain. Are the first few lines in the scenario really asking Julie a question and offering her a real choice, or is Sue just telling her to get in this car *now*?
- Is it easier sometimes to 'hope for the best' rather than have a confrontation?
- Does anyone have the right to make someone else feel like that or put someone else at risk or in danger?
- If Julie didn't want to take the lift, what could others have said and done differently to help her make her own decision?
- How would Sue have felt if Julie had continued to 'stand there in the rain' and refused to get in? How would you feel in Sue's shoes if someone made a stand in that situation?

Extension questions

Questions to explore the past:

- Why was Matt driving like that?

Look for:

- Inexperienced
- Distracted
- Influenced by alcohol/drugs.

- How do you think Julie felt being driven like that?
- If the driver had been drinking with friends who let him drive home, how are they feeling now?
- Why might Nathan say he thought Matt was safe to drive?

Look for:

- Honestly thought he was safe
- Not wanting to confront the reality that he knew he wasn't but not sure how to handle it.

If I told you that one of the first things alcohol does to our brain is shut down the part that helps us assess risk, do you think this could have contributed to the accident? *Perhaps emphasise that the more we drink the less drunk we think we are – everyone else, however, usually knows – unless they are equally drunk.*

- If Matt's friends had been drinking alcohol, how would that have affected their ability to assess Matt's ability to drive safely?
- When they said he was OK to drive, might they have honestly believed they were right?
- In what way might this have influenced the pressure they put Julie and her friends under to get in the car with him?

Questions to explore the future:

- What did the two drivers' families feel when they heard the news?
- What did the police and ambulance/paramedics feel – especially if they had to break the news to the families?
- If Matt, Julie and Sue could have seen into their futures and known this was going to happen, what might they have done differently? At what point in the timeline would this change have started?
- If they had believed this accident was likely to happen, how would each of the others have behaved differently?
- Can you estimate how many lives have been ruined?

If the climate in your class makes it safe to do so, you can increase the introspection of individuals by shifting the questions to 'you' – first as a witness, then as the person being offered the lift. How would you feel:

- if you had been a witness
- if you had to break the news
- if you were their friend?

Reflection

Have you ever been in a position where you have made a decision that you know is wrong, risky or one you really didn't want to make? What pressures were you under? Were they from outside of you or from inside of you? Can you suggest ways to manage pressure like this?

Does anyone have the right to put other people at risk? How much responsibility do we have for other people's feelings?

A question of media treatment of drugs issues

D4

Why do I think we hear so much about *illegal* drugs in the media, on the news and in films?
If I read, watch, listen carefully to the media, can I find examples of local and national concern about legal drugs, too?
Do some of these concerns relate to the health of users of these legal drugs?

To the teacher

It is quite common for young people not to listen to valid and significant information about illegal drugs, particularly when it relates to dangers. This may be for a number of reasons:

- They do not believe the information.
- They do not trust the information-giver, or the route of delivery (government, school, parent, newspaper).
- It suits them not to 'hear' information they don't want to believe.

In part, this may also relate to the very illegality of the drug or drugs. It is this factor that has, at least as much as others, helped the mass media to perpetuate feelings such as fear and loathing. This may help sell newspapers peddling shock and horror, but may do little to inform, and even less to inform in the calm, objective and balanced way that is vital in education. It is important for us, and for students, to distinguish clearly between danger and disapproval. Even when we are right to disapprove, it doesn't change objective facts about drugs, which good practice dictates should be delivered in both a dispassionate and a credible way.

It can be interesting to note differences in media treatment of young people's use of alcohol and their use of illegal drugs. The word 'criminal' and its attendant adjectives are often absent from alcohol reporting, but a similar focus on associated dangers may be accompanied in the writings of columnists by expressions of bewilderment about a young binge-drinker's mindset. It is much easier to disapprove of illegal behaviour – there is no need for detailed understanding, explanation or justification of the stance. In fact, binge drinking might be a lot easier to write about if it *was* illegal to drink, because then journalists and reporters would not need to try to understand why young people behave as they do.

This session is aimed at helping students recognise bias and emotive delivery in media treatment of drugs issues, and to be able to seek, instead, accurate and unbiased information whenever it might be helpful. You will need to forewarn the class to collect newspaper cuttings and it may be helpful if you can augment these with some you have collected yourself. Multiple copies will assist scrutiny in small groups.

To the students

This session explores the way newspapers and magazines deal with drugs issues – illegal drugs in particular. It may be possible to locate sound information in the press, but how easy is it to find? How can you recognise when information is sound? You will need several press cuttings – the more you can see, the more valid any conclusions you draw. You might collect them yourself, cutting them from papers or magazines, or printing online versions of the papers. (Remember, this isn't an internet research exercise – there's plenty on the internet that has no relation to newspapers, and that's another subject entirely.)

'I don't get it,' Josh said. 'It says here drug use is rampant among young people.'

'Where?' Joe replied.

'Look, this newspaper article,' said Josh, holding the paper up.

'Well, maybe I lead a really boring life, but I don't know anyone who uses drugs,' said Joe. 'I suppose it depends what you mean by drugs. If you count medicines and alcohol, I guess we all do.'

'Somehow I don't think it means medicine,' Josh answered, then paused. 'But you have a good point about alcohol.'

'So what does it say then?' asked Joe.

'Well, according to this, lots of young people are probably going to die horrible, deaths and be locked up for years,' Josh replied.

'So, die first then get locked up … saves on the food bill I guess!' Joe joked.

'But that's the problem, isn't it? Of course drug use can be risky, but if I really want information, the sort I might need to have to stay safe, who can I trust?' asked Josh.

Focusing

What are the main tasks of reporters?

Look for:

- report
- excite
- horrify
- surprise
- inform
- sell newspapers.

How well do you think reporters do each of the things on the 'Look for' list? Is it their job to 'inform' readers about drugs? Do you think their role 'to inform' amounts to a responsibility 'to educate'?

Take feedback from the class and discuss the ideas presented. You may find a distinction is naturally drawn between 'red-top' and 'quality' papers. Ask which reach a wider audience.

Into action

Share cuttings from newspapers and magazines in groups of four. In your group, read them and look for evidence of how the paper or magazine generally treats the subject.

Look for:

- Words or phrases that reveal the newspaper or magazine's attitude to drugs, drug use or drug users (positive, negative or neutral)
- Any detailed information about drugs that could be taken by the reader as 'fact' (ignore whether or not it's correct)
- Adjectives applied to a drug or to a drug user
- Anything else that seems to indicate the attitude of the writer, or that seems to presume the attitude of the reader.

Collect feedback from the groups and identify common threads.

Are newspapers a good source of information about drugs? What about magazines? Does it depend what age they are aimed at? Is the role of the printed media responsibly handled? What tells you this? Or do there seem to be unhelpful generalisations (drugs kill, drug users steal to pay for drugs, criminals are a danger to us all)?

How can you tell whether printed information about drugs is:

- true or untrue
- selective or comprehensive
- up to date or out of date
- balanced or misleading
- biased or objective?

Look for:

- Understanding the need to check with trusted sources.

Point out some sound sources of local information. Mention the DrugScope website – probably the best repository of accurate, up-to-date and objective drugs information in the UK (though mostly not *aimed* at young people).

Go to: http://www.drugscope.org.uk/, click on 'Resources' and then 'DrugSearch' to view a comprehensive glossary.

Reflection

Think about how the press 'informs' its readers, and how it may create, perpetuate or challenge attitudes – which may not be helpful. Think about the kind of reader each paper is aimed at, who they are trying to please, and what role money and politics might play in how they treat the subject.

How confident do you now feel about seeking and checking drug information to ensure you have the best information you can get?

A question of attitudes to alcohol and drug use

D11

Do I think the opinions of others around me are changing about alcohol or drug use?
Why do I think this?
Do I think people of my age are using alcohol or tobacco more regularly?
What do I feel about this?
Are my feelings about the consequences changing?
Do I know for sure whether those (my age) around me are, or are not, using drugs?
What do I feel about those making the same choices as me?
What do I feel about those making different choices from me?

To the teacher

Research shows that young people pretty consistently guess incorrectly about the drug and alcohol consumption of those their own age and immediately above, presuming this to be greater than it is. Consequently, their idea of the 'norms' for their age group are usually wrong, often significantly. As the perceived (normal) behaviour of peers affects young people's choices about trying and using alcohol and other drugs, it makes sense for their perception to be based on reality rather than guesswork.

This session will encourage interchange about attitudes and perceptions among class members and support independent thought before decisions. The session starts with smoking, progressing to alcohol. Decide whether you want to extend it into the arena of controlled drugs and, if so, which. Only cannabis is specifically mentioned here.

We suggest that some local research in the upper school can be very illuminating. However, the managerial 'climate' in the wider school needs to be conducive to such research, and the students need to be convinced of the purpose, to trust the process and believe the anonymity promised to responders. One spin-off is that all classes and year groups could benefit from the findings, which may contribute to more reasoned decision making. Another is that there may be learning for the staff and an improved 'climate' for drug education. Clearly, the choices of how research findings are to be used by the school are a matter for you and your colleagues.

In this session, beware of any mistaken belief by students that the session is intended to get them to change their behaviour. Reassure, if necessary.

To the students

How many smokers are there in the class? How many have just tried smoking? How many have thought about trying it? How many drink alcohol at least once a week? A show of hands might tell you these answers, but some nervous hands may stay down. What about cannabis? No, perhaps it's unfair even to ask anyone to openly declare an illegal activity.

This session aims to find ways to explore how attitudes in the class to drug and alcohol use have changed, and what those who *do* use think about those who *don't* (and vice-versa).

Are these examples of self-talk realistic?

- 'Everyone has tried it except me.'
- 'I bet I am the only one who hasn't done …'
- 'Everyone says they have by my age … but I haven't, I must be odd.'
- 'They say all young people do … but I haven't.'
- 'I did … because I felt I was missing out.'

Focusing

What do you think about people who smoke? Answers to this may depend on whether you smoke. What do:

- non-smokers think about smokers
- light smokers feel about heavy smokers
- smokers think about non-smokers?

Instead of answering these questions, discuss, in pairs, how you could find out, and ensure that you get honest answers from the others in your class. *It may not feel too threatening simply to talk openly in class, as long as the ground rules are sound and working. (Do they need checking, reinforcing or amending?) Or perhaps there's a better way.*

Widen your pairs discussion to include similar questions about alcohol and cannabis. *The 'open discussion' option may not seem quite so appealing on this occasion, even if it was earlier. Collect some alternative feedback suggestions. Are they feasible? Do they attract support from the whole class?*

Look for:

- Written (anonymous) responses – perhaps collated by the teacher or a trusted class member
- Questionnaire
- Open discussion in small, friendship group, with generalised 'findings' presented by spokesperson
- Could answer all the questions except the one addressed to cannabis users.

Perhaps the questions themselves need editing. In any event, care will be needed to ensure any ground rules and assurances about anonymity or confidentiality are adhered to.

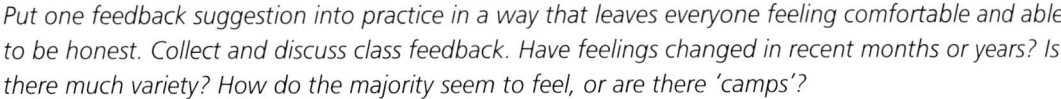

Put one feedback suggestion into practice in a way that leaves everyone feeling comfortable and able to be honest. Collect and discuss class feedback. Have feelings changed in recent months or years? Is there much variety? How do the majority seem to feel, or are there 'camps'?

Ask the class to suggest how many drinkers, smokers and drug users there are in the upper school. Refine and extend these questions to ask about frequency/heaviness of use and age. Is there general agreement? Can the students come to a consensus about how many are involved, and broadly from what age(s), or does consensus seem unlikely? Whether or not there is a consensus, how might their estimations be checked in reality?

Ask the class to discuss in small groups how this might be done for all the students in Year 11, or if you have a sixth form, Year 12. (If it accords with the current needs of the school, this could be extended to Years 10 and 13.) The suggestions will probably take the form of a survey or written questionnaire.

Groups may be encouraged to think about:
- how they could guard against dishonest responses
- how they could protect anyone asked about illegal activity
- how to identify and discount false answers
- what to do if someone refuses to take part
- what might be done with the results
- who would be allowed to see any written records/responses
- what would happen to records/responses after the research was complete
- what the head teacher might say about the idea
- how they could reassure parents.

If you want to emphasise the research process, consider introducing or re-introducing the concepts of:
- hypothesis – a statement we make that we can test through our research – we prove it or disprove it
- data – the figures we gather, which is different from information, or the conclusions we draw from it. (We interpret data to become better informed.)
- validity – is our approach going to gather really accurate or valid data?
- reliability – assurance that our research tool will always work with a similar group of young people so we can compare results between groups
- generalisable – the degree of confidence that, whatever our conclusions are, they generalise to other young people of a similar age.

Pursue this activity if all the conditions that emerge seem favourable. Encourage the class to identify tasks, and decide who would undertake them. Discuss timing and the detail of carrying out the project and processing the results.
- What could we do with the data?
- How confident are we that our data is accurate?
- Are our results as we expected or surprising, reassuring or alarming? If so, in what way?
- Are there any contradictions? Why might this have happened?

How would maximum value be extracted from the exercise once the results were collated? What messages might it be useful to publicise within the school?

Into action

The vital need to follow up this data-gathering exercise to check out expectations against outcomes, and explore both findings and feelings, is evident. However, we have not suggested how you might conduct this.

One thing we do suggest is that, after the research findings are understood, students can be invited to look back at the self-talk examples given earlier on page 156 to see whether their feelings about them have altered. Perhaps those examples might now be tagged: 'Before I really investigated this I felt …' Can the students give examples of self-talk that might follow this: 'You know, once I really dug into this, it turns out …'? Are any of the following now more realistic?

'I feel sometimes that everyone has tried it except me … but maybe I am wrong.'

'I would have bet I am the only one who hasn't done … but turns out I would have lost!'

'Everyone says they have by my age … I haven't and I thought I must be odd. Turns out I was the same as virtually everyone else.'

'They say all young people do … but I haven't. Turns out hardly anyone of my age has.'

'I'm glad I didn't … because I might have been the only one …!'

Reflection

Are you aware of how the attitudes of others in your age group (your friends in particular) affect your decisions and behaviour about tobacco, alcohol and drug use? Do you feel better informed about what others think? Are your own views now more clearly formed (and have they changed)? Are you able to make your own decisions regardless of others' views?

Think about how you make decisions. The inner 'parent' in you might be telling you what you must or must not do. Your inner 'child' might be telling you what it wants or doesn't want you to do, and how strongly it feels about it – even that it doesn't want to be (or feel) left out. While your inner 'adult' is capable of listening to both, taking into account the data you have collected and making up its own mind.

A question of change

R3
How might relationships help or hinder my learning?
How might they affect my plans for the future?

R19
Do I expect relationships to go on, to change or to stop?
How do I feel about breaking up with someone I care(d) about?
How would I feel if someone I cared about or still care about now wants to be close to someone else?

To the teacher

This session links the above two content boxes and two of the three strands. It explores how, as the individual develops and goes through life changes, this can impact on their relationships – and how relationships, in turn, can impact on their life choices and decisions. It also links with Year 11, R18, which deals with pressures.

The session sits within the broad theme of 'life changes' that we have identified as particularly apt for this age group. It encompasses some of the situations concerned with relationships and sex that older teenagers might encounter, along with their potential pressures: changing expectations; differing levels of commitment, risk and contraception use in longer-term relationships; being away from home, etc.

This session aims to raise students' awareness of how expectations might differ and change between people in a relationship as they get older and make different life choices, and the pressures that can be experienced as a result of this. It is also about helping students to begin to develop strategies and skills for dealing with these pressures.

Note: The second (alternative) scene with Nathan and Becky could be more appropriate if your school does not have a sixth form.

To the students

This session is about how people's expectations might change as they get older and have to make different life choices, which might be exciting, scary or both. The session looks at how relationships can change; how the choices people make can affect relationships; and how relationships can affect choices. It is about the pressures this might bring and how people might deal with this.

Josh's friend Joe has been going out with Karen for quite a long time. They are talking about what they will do when they leave school.

'I'll probably leave after my GCSEs,' said Joe. 'I'm going to go into the navy when I leave school – I've always wanted to do it.'

'But you can't! It'll mean you going away … it'll be terrible!' Karen was obviously upset.

'Oh, come on, Karen. I've often talked about it … don't be so daft,' said Joe.

Jack's friend Nathan and his girlfriend Becky have been going out together since Year 11. They will soon finish their A Levels. They are talking about future plans.

'Why do you have to apply to that university? It's hundreds of miles away. That means I'll never see you – you know I need to stay local because of the family situation.' Nathan looked very unhappy.

'Look, Nathan, everyone says it's the best place for my course,' said Becky firmly. Nathan just shook his head and wouldn't answer.

'Oh, come on,' Becky sighed. 'We've talked about this – I need the best course and it'll be good for my CV if I want to succeed in that field of work. I've got to do what's best for my career.'

'Yeah, but what about us? I thought you loved me – but I suppose you'll soon forget about that if you're that far away …' Nathan managed to look angry and miserable at the same time.

Note to teacher: The following alternative scene with Nathan and Becky could be more appropriate if your school does not have a sixth form.

Jack's friend Nathan and his girlfriend Becky have been going out together since Year 11. Becky has been working with her company since they left school and has just been offered a fantastic job opportunity – there's just one problem …

'You've got to go where?!' Nathan exploded, 'But that's hundreds of miles away – I'll never see you …'

'Look, Nathan, it's an amazing career opportunity – it's tons more senior than what I do now,' Becky said, more than a bit exasperated. Nathan just shook his head and wouldn't answer.

'I thought you'd be really pleased for me,' Becky sighed. 'I thought you wanted me to succeed.'

'Yeah, but what about us? I thought you loved me – but I suppose you'll soon forget about that if you're that far away …' Nathan managed to look angry and miserable at the same time.

Focusing

Prompt some immediate reactions and discussion by asking these questions:

- What do you think about the situation with Joe and Karen? Why do you think she doesn't want him to go?
- Do you think Joe should respond to Karen's feelings and not go, or follow what he's always wanted to do?
- What do you think will happen if Joe goes?
- What do you think will happen if Joe doesn't go?

- What about Nathan and Becky? Why do you think he doesn't want her to go?
- Do you think Becky should respond to his feelings and not go, or follow what she wants to do with her studies and/or career?
- What do you think will happen if Becky goes?
- What do you think will happen if Becky doesn't go?

Into action

In small groups, choose one of the scenarios – either with Joe and Karen or Nathan and Becky:

- What are the pressures in this situation?
- Decide what should happen *immediately* in the short term? Decide what they should say and do right *now*.
- Is there anything that needs to happen in the future to solve the situation? Decide what else they should say and do.

Look for:

- Being torn between the need for the other person in the relationship and the need to follow ambitions
- Different expectations from the relationship – different ideas about what's important, and where priorities lie
- Fears about breaking up – that the other person will move on and find somebody new – or just 'grow away' from him or her
- Ways of being assertive about our own needs without rejecting the other person
- Understanding that one person might resent the other if they abandon what's important to them
- Ways of reassuring the other person
- Acknowledgement of the possibility that relationships will break up
- Realisation that it can be difficult to deal with the feelings that come from this.

Into action continued

Discuss the fact that in 'healthy relationships' you can do things separately as well as together – both people can have freedom to pursue their interests, ambitions, etc. and still care about each other. However, it's also important to recognise that where people's expectations/needs and ideas about what's important differ or change substantially, it might mean that the relationship needs to change or end and that this might not be easy.

Reflection

What do you think you would have done in any of these situations? You don't have to share your thoughts, but have any of your ideas about what's important to you changed in the last year? Are any relationships changing? Are there conversations you now feel you need to have?

A question of being yourself, and becoming an adult

R8

Am I aware that people's feelings of sexual attraction, their sexual behaviours and their sexual identity are not necessarily 'fixed' throughout their life?

Do I understand that, for a variety of reasons, these three things might not always coincide and that trying to fit people to stereotypes and labels is not helpful?

How do I feel about this in relation to me and other people I know, or groups of people?

Do I feel comfortable with my own sexuality and other people's?

R17

How does my family feel about me becoming an adult and forming new types of relationships?

What do they expect from me?

Do other people or groups have expectations about how I should behave?

How do I feel about that?

Do I agree?

To the teacher

This session links the above two content boxes – one from the 'Becoming everything I can be' strand and the other from the 'Managing my changing relationships' strand. The session focuses on the developing individual and their sexual orientation – attraction, behaviour and identity. It tackles a number of issues and could also link with content box R18, which looks at relationship pressures.

This session explores pressures that might be experienced by young lesbian, gay or bisexual people. It does not specifically address the needs of transgendered young people; should such issues arise in discussion, some supporting notes have been provided on page **279**.

All too often lesbian/gay/bisexual young people have to make sense of relationships and sexual issues in SRE sessions by 'translating' and applying material geared to heterosexual young people. In a way, this session reverses that process. The broader issues explored here, initially through a situation facing a lesbian couple, actually have relevance for all young people.

To the students

This session is concerned with issues related to sexuality and sexual orientation. It's also about the different types of situations you might encounter as you get older, the pressures these situations might bring – such as dealing with changing relationships, including your relationship with your family – and how you would deal with them.

'There's just no way I can do it, Hannah,' So Sen said, shaking her head. 'I wouldn't know how to start – they have no idea – they've always thought she was just my really close friend – like you. They'd be so shocked – I don't know what they would do.'

Hannah wasn't sure how to advise her friend. So Sen had been in a relationship with another girl, Nikki, for a year – but they had kept it hidden. Now they were 18 they were talking about living together and So Sen's girlfriend had said they should tell their families about their relationship.

'Surely Nikki understands how you feel,' Hannah said.

'Sort of,' So Sen said. 'But she says we're adults now and it's stupid to hide who we really are – we need to be ourselves – she even asked if I was ashamed of her,' So Sen said, miserably.

*'Well, you managed to tell **me** last year that you were gay – and that was all right, wasn't it? I was really glad that you told me. I couldn't believe you'd kept it hidden for so long – you even went out with Simon when we were in Year 11, remember?'*

*'Well, he was nice – and I suppose I was also doing what everyone expected – but I guess I always knew I preferred other girls really. Anyway, telling you is **not** like telling anyone else – I haven't told anyone else! Oh, Hannah, what shall I do? I know Nikki is right, and I'm **not** ashamed of her – I love her.'*

Focusing

Prompt some immediate reactions and discussion by asking these questions:

- What do you think So Sen is worried about?
- Do you think Nikki is right?
- What might happen if So Sen tells her family?
- What might happen if they 'come out' publicly?
- What might happen if they don't?

A variety of issues could be raised at this point, including things like fear of rejection, pressure from family and peers, how people want to be accepted, being able to be independent as you get older, being able to love who you want to, being open about who you love, possible break up of the relationship. Use these to lead into the following activity.

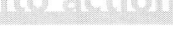

Divide the class into groups. Give each group a copy of the statements in the table below to discuss and decide their response as a group. Ask each group to appoint a spokesperson.

Draw an empty recording grid, like the table below, on the board. When the groups have finished their discussions:

1   *read out each statement*

2   *ask each spokesperson to raise their hand to show their group **agrees**, **disagrees**, or is **not sure***

3   *record the votes on the grid*

4   *discuss the responses for each statement, exploring the issues raised.*

Note: A photocopiable handout of these statements can be found on page 188.

	Agree because ...	Disagree because ...	Not sure because ...
1 If an adult has only ever been attracted to the opposite sex, they are definitely heterosexual ('straight').			
2 If a man has had both male and female sexual partners, he must be bisexual.			
3 If a woman has had both male and female sexual partners, she must be bisexual.			
4 A girl who has a sexual experience with another girl at school is a lesbian, even if she marries a man later.			
5 A boy who has a sexual experience with another boy at school is gay, even if he marries a woman later.			
6 A married man who has sex with other men without his wife knowing is pretending to be straight, but is really gay.			
7 A woman who fantasises about sex with other women is definitely lesbian.			
8 Somebody who has been married to somebody of the opposite sex for most of their adult life *can't* be gay.			

With some statements, there may be more variation than others. As you progress through the statements and issues are discussed, some groups might begin to change their minds about earlier responses. For example, groups might respond to statements 2 and 3 by agreeing that they are 'bisexual' and then disagree with statements 4 and 5, suggesting that the people concerned were 'just experimenting'. What if the people in these four scenarios turned out to be the same people?

Sexuality is said to have three elements: feelings (of attraction, etc.); behaviour (what we actually do); and identity (who we feel/say we are). People's feelings, behaviours and identity do not always coincide – and this can even change over time.

Consider raising these questions:

● Why (or under what circumstances) might somebody be attracted to people of the same sex (feelings), but only have opposite sex relationships (behaviour)? Or why might somebody have feelings for the opposite sex but have same-sex relationships?

- Why might somebody be attracted to people of the same sex (feelings), but describe themselves as heterosexual (identity)? Or actually have sex with somebody of the same sex (behaviour) but describe themselves as heterosexual (identity)?

Factors such as these may be at work:

- Common social and cultural views.
- Possible 'internalised oppression' resulting from this – this is where people take on board others' prejudiced views of themselves.
- Sexual opportunity – or lack of it. (For example, groups often raise the issue of single-sex environments like prisons.)
- Strength of feelings.
- Level of self-esteem, how secure or confident we feel.

Sexuality is not necessarily permanently 'fixed' throughout our lifetime. Applying labels to people is not necessarily a good – or accurate – way of describing them or understanding them.

Note to teacher: *Although some young teenagers might 'experiment' with same-sex experiences (as indeed might adults), many are also clear from an early age that they are lesbian, gay or bisexual and we should not be dismissive of this. Note also that people who say young people's same-sex experiences are 'just a phase or experiment' would almost certainly not say that about young people's heterosexual experiences.*

Point out that it is only natural that we all have our own feelings about sexuality and sexual orientation. This may mean that we find it hard to understand a person whose feelings, behaviour or sexual identity are different from ours. However, whether or not we can understand another person's feelings or alter our own views, every person has the right to be treated with respect.

However, this session has not just been about sexuality and sexual orientation. Thinking back to the scenario with So Sen talking about her girlfriend and her family, it's also been about becoming an adult and being ourselves – and how we might feel about other people's expectations of us – especially our own family.

So Sen had not actually discussed anything with her family – can she know for sure how they will react?

Reflection

Thinking back to the scenario with So Sen talking about her girlfriend and her concerns about her family, could a situation like this also be possible if she'd been talking about a boyfriend?

Could similar pressures apply to most young people as they become adults? Do you think that the expectations of family and friends create pressures? Keeping your thoughts to yourself, how important is it what your family and friends think of you? Has that changed at all in the last year?

A question of opinions, a question of feelings

R9

Are any of my views and feelings about relationships and sexual issues changing as I get older?

Am I able to help others explore and discuss their views and feelings?

R22

What are my views on termination of pregnancy?

How do I respond to people whose views might be different from my own on this and other controversial issues?

How would I handle differences like this with a boyfriend or girlfriend?

To the teacher

This session is about enabling students to explore and develop their views, awareness and knowledge of a range of issues about sex and relationships and sexual health. It encourages students to facilitate other students in discussion. This will develop their facilitation skills and their openness to diverse points of view. It will also encourage them to distinguish between fact and opinion, and make informed choices between their own and others' opinions.

By its very nature, this session 'skims' a broad range of issues rather than exploring one or two in depth. This is because the process and the broad principles are almost more important than the content. If you wish to allow more time for students to facilitate discussion, you might wish to split this session into two. You could take any single topic raised here and expand it into a session in its own right.

To the students

This session is about figuring out your views and feelings on things to do with relationships, sex and sexual health. It's also about deciding when you agree with other people's opinions on these things – and when you don't. It's not always easy to decide whether we are hearing facts or just other people's opinions. It can be particularly difficult to respond to people whose views are very different from our own, and sometimes those differences can have a big impact on us – such as when we have to decide on something important that's happening to us in a relationship. Helping other people think things through is also a real skill and it can often help us to sort things out for ourselves.

'There's no way I could ask Dad about that stuff,' said Josh. Josh and Emma were discussing a Sex and Relationships lesson they had been to, and Josh's friend Joe had said that his dad had taught him ages ago how to put on a condom.

'Well, I can talk to Mum about stuff,' said Emma (thinking, 'Well, some stuff').

Hannah came in at that point and asked what they were talking about.

*'Yeah, I used to talk to Mum a bit when I was your age,' she said. 'Mind you, although she would tell me **some** stuff, she always used to say things like, "Well, you won't have to worry for a while, you're way too young, it's not even legal". It used to drive me mad … but at least she wasn't like Becky's mum and dad.'*

Hannah was remembering last year when Becky had thought she could be pregnant. She was terrified of telling her parents, they were so strict – you can't even mention sex in their house – and Becky was thinking about having a termination. Mind you, she wasn't even sure how her boyfriend, Nathan, would have reacted to that. Becky didn't think he believed in it – not that it was up to him, was it?

'Anyway,' Emma said. 'I don't think you could go and get condoms.'

'Yes, I could!' said Josh (thinking, 'She's probably right').

'Well, even if you could, you haven't got a regular girlfriend,' Emma said smugly.

'So what – you never know when you might just get lucky!' Josh answered with a grin. He had just read this really good magazine.

'Typical boy!' said Emma. 'There's no way I'd just do it with somebody I wasn't in a relationship with.'

Focusing

Obtain some initial reactions from the class.

What do you think about the things that Josh, Emma and Hannah were saying and thinking about:

- Joe and his dad
- talking to their own parents
- it not being 'legal'
- what happened with Becky and Nathan
- Josh's magazine and about relationships?

What happens if two people in a relationship have really different views about something major – such as terminating a pregnancy?

Into action

*Tell the class that they will have the responsibility for running the rest of the session themselves. They will work as a team to **plan** and then **run a short discussion** on **one** of the concerns that have just been raised.*

Divide the class into teams of four or five, and tell them that each team will be given a broad question for discussion:

1 Do parents have a role to play in teaching their children about sex and relationships? If so, what should this role be?

2 Do you think there are things that should be done to make contraception more easily available to young teenagers?

3 Some people say that the age of consent is meaningless and should be scrapped – what do you think about this?

4 Who do you think should be involved in the decision to terminate a pregnancy?

5 Do you think that the media gives responsible messages around sexual health and behaviour?

6 Do you think that sex is special and better in a committed relationship?

Before discussing their topic, ask students to decide in their groups what issues they need to think about and how they can make sure that there is a really good class discussion. They should try to involve the whole class and encourage people to form their own opinions.

- *Have the discussion topics ready in envelopes and tell the class that each envelope also contains some 'tips' for discussion – questions they could ask and perhaps ideas to look for.*
- *Ask one person from each team to pick an envelope.*
- *Once they have their topics, tell the groups that they will have a maximum of ten minutes to prepare to lead a five-minute discussion with the rest of the class.*
- *Tell them that you will circulate and help the teams.*

*Some useful **general prompts** you could give students:*

- How will you make people think/get them talking? How will you start the discussion? With the main topic question, a related question or both?
- Will team members contribute or just encourage others? Will you highlight different (opposing) points of view? For example, 'Some people are saying … but others are saying …'
- Will you note points on the board?

*Remind students that they only have **five minutes**, so they may not be able to ask every question they think of.*

Discussion tips for the teams to be included in their envelopes

(Note: Questions the team could raise for every topic are included. Some 'Ideas to look for' have been given for the first topic only. You may wish to develop similar ideas lists for other topics.)

1 Do parents have a role to play in teaching their children about sex and relationships? If so, what should this role be?

- Has the parental role become less important now that young people can get information from so many different sources?

    Ideas to look for (sources of information):
    - The internet (including a number of websites dedicated to sexual health information for young people).
    - Magazines.
    - Television.
    - School sex and relationships sessions like this one, and science.
    - School nurses.
    - Youth workers.
    - Advice centres and clinics – including specific young people's clinics.
- Or has the parental role become more important? Do other sources give young people everything they need?
- If parents do have a role, what is it? If not, why not?

2 Do you think there are things that should be done to make contraception more easily available to young teenagers?

- How difficult is it for young teenagers to access contraception? Where are the local sources?
- What could make it difficult? What could make it seem difficult?
- Do we believe that it should be made easier? If yes, why? If no, why?
- If it should be made easier, what should be done?

into action

3 **Some people say that the age of consent is meaningless and should be scrapped – what do you think about this?**
- Does everybody know what the age of consent is? Is it the same for everyone?
- Is it the correct age? If no, what do you think it should be and why?
- Why do you think we have an age of consent?
- What do you think would happen if we didn't?

4 **Who do you think should be involved in the decision to terminate a pregnancy?**
- Who actually has the say in whether a termination happens? Does the boy involved have a choice if a girl gets pregnant and wants to have a termination?
- Who do you think is most affected by a pregnancy? Why?
- Who do you think is most affected by a termination of pregnancy? Why?
- What effects would you say it has on the various people involved – girl, boy and their families?
- What do you believe are the main things that influence whether somebody has a termination or not?

5 **Do you think that the media gives responsible messages around sexual health and behaviour?**
- Do some teenage magazines give the impression that 'everyone is doing it'?
- If yes, what effect might this have on readers?
- What about the role of television, such as the soaps? What sorts of storylines do these feature? How realistic do you think they are?
- Are there any messages being given out that are responsible? For example, how much do they highlight risks and consequences?

6 **Do you think that sex is special and better in a committed relationship?**
- Should sex only be part of a committed relationship, or is it OK to just do it for fun? Is it the same for boys and girls?
- In what ways might it be better in a committed relationship? In what ways might it be not so good?
- Some people give 'being in love' as a reason to have sex. Is it a good reason?
- What does being in love mean? Can you be in love without having sex?

When the teams are facilitating their discussions, act as timekeeper and help the session stay on track, but let the students keep control. Pick up on important factual details that need adding/correcting. For example: age of consent is the same for everyone; you can access advice and contraception 'under age'; the younger the teenager, the less likely they are to use contraception in first sexual experiences; the man has no control over termination even if married to the woman, etc. Check with your school nurse or other health professional before the session if there are points you need to clarify. You can take opportunities to 'signpost' local services.

Reflection

Have any of your own views changed on the topics we've discussed since:

- you've got older
- the beginning of this session?

How easy was it to hear views that were different from your own and not to respond? What do you think you would do if you were in a relationship with somebody and they had very different feelings about something important, such as having sex, using contraception, terminating a pregnancy, etc.?

A question of 'adult' situations

> **R6**
> Do I know that I have a right to only do what I feel comfortable with?
> Do I know that I have a responsibility to protect others' rights to be safe and feel comfortable?

> **R18**
> What different pressures could be involved in my relationships as I am getting older – now or in the near future?
> How will I handle these?

To the teacher

This session aims to address some of the sex and relationships pressures that teenagers might encounter as they get older. It focuses on some of the potential 'pressure situations' older teenagers might face: changing expectations; risk and contraception use in longer-term relationships; being away from home; etc.

It is intended to help young people think through the sort of pressures that they might experience, and which may seem more complex than those they have previously encountered, and to develop strategies and skills for dealing with these pressures. Some of these pressures will arise from other people making demands that take them out of their 'comfort and safety zone' and this session also explores 'rights and responsibilities' in this respect. We know, for example, that sexual pressures for teenagers might not just be about whether they have sex or not, but also, particularly with easy access to pornographic material, might be about the kind of sex they have or think is 'the norm'. These sorts of issues need to be addressed.

Note: A photocopiable handout of the situations below can be found on page 189.

To the students

As teenagers get older, they tend to broaden their experience of relationships and life in general – they simply encounter different things. This session is about some of the situations that people might experience, the pressures that those situations might bring and how people can deal with them.

Situation 1

Sean was really starting to moan at Sara. 'Why not?' he asked looking sulky. 'We've been going out for ages now and you're on the pill – we just don't need to use condoms any more.'

'Look, Sean,' Sara said. 'After that scare we had, I would have thought you'd have given up trying to persuade me to do stuff I don't really want to do.'

*Sean looked gloomy. Sara would probably never let him live down how they started to have sex in the first place – drunk at a party when he persuaded her to do it with no condom. The school nurse had helped Sara get emergency contraception and, ever since then, they had used the pill **and** condoms. 'Double Dutch' the nurse called it.*

'Yeah,' he said. 'But I just don't get it. Why do I need to keep on using condoms if you're on the pill? It's not like we'd only just started going out.'

Situation 2

Emma and Sara were talking about their friend Jodie and her boyfriend Dan.

*'Well, I think she's really lucky,' said Sara. 'Having an older boyfriend like Dan who's not only totally gorgeous but **really** generous.'*

Dan had said that he wanted to take Jodie on holiday and, because he was working, he'd offered to pay for her.

'Hmm,' said Emma, with a doubtful expression on her face. Sara often told her that look reminded her of her mum when she was going to tell Sara she couldn't do something. 'He is really nice – but I'm still not sure she should do it.'

*'That's what Jodie said!' Sara shook her head. 'She's not sure! I think you're **both** mad – **I'd** go!'*

Situation 3

Jane is 17 and her boyfriend, Ian, is 18. They have been going out for a long time and have been having sex for some time. Jane knows Ian watches quite a bit of porn. Now he wants to try something different.

'Come on, it'll be really good,' he said.

'It could hurt,' Jane replied.

'No, it won't. I'll do it carefully,' he answered. 'Look, it'll be great – and we won't have to use a condom if we do it that way 'cos you can't get pregnant, can you?'

'Look, I know you've been watching all that stuff on the internet…' She wasn't sure what to say next.

Focusing

Prompt some immediate reactions and initial discussion by asking the class to think about the three situations they have just read. Ask students to consider whether, although they are obviously different situations, there any common features.

Look for:

- One person feeling unsure/anxious about, or uncomfortable with, what is expected of them by the other
- Feeling pressure, and perhaps also potential risks of the situations.

Into action

Divide the class into small groups and give out transcripts of the three situations.

Ask at least two groups to work on the scene where Sean is talking to Sara about not using condoms any more:

- Why do you think Sean has suggested this?
- Do you think Sean is right? If yes, why? If no, why?
- How do you think Sara might be feeling about this? What worries might she have?
- What could happen if Sean and Sara stop using condoms?

Ask another two groups to work on the scene where Emma and Sara are discussing Dan and Jodie going on holiday:

- What sort of thoughts and feelings do you think Jodie might be having?
- Do you think it is a good idea for Jodie and Dan to go on holiday together?
- What would be good about it?
- Could there be any worries or problems? What might Emma's view be? What might Jodie's view be?

Ask another two groups to work on the scene where the young man (Ian) is asking his girlfriend (Jane) to experiment sexually:

- What sort of thoughts and feelings do you think Jane might be having?
- Would it be OK to do what Ian wants?
- Is Ian right about not needing condoms?
- What do you think will happen if Jane says 'no'?

For their specific situation, ask all groups to consider the following and present back to the class:

- What are the pressures in the situation you have examined?
- What is your solution? What should happen *immediately* in the short term? Decide what the characters should say and do right now. *(If the groups wish, they can try writing a few more lines of script.)*
- Is there anything that needs to happen *in the future* to solve the situation? Decide what else, if anything, the characters should say and do.

As groups feed back ideas on how to handle their situation, ask the rest of the class whether they agree or have different ideas. Raise the broader issues. Explore how 'healthy' students think the relationships in the situations are. For example, are the couples able to trust themselves and the other person? Talk about the importance of respecting each other's sexual 'stopping points' and need for safety. Does the need for safer sex go away just because people have been going out together for a while?

Suggest that people who care about each other will want to protect each other. Suggest that when you say 'no' to something you don't want to do, you are also saying 'yes' to yourself and your own importance. Are there different standards for boys and girls as to how much respect or freedom they get in a relationship? What about in a gay relationship? Do people's expectations of relationships change as they get older?

Reflection

Think privately to yourself about whether you are experiencing different situations and perhaps different pressures in relationships as you get older. Do you know who you can speak to about any concerns if you need to?

A question of knowing your ABC

> **S5**
> Am I aware that stress can result from what we believe about a situation and that changing my thoughts about something can change my feelings?

To the teacher

This session is about helping students manage stress by using what might be described as a 'rational-emotive' approach. We create a good deal of 'destructive stress' inside us because of how we react to events and to our own thoughts. A certain situation or incident may trigger a negative reaction and cause us to feel stressed because of the beliefs we hold about the situation – the notion that 'negative thoughts create negative feelings' and vice versa. Frequently, we engage in 'mind reading' other people and/or predict unpleasant consequences based on little or no evidence – creating an unpleasant future for ourselves and living in it. We may hold irrational expectations for ourselves and others.

This session teaches a simple approach to changing those reactions and, thereby, managing stress. We are tackling stress at one or more three fundamental levels:

1 **Removing or reducing** the demand on us (for instance, the stressor).
2 **Changing our perception** of the demand.
3 **Changing belief about our ability to cope** (see Focus on stress, page 266).

Note: A photocopiable sheet of the situations below can be found on page 190.

To the students

This session is about how we often get stressed because of what we think about something that is happening and that makes us feel bad. Often, this is because we try to read other people's minds or predict the future and we can end up feeling stressed because of something we just *think* is happening or will happen. Sometimes our beliefs lead us to expect things of ourselves, or other people, that we needn't expect – and that gives us unnecessary stress.

Situation 1

Josh came in looking really miserable. He slammed his bag down on the floor and slumped into a chair.

'What's the matter with you?' Emma asked. 'You look like you've just heard the world will end at teatime!'

'Joe just walked past me and totally blanked me – ignored me completely like I wasn't there.'

Joe was Josh's best mate – they'd been friends right through school, had always played football together, played computer games together, sorted out each other's 'girlfriend problems', helped each other with homework and just generally had a good laugh and a good time hanging out together.

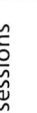
'He's obviously not talking to me – I must have done something to upset him.'

'How do you know?' asked Emma. 'Has he said anything? Do you remember anything happening? Have you spoken to him?'

Josh did not appear to have heard Emma at all. He was still mumbling stuff to himself.

'Great. Great time to lose your best mate – just before we have to play in a match together.'

Situation 2

Becky had been sitting staring at the same bit of paper for about ten minutes. 'There is just no way I'm going to get these grades,' she said miserably, for about the tenth time.

'Becky, that's just silly. You don't know that – whyever shouldn't you manage it? You're really clever and you work really hard.' Nathan, her boyfriend, was beginning to look almost as upset as she was.

'That test result I got was **so** bad, I **shouldn't ever** do badly in a test like that,' she groaned. 'I just **know** I'll get a bad grade in the A Level.'

'Becky, it's just **one** little test – and it wasn't that bad – and think of all the other stuff you've got brilliant marks for.' Nathan was doing his best.

'… and when I don't get good grades, I won't get into the place I want – and I **must** get in – it's really the only place that's any good if I want to succeed in that field of work. I'll probably end up in some dead-end job.' Becky just carried on as if Nathan hadn't said anything.

'Becky, for goodness sake, it's just one test! Anyway, what if you did have to go somewhere else? Which you probably won't of course – but it doesn't mean that you'll fail,' said Nathan.

Becky turned around and snapped at him, 'Well, **you** don't want me to go to that university anyway 'cos it's so far away!'

'Oh, I give up!' Nathan growled. 'I'm going round to see Jack and Hannah!' He slammed out of Becky's house. Becky burst into tears.

Focusing

Situation 1

- What does Josh believe? How does that make Josh feel?
- Why do you think Emma asks the questions that she does?
- Can you think of any other explanations for Joe's behaviour? How might Josh feel if any of the alternative explanations were the case, rather than the situation he's imagining?

Situation 2

- What about Becky – do you think she needs to feel as stressed as she does?
- What do you think about what Nathan said to her? Was he making sense? Why do you think he wasn't getting through to Becky?

Explain to the class that what Josh and Becky were doing is something that most of us do to some extent – mind reading and predicting the future. We get irrational/illogical beliefs about something that happens, such as:

- What other people are thinking and feeling.
- Our abilities (or lack of them).
- What we **must** do, **should** do or **must** have.

We also worry about how awful it will be if things don't work out the way they should … and this gets us really stressed. In reality, the 'musts' and 'shoulds' are not really absolute necessities – and how awful would it *really* be if they didn't happen? We also do things in our heads like 'playing things down' when we do well and blowing up what didn't go so well – just like Becky's results.

Josh and Becky had really negative thoughts, which were giving them really negative feelings and behaviour. What Emma and Nathan were trying to do was challenge how Josh and Becky were thinking, and help them to **think** differently so they could **feel** differently – and not be so stressed. In other words, **positive thoughts for positive feelings**. There's actually a good way to do this for yourself – you might call it the 'ABC' of being positive and less stressed.

Write up on the board:
Actual event (which **A**ctivates the beliefs and consequences).
Beliefs about it (possibly wild and imagined).
Consequences (feelings, behaviour).
Beliefs that we *could* have instead (**B**etter because it allows for more possibilities).
leading to …
Consequences that are more positive.

So, as an example, the **A**ctual event is that my best friend walks past me without speaking. What *could* I **B**elieve about it? He's not talking to me any more! I've done something to upset him …

Consequences: I feel miserable and stressed. Why? Because I'm mind reading. I could make it even worse and believe that I've done something to upset him, and he'll never speak to me again and I won't have a best friend…

Consequences: I feel even more miserable and stressed. OK, now I'm mind reading and predicting the future based on this. But I don't *know* what's going on in his mind. I'm creating my own stressful version of the situation in my head.

Explore and modify my beliefs: What could I **B**elieve about it instead? Maybe he didn't see me – he's got a lot on his mind – or maybe he's not wearing his contact lenses. Or … what else? Perhaps I just don't know and I need to talk to him…

Improved **C**onsequences: I feel much better and I'll probably go and talk to him.

Tell the class to try out the 'ABC' method with some of the situations below. Divide the class into groups and give each group a different situation to work on. Give students time to discuss and generate some ideas, and then get each group in turn to read out their situation and feed back what they discussed.

Note: A photocopiable handout of these situations can be found on page 191.

Situation 1 (the Becky scenario)

Actual event: Becky gets a test result that's not as good as she wanted.

Beliefs: She's a failure because she **shouldn't ever** get lower marks. It means she'll get a poor grade at A Level, she won't get the university place she wants. She **must** go there or she'll end up in a dead-end job. No other university will do. Also, Nathan doesn't really care.

Consequences: Becky's stressed and unhappy. She snaps at Nathan and they have an argument.

Situation 2

Actual event: Joe misses a penalty shot in an important match, although he usually scores lots of goals.

Beliefs: He has lost his skills, all his team will think he's a rubbish player, he'll be dropped from the team and that will be a complete disaster.

Consequences: Joe's stressed and depressed. He becomes quiet and withdrawn.

Situation 3

Actual event: Emma's friend, Sara, and her boyfriend, Sean, have been going out for ages and they usually see each other a lot. Sean tells Sara that he can't see her tonight, as he's too busy.

Beliefs: He doesn't want Sara any more and he's going to dump her.

Consequences: Sara gets scared and puts pressure on Sean and he gets cross about it. She's convinced he'll dump her now. She's stressed and miserable and goes off her food.

Situation 4

Actual event: Sean has been going out with Emma's friend Sara for ages. At lunchtime he sees Sara in the queue for food, really close to their friend Jay. Jay is smiling and Sara is looking up at him, laughing.

Beliefs: Sara **shouldn't** ever look like that at anybody but Sean. Sara looks like she fancies Jay. She's flirting with him. Jay looks like he's chatting her up and she will want to go out with him.

Consequences: Sean feels really jealous and a bit sick. He pushes into the queue next to them. When Sara says, 'Hi, Sean!' Sean glares at her.

Situation 5

Actual event: Emma has just auditioned for the next school play. She really loves acting and singing and this is a musical she's always wanted to do. She notices the director and assistant director talking and shaking their heads. They say they'll let everyone know the next day.

Beliefs: She did badly and they don't want her. She won't get a part and that would be totally awful.

Consequences: Emma feels really miserable and stressed. She wants to cry.

In each situation, ask the groups to consider how the main character could see things/interpret the event differently, and what they could believe instead that could lead to better consequences (how the people feel and/or behave).

After each group's feedback, invite discussion, more options and praise for good ideas. Comment on any creative and positive thinking.

Reflection

Keeping your thoughts to yourself, how often do you get stressed about what you *think* people are thinking, or what you *think* is happening or is going to happen? Could you try the ABC method next time you sense that is happening? Try saying to yourself, 'The *actual* situation is … Right now, I believe … As a consequence, I feel … but, instead, I **could** believe … (see it differently). **Now** I feel …'

---

* This session is adapted from 'Stop Stressing' and various stress training materials by Alan Van Loen, Aware Consultancy.

A question of feeling ready to become a parent

P3

How will I know I am ready to become a parent?
Are there experiences I want to have first?
Are there things (for example, knowledge, skills, attitudes of mind) I would need to bring a child up safely and healthily that I don't yet have?
How can I make sure I have these when I need them?

P9

Do I understand that biologically ideal times and socially ideal times can be different?
Do I understand the risks of having children very early in life and the risks of leaving it too late to try to become a parent?
Do I know that the biological risks are different for men and women?

To the teacher

There is an old saying that you are probably never completely ready to become a parent. Perhaps the only people who are fully trained are those whose kids have grown up and left home. Simply working out the financial implications might give many of us pause for thought.

This session recognises that the decision to have a planned child with someone is not always a rational or logical decision. The decision to have a child with another human being is almost certainly more connected with our feelings towards them, rather than our respective bank accounts. We need to ensure balance. The biology of conception is not an 'equal opportunities' issue and we need to explore the issues for both males and females.

Becoming a parent when you are young has both advantages and disadvantages, especially for women. However, leaving the decision to become a parent until later in life (perhaps after developing a successful career) can also bring difficulties, especially with conceiving. What is the ideal time to have a baby? Biologically, it is between 20 and 35. Young people may believe fertility treatment is available and will always work, but this is currently far from the truth. It can help, and techniques are constantly improving, but it is still frequently unsuccessful. At the time of writing, the average age of becoming a mother for the first time is around 27 years.

Some people make a deliberate choice to have a child when they are very young. This decision can be made for a variety of reasons but, without a network of consistent support, it can be a tough challenge.

It is important to give students an opportunity to explore whether finding someone sexually attractive, and perhaps having a sexual relationship with them, is the same as wanting to have a child with them. For some people it will be, for others it won't. The first few months of any new relationship may be emotionally and physically very intense. Although portrayed as romantic, it is actually hormonal and can often wear off: 'What did I ever see in him/her?'
In addition, our capacity to judge a partner's suitability as a lifelong companion, or prospective fellow parent, can be impeded at this time.

Relationships are complex. This session focuses on different-sex couples. The same questions, however, are equally appropriate to same-sex couples or individuals who plan to become parents. This resource takes the position that 'every child should be a wanted child', which is not quite the same thing as a 'planned child'. Many pregnancies are not planned. Some come as a wonderful and welcome surprise; others don't and may take a person's life in an unexpected and unwelcome direction. The purpose of this session is, therefore, simply to offer students an opportunity to reflect on what would need to be true for them before they felt ready to become a parent.

This session has two separate themes: the first focuses on the student's own wants, needs, ambitions and aspirations and the impact being a parent might have on those; the second focuses on what students feel they will need to have in place – both externally, for example home, a stable income, support, etc., and internally in the form of the knowledge and skills necessary for a child to thrive. This session offers an opportunity to explore both personal and economic wellbeing.

This is a sensitive subject as students may themselves have experienced a range of parenting.

To the students

Deciding to become a parent is probably one of the biggest decisions you can make. The purpose of this session is to give you a chance to think about when it might be right for you to become a parent. You need to consider two things:

1 What would be the consequences for you if you had a child?
2 What knowledge and skills would you need to be a really good parent?

Situation 1

'I can't wait to be a mum!' Sara said. A young woman had just walked by carrying a baby.

'Yeah, it would be great one day,' Emma replied. Sara always went a bit soppy around small children.

'Don't you want one of your own? They are so adorable!' Sara said in that squeaky voice she used at times like this.

'Well, yes, some are … Of course, they also cry a lot, especially at night, need feeding, changing, dribble and want constant attention,' Emma replied.

'I know, it's great!' said Sara.

'What do you mean, you know? The last time you babysat for someone you'd only been there ten minutes when you phoned me in a complete panic because the baby wouldn't stop crying!' exclaimed Emma.

'Mine wouldn't be like that! Mine would be perfect – like his or her mummy!' said Sara.

'If your child is just like you, you are in so much trouble! Anyway, there's loads I want to do before I have children. Think of all the things you would have to give up or miss out on. Not to mention how much a baby costs! Anyway, the other thing is … you need a bloke to be the dad!' Emma said.

Sara had not had a serious boyfriend since breaking up with Sean last year, and it was amazing how quickly he had gone from being her 'lifelong, one-and-only, irreplaceable soul mate' to 'totally dumped', when Sara had found out he was also seeing two other girls!

'I know, but Paul and me ...' Sara stopped herself.

'PAUL!' Emma shrieked.

'What?????' Sara replied.

'One, Paul is a really sweet guy, but spending a major chunk of your life with him??? Two, his idea of an ambitious career is working on the burger stand on the market. Three, he missed your last date because he thought Monday was Tuesday so nought out of ten for reliability and, four, that was going to be the second time you went out together, which makes one actual date in total to see, if I remember rightly "Return of the Star Pirates of Mars"! Just think, your baby could be a "mini Paul"!'

'All right all right ... he's not that bad. He wants to take me to "The Blob 2" on Friday,' Sara replied.

'Oh, how romantic! Besides, there are loads of things I want to do before I have kids.'

'Oh, let me guess, go to university, have a big house, a job with loads of money and a trip round the world!' Sara said.

'No ... well ... yes, I do want to do some more studying, get a job I really enjoy and I would like to travel a bit. But what I want is to be able to go shopping when I want, go clubbing in the evening if I like, spend the money I earn on me, go away when and where I want and generally have some fun for me, at least for a while,' Emma replied. 'Not only that, if I had a child with someone they would have to be very, very special and I'd want to be sure they would be around all the time to support me. It must be really hard to raise a child on your own.'

I wonder if boys ever think like this, Emma wondered to herself.

Situation 2
'I overheard Emma talking about having kids with Sara,' Josh said to Joe, as they watched television.

'Not sure that's biologically possible and, if it was, not sure it would be a good idea,' Joe replied, without taking his eyes off the screen.

'Idiot!' said Josh, hitting him with a cushion. 'Do you ever think about having kids?'

'Er ... nope,' Joe replied.

'Me neither,' said Josh.

Odd, Josh thought to himself. I think about sex all the time, but never actually about having kids. Most of the time I think about how to have sex without having kids! Of course, actually having a girlfriend might help ... Still, one day I guess kids could be nice, but definitely not yet. I wonder if it is different for girls, Josh wondered.

Focusing

● What do you think about being a parent in the future? Do you think anything at all about it?

- Think about the dialogue in Situation 1 above. Do you think many young people really think like Sara?
- Do you think young men and women feel differently about having children?
- What might encourage someone to make the decision to have a baby when they are still young? (Having 'someone to love'; fear of being 'left on the shelf'; to make someone else happy; to get out of the children's home and prove they are grown up.)

Into action

In pairs or groups, ask students to discuss the following:

- Think about your current lifestyle and all the things you do and enjoy. Write these activities on to sticky notes. Now, imagine you suddenly were the parent of a young child. What would you still be able to do? What would you only be able to do sometimes? What might you have to give up, perhaps completely? Reorganise your sticky notes under these headings, or remove them altogether. Why might you have to give up some activities?

Look for:

- Lack of money
- Demanding baby to look after
- Need for short- or long-term child care
- Being simply too tired.
- What are all the things that you imagine you might like to do over the next few years? What experiences would you like to have or enjoy? Think about education, employment, leisure, hobbies and interests, fun, etc. How might these be affected by having a young child?
- What qualities would a person need to have before you would consider having a child with them? Is being physically attracted to them enough? What else would you want?

Having separate boy and girl group discussions and then comparing the lists of qualities can be interesting and illustrate real differences between the sexes. Young women's expectations are often far more practical than young men's, and often represent very different priorities for a long, close relationship. Why is this? Is it partly because young women are often more mature than young men in Year 11, or is it because of a genuine difference between the genders? Perhaps both? An extension can be to rank their chosen qualities in order of importance before comparison.

- Do you think people make the choice to have children with someone this logically? What else might influence their choice – is this OK? Is this a time when we should always follow or question our feelings? How easy is this?
- Either:
  - What do you think you would need to have in place before you would consider having a child with someone?

  Or:
  - What would parents need to provide for a baby to ensure that he or she grows up healthy and develops well?

Think about three lists: physical things (safe comfortable home, money); the type of relationship that you would want to be in; and the skills that you and your partner would have.

Reflection

Imagine that someone of your age said they were considering having a baby. Out of everything we have talked about in this session, what three things would you encourage them to consider? Why would you choose these three over any others?

Extension: a question of balancing children and career

This session could be enriched with visitors such as personnel officers from local businesses explaining maternity policies, or parents who have to juggle a career with raising a family. Invite them to talk about how they made their decisions and the implications of their choices.

To the students

Although we would encourage any young person to think carefully before deciding to have a child, it is also important to recognise that it is possible for a woman to leave it until it is too late biologically to easily conceive. Nature has not made this an equal issue. A man can biologically continue to father children until very late in life, but for a woman it can become increasingly difficult to have children past 35 years, and for some women sooner. This can present difficult choices, especially if a woman (or her partner) has a career where further advancement might be affected by a break to have and bring up children. Child care is available, but it can be very expensive and, of course, there is no reason why the father should not take a career break to help raise their children. No one can tell you when it is the right time to have children, although we might strongly suggest a stable relationship, comfortable home and steady income would all be very good ideas.

'I always thought Uncle John and Aunt Mai would have been great parents.' Josh and Hannah were helping their stepfather, Ray, clear up after dinner.

'Well,' Ray replied. 'They always intended to have kids, but sort of never seemed to get round to it. John had his business to develop and Mai had her career to think about. It just never seemed the right time. When they did finally try for a baby, I guess it was a bit too late. I know they tried to get some medical help, but it didn't work out.'

'Weren't they upset?' Hannah asked.

'Well, they both were really disappointed when the doctors couldn't help, so I guess the answer is yes,' replied Ray.

'It must be difficult. I know John was working really hard to keep the business going and Mai was really successful, and I guess taking time out could have been a problem. It must be easy to keep putting it off ...' Hannah said.

'Well, some people don't want kids,' Josh said. Actually the thought of being a dad was really weird. He guessed it might happen one day.

'Well, yes,' Ray replied. 'But I suppose there is a difference between deciding that you don't want kids, and sort of expecting to have them one day and suddenly finding that you can't, and probably never will.'

Focusing

- How do you think Mai and John felt when they discovered they could not have their own children?
- How might you feel if you discovered the same issue (for any reason)? What options are available to you?

Into action – if you have visitors

If you have a parent visitor, invite them to talk about how they made their decisions.

If you're a mother who is an employee, you have the statutory right to a minimum amount of maternity leave. An employer may also offer their own maternity leave scheme. If you're a dad who is an employee, you may be eligible for paternity leave when your child is born or when you adopt a child. Maternity and paternity leave aren't the same as parental leave, which is unpaid leave that working parents can take to look after children under the age of five. If you have a visitor from business, invite them to talk about how their company supports employees wanting to start or extend a family. Ask about how these arrangements affect pay and pensions.

Into action – if you don't have visitors

Working in pairs, produce a short dialogue, which you could 'play' to the rest of the class, or for another pair of students. One of you chooses to be either Sara or Joe, and the other chooses to be either Sheila (mother to Hannah, Jack, Josh and Emma) or Ray (their stepfather). Use the dialogue to explore how these parents came to have children when they did. Would they do things differently if they could have their time over again? Remember, Ray and Sheila have a son, Leigh, in infant school, and the father of Sheila's bigger children is Phil, from whom Sheila is now divorced.

Explore the issues raised in these dialogues. Getting several pairs to 'play' their dialogues simultaneously, each to just one other pair of students, can increase activity and reduce stage fright. Audiences and players can then swap roles.

As they watch, ask audiences to think about the following:

- What do you think were the critical issues that led to a decision?
- If a character had asked your opinion, what would you have said/advised?
- Would these be important considerations for you? If not, what would be important? What advice might any of the characters have for you?

Ask players and audiences to feed back to the class what they have learned from this activity and from the thinking, actions (and any regrets) of these characters.

Reflection

How important is it for you to think *now* about children? Perhaps it's not high on your list at the moment. So when *may* it become important – when you leave school, when you think you've met the 'right' person, when you start to make long-term plans for yourself? Ask yourself how useful it might be to file away what you've covered in today's session until you need it.

How do you think you will feel about having children in two years' time? How do you think you will feel about having children in five years' time?

Reflect on how important it may be to have a plan to help ensure you don't have children earlier than you mean to, nor leave it too late.

Recall some of the things you said you'd like to do, to have, or to be in place before you'd feel ready to have children.

A question of moving on ...

M6
Do I like myself?
Do I like who I am becoming?
Would I choose myself as my own best friend?
Am I proud of me?
Would I swap places with myself?
How do I hope people think of me?
How do I hope they will remember me?

M7
Is there anything about me I want to leave behind when I move on?
Are there changes I want to make in me, things I want to do differently, especially if I am moving on to a new place with new people?

To the teacher

While young people will continue to learn beyond the age of 16, this is a time of transition. This session offers an opportunity to reflect on the past five years. At any period of transition there are opportunities for us to change. Some parts of us we may feel really good about and want to take forward, some parts of us we might want to leave behind, some memories we might want to treasure and some we might sooner forget. It is important to give people a chance to reflect, take stock and make any choices they want. You might want to use Invitation 1: Looking back/Looking forward on page **204**. If you want to carry out a validation exercise (see reflection on page **184**), you will need the appropriate material.

It is assumed that this is the final session in the programme.

To the students

The last five years at secondary school are almost over and it's time to move on. This session will allow you time to just reflect on what has been good about the last five years, and what's been not so good. It is a chance to think about anything you will miss, the qualities and strengths you have built up, and perhaps anything you want to change about yourself next year.

'So, that's it then,' Josh said. They were walking home at the end of their last day.

'Hardly, we get a long summer break, with the exam results in the middle to give us something to worry about, then its back to it!' Emma replied. 'But it feels different this time, like something will change next year.'

'Well, it will. It is more school but it isn't ... sort of ...' Josh said. He and Emma had decided to stay on in the sixth form.

'Well, there will still be classes and exams, so nothing new there then but, you're right, it will be more different for us,' Joe replied. He and Sara were going to the local college.

'You know, it will be good to start somewhere new where lots of people won't know me, but it's odd, I think I actually might miss this place ... er ... just a bit ...' Sara said, slightly embarrassed that she had almost admitted that she would miss their school.

Whilst college sounded good and Sara was certain it was right for her, it didn't stop her feeling a bit odd. A mixture of excitement and nerves. At least she wasn't going on her own, but she was sad Emma wasn't going with her ...

'Well, we are staying on so everyone will know us. I sort of envy you going somewhere new,

but I still like it here,' Emma replied. It would be odd not having Sara around. Sometimes Sara could be a complete nightmare, but they had always been there for one another. She had almost been tempted to go with her, but she knew the sixth form was right for her.

'I still can't believe it is five years since we first came here!' Josh said, looking back at the school.

'Remember our first day ...?' Emma asked.

Focusing

Can you remember your first day in your school? Does it feel like it was five years ago? Can you remember how you felt to be somewhere new?

Looking back, what have been the real high points of the last five years – what do you remember that you really enjoyed?

Collect feedback from the class – what do students have in common?

Into action

When you go on to somewhere new or something different, there is a chance to stop and have a think. In pairs or small groups, think back over the last five years. Only share feelings and thoughts you are comfortable with, feel free to keep any thoughts private. You might find these questions useful to start your thinking:

- How have you changed physically? What have you become good at? What do you feel that perhaps you didn't before? How have your friendships or relationships changed?
- What do you like about being you now?
- What are you proud of?
- If you could, would you be your own best friend?
- If you were your own best friend, how would you describe yourself? What do you like about yourself? What, if anything, would you change or would you do differently?
- If you are moving on to somewhere new, how do you think people staying at the school will remember you? Is this how you want to be remembered?
- If you are moving on, what, if anything, will you miss? Who will you miss?

Looking forward to the next couple of years:

- What are you looking forward to?
- If you are moving on to somewhere new, how do you feel? Is it similar/different to how you felt when you started here?
- What do you hope the next few years will be like?
- What opportunities do you hope for or expect?
- Are there any challenges, things you need to be ready to manage?
- What strengths are you taking with you?
- Do you want to be the same person next year, or are there characteristics you think you might need to leave behind?
- Are there parts of you that you would like to change? Is now a good time to make these changes?

Reflection

To the teacher

There are powerful ways of ending the formal meetings of any group. Even with promises to keep in touch, many groups have a natural life and gradually break up, but the feelings at the 'parting point' are often very strong, and need to be recognised and valued. Some relationships lose none of their strength and last a lifetime; others gradually move apart, leaving behind a small mutual connection that can be suddenly re-energised when students meet again, perhaps in many years' time.

Ending 'rituals' can offer a conclusion to the formal meetings of a group. A powerful way to end a final session is though a 'validation' activity. Be aware that these are very powerful and you need to feel confident your group will respond supportively to one another.

It is worth establishing a ground rule that only honest and supportive comments are appropriate in this session, though it is very unusual for negative comments to be written by students who have been members of a strong PSHE group.

A validation provides each member of the group an opportunity to send a message to every other member, perhaps thanking them for working with them and telling them something they have really valued about working with them. You could offer a sentence opening, for example:

'Something I have really valued about you is …'
'I have really enjoyed working with you because …'

These can be collected up in a variety of ways. One is to attach a sheet of flip-chart paper to everyone's back with masking tape, a little like a cloak. Give everyone a pack of sticky notes (fun shapes are good). The group then circulates, writing and putting at least one comment on everyone else's back. This keeps an element of anonymity if people wish it. Another variation is to provide each student with a small notebook with their name on it and circulate it. At the end, each student should leave the session with approximately 30 positive comments about themselves.

Remember that you are part of the group, so add your contributions. Many students want the opportunity to share their thanks and have the chance to validate you.

To the students

This may be the last of these sessions, and the group may not meet again in this form. What are you feeling? What are others feeling about themselves, about the class, about you? The final activity invites you to reflect and offer positive feedback to your class colleagues. Your teacher will show you how this 'validation' activity works.

There are two rules: what you offer to each person must be *honest* and it must be *supportive*. This is not a time to challenge each other. The aim is for you to take away honest, personal reflections from your class colleagues, and for them to do the same.

Good luck in your future lives!

Part 3

3.1 Session support worksheets

These sheets are grouped together to make them easy to find, and to emphasise that some are generic and may be used in more than one session.

Worksheet	Supports	Session	Year
A Page 187	S1, S2, S4	A question of coping with stress on page 115.	10
B Page 188	R8, R17	A question of being yourself, and becoming an adult on page 161.	11
C Page 189	R6, R18	A question of 'adult' situations on page 169.	11
D Page 190–192	S5	A question of knowing your ABC on page 172.	11

'Can I learn from others?' (page 193) is a generic activity. It could be used whenever it seems to make sense for your students to try to discover the experience, perspective, learning (and mistakes) of an older person, and to learn from them. It is placed here because, unlike the sheets in the Invitations section, it is not a worksheet in itself. However, because of its occasional, possibly widespread application, it's an activity to have up your sleeve, so to speak.

Worksheet A

Script for Year 10 session: A question of coping with stress (S1, S2 and S4) on page 115.

Narrator: Josh was sitting struggling with his maths revision, scratching his head, wishing he was playing football and wondering whether it was time to take a break for a small snack (which would only be his third since he got home). His concentration (which wasn't that great anyway) was suddenly broken by a crash in the kitchen, followed by swearing, followed by the unmistakable sound of his sister, Emma, crying. Josh was in the kitchen faster than a penalty shot.

Emma was sitting on the kitchen floor sobbing, surrounded by a broken mug and a pool of coffee. She was attempting to pick up sticky wet pieces of mug. Josh breathed a sigh of relief.

Josh: I thought you'd really hurt yourself.

Narrator: Josh stopped and looked at her with a puzzled expression.

Josh: Whatever's the matter, Emma? It's only a mug and a drop of coffee. Why are you crying? Is it, you know, that time of the month?

Narrator: Josh thought his last question was quite helpful. Emma's expression suddenly made maths seem like a really good option.

Emma: (*Shouting at him*) No, it's not! Why do boys always think girls aren't allowed just to be really upset and angry – just because they are!!

Narrator: Then she started crying again.

Emma: (*Tearfully*) I thought twins were supposed to understand each other.

Narrator: Josh thought it would be a good idea not to say anything else; he just put his arm round his sister. After a moment or two Emma spoke again.

Emma: Oh, I'm sorry, Josh. I've had such a rotten day. I was late for the bus, I forgot to take my books for the library and now they're overdue, Miss Beale was in a funny mood and I had a row with Sara about our project. Now we'll probably make a mess of that … I just want to run away … the coffee was just the final disaster!

Narrator: Josh didn't think any of it sounded like a disaster to him, but wisely didn't say so.

Josh: It's OK, Emma. You take a deep breath and sit down. I'll do this, and then we can think about the other stuff together …

Narrator: He bent down and starting picking up bits of broken mug.

Josh was still feeling puzzled, though. His sister usually coped with much bigger stuff – she seemed to thrive under pressure. Like when she helped organise the school play **and** acted in it – there was so much involved and a deadline to meet **and** being on stage. It would have got **him** stressing like mad, but she was just buzzing.

Worksheet B

Handout for Year 11 session: A question of being yourself, a question of becoming an adult (R8 and 17) on page 161.

	Agree because ...	Disagree because ...	Not sure because ...
1 If an adult has only ever been attracted to the opposite sex, they are definitely heterosexual ('straight').			
2 If a man has had both male and female sexual partners, he must be bisexual.			
3 If a woman has had both male and female sexual partners, she must be bisexual.			
4 A girl who has a sexual experience with another girl at school is a lesbian, even if she marries a man later.			
5 A boy who has a sexual experience with another boy at school is gay, even if he marries a woman later.			
6 A married man who has sex with other men without his wife knowing is pretending to be straight, but is really gay.			
7 A woman who fantasises about sex with other women is definitely lesbian.			
8 Somebody who has been married to somebody of the opposite sex for most of their adult life *can't* be gay.			

Worksheet C

Handout for Year 11 session: A question of 'adult' situations (R6 and R18) on page 169.

Situation 1

Sean was really starting to moan at Sara. 'Why not?' he asked looking sulky. 'We've been going out for ages now and you're on the pill – we just don't need to use condoms any more.'

'Look, Sean,' Sara said. 'After that scare we had, I would have thought you'd have given up trying to persuade me to do stuff I don't really want to do.'

*Sean looked gloomy. Sara would probably never let him live down how they started to have sex in the first place – drunk at a party when he persuaded her to do it with no condom. The school nurse had helped Sara get emergency contraception and, ever since then, they had used the pill **and** condoms. 'Double Dutch' the nurse called it.*

'Yeah,' he said. 'But I just don't get it. Why do I need to keep on using condoms if you're on the pill? It's not like we'd only just started going out.'

Situation 2

Emma and Sara were talking about their friend Jodie and her boyfriend Dan.

*'Well, I think she's really lucky,' said Sara. 'Having an older boyfriend like Dan who's not only totally gorgeous but **really** generous.'*

Dan had said that he wanted to take Jodie on holiday and, because he was working, he'd offered to pay for her.

'Hmm,' said Emma, with a doubtful expression on her face. Sara often told her that look reminded her of her mum when she was going to tell Sara she couldn't do something. 'He is really nice – but I'm still not sure she should do it.'

*'That's what Jodie said!' Sara shook her head. 'She's not sure! I think you're **both** mad – **I'd** go!'*

Situation 3

Jane is 17 and her boyfriend, Ian, is 18. They have been going out for a long time and have been having sex for some time. Jane knows Ian watches quite a bit of porn. Now he wants to try something different.

'Come on, it'll be really good,' he said.

'It could hurt,' Jane replied.

'No, it won't. I'll do it carefully,' he answered. 'Look, it'll be great – and we won't have to use a condom if we do it that way 'cos you can't get pregnant, can you?'

'Look, I know you've been watching all that stuff on the internet …'She wasn't sure what to say next.

Worksheet D

Script for Year 11 session: A question of knowing your ABC! (S5) on page 172.

Situation 1

Narrator:	Josh came in looking really miserable. He slammed his bag down on the floor and slumped into a chair. Emma looked at him.
Emma:	What's the matter with you? You look like you've just heard the world will end at teatime!
Josh:	Joe just walked past me and totally blanked me – ignored me completely like I wasn't there.
Narrator:	Joe was Josh's best mate – they'd been friends right through school, had always played football together, played computer games together, sorted out each other's 'girlfriend problems', helped each other with homework and just generally had a good laugh and a good time hanging out together.
Josh:	He's obviously not talking to me – I must have done something to upset him.
Emma:	How do you know? Has he said anything? Do you remember anything happening? Have you spoken to him?
Narrator:	Josh did not appear to have heard Emma at all. He was still mumbling stuff to himself.
Josh:	Great. Great time to lose your best mate – just before we have to play in a match together.

Situation 2

Narrator:	Becky had been sitting staring at the same bit of paper for about ten minutes.
Becky:	(Miserably) There is just no way I'm going to get these grades.
Narrator:	This was about the tenth time she'd said this. Nathan, her boyfriend, was beginning to look almost as upset as she was.
Nathan:	Becky, that's just silly, you don't know that. Whyever shouldn't you manage it? You're really clever and you work really hard.
Becky:	(Groaning) That test result I got was **so** bad, I **shouldn't ever** do badly in a test like that. I just **know** I'll get a bad grade in the A Level.
Nathan:	Becky, it's just **one** little test – and it wasn't that bad – and think of all the other stuff you've got brilliant marks for.
Narrator:	Nathan was doing his best.
Becky:	… and when I don't get good grades, I won't get into the place I want – and I **must** get in – it's really the only place that's any good if I want to succeed in that field of work. I'll probably end up in some dead-end job.
Narrator:	Becky just carried on as if Nathan hadn't said anything.
Nathan:	Becky, for goodness sake, it's just one test! Anyway, what if you did have to go somewhere else? Which you probably won't of course – but it doesn't mean that you'll fail.
Narrator:	Becky turned around and snapped at him.
Becky:	Well, **you** don't want me to go to that university anyway 'cos it's so far away!
Nathan:	(Angrily) Oh, I give up! I'm going round to see Jack and Hannah!
Narrator:	He slammed out of Becky's house. Becky burst into tears.

Handout for Year 11 session: A question of knowing your ABC (S5) page 172.

Situation 1 (the Becky scenario)

Actual event: Becky gets a test result that's not as good as she wanted.

Beliefs: She's a failure because she **shouldn't ever** get lower marks. It means she'll get a poor grade at A Level, she won't get the university place she wants. She **must** go there or she'll end up in a dead-end job. No other university will do. Also, Nathan doesn't really care.

Consequences: Becky's stressed and unhappy. She snaps at Nathan and they have an argument.

- How could Becky see things/interpret the event differently? What could she **B**elieve instead that could lead to better **C**onsequences for her (how she feels and/or behaves)?

Situation 2

Actual event: Joe misses a penalty shot in an important match, although he usually scores lots of goals.

Beliefs: He has lost his skills, all his team will think he's a rubbish player, he'll be dropped from the team and that will be a complete disaster.

Consequences: Joe's stressed and depressed. He becomes quiet and withdrawn.

- How could Joe see things/interpret the event differently? What could he **B**elieve instead that could lead to better **C**onsequences for him (how he feels and/or behaves)?

Situation 3

Actual event: Emma's friend, Sara, and her boyfriend, Sean, have been going out for ages and they usually see each other a lot. Sean tells Sara that he can't see her tonight, as he's too busy.

Beliefs: He doesn't want Sara any more and he's going to dump her.

Consequences: Sara gets scared and puts pressure on Sean and he gets cross about it. She's convinced he'll dump her now. She's stressed and miserable and goes off her food.

- How could Sara see things/interpret the event differently? What could she **B**elieve instead that could lead to better **C**onsequences for her (how she feels and/or behaves)?

Situation 4

Actual event: Sean has been going out with Emma's friend Sara for ages. At lunchtime he sees Sara in the queue for food, really close to their friend Jay. Jay is smiling and Sara is looking up at him, laughing.

Beliefs: Sara **shouldn't** ever look like that at anybody but Sean. Sara looks like she fancies Jay. She's flirting with him. Jay looks like he's chatting her up and she will want to go out with him.

Consequences: Sean feels really jealous and a bit sick. He pushes into the queue next to them. When Sara says, 'Hi, Sean!' Sean glares at her.

● How could Sean see things/interpret the event differently? What could he **B**elieve instead that could lead to better **C**onsequences for him (how he feels and/or behaves)?

Situation 5

Actual event: Emma has just auditioned for the next school play. She really loves acting and singing and this is a musical she's always wanted to do. She notices the director and assistant director talking and shaking their heads. They say they'll let everyone know the next day.

Beliefs: She did badly and they don't want her. She won't get a part and that would be totally awful.

Consequences: Emma feels really miserable and stressed. She wants to cry.

● How could Emma see things/interpret the event differently? What could she **B**elieve instead that could lead to better **C**onsequences for her (how she feels and/or behaves)?

'Can I learn from others?'

This activity can be used to help young people learn from others, particularly those who are older. It is designed to encourage students to open a dialogue with parents and carers to enable them to learn from their parents' mistakes. The older person may be able to pass on learning that they found useful later on in life, but perhaps hadn't learned quite early enough.

You and your students will need to judge when it is appropriate to use this activity.

Its principal use may well be to encourage a parent–offspring dialogue, where the sharing of values, feelings, ideas and experiences may be of worth by itself. But it may also provide reassurance to know that the issues with which today's young people tussle may not be new at all, and talking to someone who has faced them before can be supportive. Besides, it may not occur to many 14 or 15 year olds that there could possibly be anything useful to learn from their parents or carers, and the reverse may be true in reality!

Situation 1

Josh stamped into the sitting room, slamming the door behind him and flopped noisily down on to the sofa, chin in his hands.

'You OK?' asked his mum. 'I've seen happier people waiting in the rain for a late bus!'

'Just great!' said Josh. 'I shouldna said what I said. And now I wish I hadn't!'

'If I'd had a pound every time I thought that at your age, I'd be a rich woman!'

'I'd pay quite a bit for the chance to unsay what I said, but I can't …'

'That's the thing with mistakes – you can't learn from them if you don't make them. Maybe the only way is to open your mouth and put your foot in it another couple of dozen times, and see what you can learn from that …'

*'OK, come on then, how do **you** manage to avoid making a prize twit of yourself? What do you know that I don't?'*

Situation 2

Emma didn't know what to do, and it was making her feel sick.

'You're a bundle of laughs today. What's up with you?' Ray asked. Emma had a lot of respect for Ray. When he offered help, it was usually worth listening to.

*'I feel terrible. It's like I'm between a rock and a hard place. Doesn't matter what I decide to do, I'm gonna upset **someone**. Why don't adults ever have those kinds of problems?'*

Ray laughed, 'Oh, we do, we do! But there's often more than one way to look at this kind of situation. What I've learned is …'

'These adults – they know NOTHING!!'

The activity itself can be used in several kinds of situation:

- It might be useful to take into the workplace on work experience, to help focus on what a 'new recruit' needs to know (perhaps to stay safe) while on their placement.

- It may follow on from a class session, when an issue is aired and explored without leading to a single, clear resolution.
- Maybe it's an insoluble dilemma. Perhaps every instance when the issue in question arises will call for individual judgement according to the circumstances; or maybe there's room for more than one point of view.

Is this a problem/issue/choice/situation/dilemma that adults you know have faced before you? What did *they* do? What did *they* learn? What do they *wish* they'd done? Uncle? Mum? Carer? Youth worker? Health visitor? The activity can be used to find out if there are lessons you could learn from the adults around you, without having to wait until faced with an issue, and possibly taking a regrettable route.

When approaching a chosen adult, the young person may start with the cynical feeling that, generally, adults know nothing worth knowing. The idea that adults are so distant from today's young people that (effectively) they 'know nothing' is one that can be tested. The following, therefore, are the sorts of questions a young person may have in mind when they open the dialogue, though they probably won't pose them in quite this way:

- Do you have a regret about something that happened when you were roughly my age – *something you did* that you might have avoided; *something you didn't do* that you wish you had?
- Can you tell me *something that you know now that you wish you had known when you were my age* that might help me avoid doing something I might later look back and regret?

The same approach can also be employed as a means to raise students' self-esteem. Invite younger pupils in the school, perhaps 12 year olds, to gently interrogate 14 or 15 year old students for advice, tips or any regrets they are prepared to share. This can feel good to a senior student who looks back at the younger age and vicariously recalls what it was like then, and how far he or she has come. Some students will enjoy giving advice.

3.2 Invitations

The invitations in this section aim to enable students to respond to virtually any issue you choose to explore. They are looser and more open to interpretation than a worksheet, which tends to be tightly focused. The invitations can be used to explore deep feelings about sensitive issues.

In our diverse society, it is important that the illustrations are appropriate to every culture and social context. The style of illustration has therefore been made as simple as possible, to help teachers working in the widest range of schools. Ideally, students should be able to relate to or 'step into' the position of any character in an illustration. You might prefer to produce your own sheets so that they are completely relevant to your students, using really simple 'stick figures' with 'speech' and 'think' bubbles.

The light structure of these invitations allows students to go where they feel they need to go. This makes them potentially very powerful tools for exploring social and emotional issues. Before using any of them, think in advance about the type of responses your group might give you and prepare accordingly. It is also worth reinforcing your ground rules before using them.

You could use the invitations in a variety of ways:

- as an individual activity for personal reflection, either to remain personal or subsequently to share with a group
- as a group activity
- as a piece of research to help you uncover the concepts and strategies that students already have, in order to refine your planning
- As an evaluation activity to explore what language, understanding and strategies students have after the completion of a session or module of work.

Some invitations are simply situations that people can explore as observers. They invite students to consider what the characters could be feeling and saying. Many have been drawn with enough space for a student to put themselves in the picture, but in a safe place. What might they be thinking, feeling and, if asked, saying?

You may want to repeat the same activity at the start and end of a module in order to enable students to see how far they have come in their understanding.

Using the invitations as research for planning

If you are intending to use an invitation as a piece of classroom research, it is important to do so with the rigour and ethics of any good classroom action research.

- Research must be inclusive. If any child is a poor reader or has poor writing skills, ensure that they have enough help to make a full response, and if necessary, provide a 'scribe'.
- Ensure that everyone knows what you are doing, how you intend to use their responses, and that they can 'opt out' if they wish.
- Ensure that, although it is not a test, you use 'test conditions' so that you get everyone's individual thoughts and not a re-telling of their friends'.
- Ensure that the students know that there are no right or wrong answers; everyone's answers are valuable.

Ideas for using the invitations

The following ideas are just a few suggestions for using the invitations; their use is really only limited by your imagination. Some invitations have been included without suggestions for their use. These are offered to support you in exploring a wide variety of possible issues.

Note: All the invitation sheets are photocopiable.

Invitation 1: Looking back/Looking forward

Based on the Roman god, Janus, who could see the future and the past, this activity offers students a chance to reflect on how they have changed or what they have learned, and to think about their future and how they feel about it. It is particularly useful for transitions, for example when moving towards work experience, final exams, sixth form, college and life beyond school. Prompts might include the following:

Looking back:

- How have I changed physically?
- How have my interests changed?
- What have I discovered I am really good at?
- How have my friendships changed?
- What have I really enjoyed?
- What am I going to miss?

Looking forward:

- What am I really looking forward to?
- What do I want to try out?
- What am I going to really work on?
- How do I think I'll cope?
- What am I a little nervous about?
- What am I really nervous about?

If the transition or forward look doesn't involve leaving school, consider collecting up the completed invitations to put away for a time. Then invite participants to revisit and reflect on their invitation after the change has occurred.

A variation is to use it as a before-and-after exercise when considering a new topic. On the left-hand side of the invitation simply state: 'Today is [date] and I think … and know …', and on the right-hand side of the page state: 'Today is [date] and I think … and know …' Invite students to record their first thoughts about a topic on the left-hand side and put the form in an envelope with their name on it; ask them to seal it and collect them in. Return them at the end of the topic and ask students to complete the right-hand side. Ask them what has changed in their thinking, what new knowledge do they have?

The following prompts can be used after an experience such as a mock examination:

Looking back:

- I did too much …
- I did too little …
- I tried hard to …
- I worked …
- I wish I had …
- I'm glad I did …

Looking forward:

- Next time I will do more …
- Next time I will change …
- Next time I will focus on …
- Next time I will try harder at …

Invitation 2: Bus stop people

Bus stop people can be used to gather students' perceptions of how they believe their peers feel about an issue. It then offers a chance for them to put themselves in the picture and reflect on what they think.

Sharing the responses can often highlight that we all believe everyone thinks very differently to us, when in fact we may all have similar feelings or concerns. For example, perhaps everyone believes everyone else is more confident than them. However, when we share our own feelings, we discover that the rest of our group shares our doubts and uncertainties.

The prompt is: 'A group of young people from our school (or our village, our community, our town) have met at the bus stop on the way home. They are all talking and thinking about …'

Issues that can be explored are virtually endless, for example:

- Bullying.
- Homework.
- Something topical in school or out of school.
- A party tonight.
- Young people carrying weapons.

It is possible to focus this further by putting words into one person's mouth, for example:

- 'I reckon you need to stick up for yourself!'
- 'I'm looking forward to tonight, there is going to be loads to drink!'
- 'I reckon everyone is doing it.'

It can be helpful to explore whether what everyone is saying is different from what they are thinking and to ask why that might be.

This activity has been used by schools to inform policy writing, especially on issues such as bullying.

Invitation 3: Adults

Use this one as a companion to Invitation 2, to gather students' perceptions of what adults think and feel about an issue – perhaps even the same issue that their peer group was talking about at the bus stop. In some instances, they may project much unhelpfully vague, critical comment on to the imagined group of adults, particularly if they are exploring behaviour that is disapproved of (comments perhaps emanating from the inner 'parent'). At other times, this exercise can help students identify what they construe as highly sensible comments, and can demonstrate extraordinary insight.

In addition to inviting students to imagine what this group of adults might be saying, this exercise can help students get in touch with their inner 'parent', both helpful and critical, and their inner 'adult'. Also, in common with drama, it can sometimes be easier and feel less threatening to project these adult-reflections on to an imagined huddle of people (or in the case of drama a character being played) than to state them 'for real' and own them, particularly if they fear they may conflict with the views of their peers.

A vital part of this activity is getting feedback, and exploring the significance of what has emerged from it.

Alongside Invitation 2, this one can be used to inform policy, and help students 'get inside' a significant issue that the school needs to prepare for responsibly and respond to competently.

Invitation 4: Draw someone of your age (or a little older than you) who ...

This one is really simple and is limited only by your imagination. Some examples include those who:

- drink a lot of alcohol
- use drugs
- smoke
- are being bullied
- have fallen out with their friends.

Around the outside of the picture, invite students to record their thoughts. Prompts for this might include:

- What risks do you think they are running for themselves?
- What might be the risks to others?
- What might people who care about them feel if they knew?

- What might happen if things stay as they are?
- How likely is it that the picture you're painting will happen?

This activity is useful for drawing out stereotypes that can then be challenged, for example:

- 'Do you have to look lonely to feel lonely?'
- 'Do all people who bully look like you have drawn them?'
- 'Do all people who use drugs look like that?'

Invitation 5: The storyboard

This is a simple version of the type of storyboard that film-makers use. In the first box there is a dialogue. You could put a prompt in the left-hand speech bubble. For example:

- I am being bullied.
- I have been invited to a party but I don't want to go.
- I am not getting on well with …
- I am finding … difficult to learn.

The task is then to invite students, in groups, to fill in the other speech bubble and the two thought bubbles with what you would be saying, what you would be feeling or thinking, and how you believe the other character would be feeling. Now complete the storyboard to a point where you all feel it's 'sorted'. (Some issues don't resolve themselves quickly or easily, so the speech bubble in the final frame has been left blank in case of unavoidably unfinished business.)

Ask groups to consider each other's strategies by bringing the groups together. (Try to avoid asking each group to share their storyboard with the whole class – many students dislike this.) Ask them to reflect on all the good things and any not-so-good things about the strategies.

Invitation 6: I'm new here!

'I'm new here, can you give me some advice about …?' is virtually self-explanatory. Simply put in the prompt you wish to explore. You can expand the context by adding a back story, for example:

'A new person has joined our class; they say to you, "Hi, I'm …"'

'A new person has moved in down your road, you meet them one morning and they say "Hi, I'm, new here …"'

Issues include:

- What to do if I get lost.
- What to do if I get worried.
- What to do if I get picked on by someone.

Or, in the wider community:

- Whether or not it is safe to go out alone around here, or with a friend, or after dark.
- Where it is good to hang out, and where it is not-so-good.
- Who I should tell if there is trouble.

A simpler variation that is subtly different is to have the new person simply ask:

'I'm new here, can you tell me about …?'

This requires a description rather than a personal opinion and the offering of advice.

Invitation 7: Bubbles

A very simple activity that can be endlessly adapted. The first character offers the prompt, and the individual or group decides their response. For example:

- 'I wish I was in your form, everyone says it's really great!'

The group then responds to two prompts you have written in before duplication of the invitation:

- In the speech bubble, have pre-written: 'Yes, it is great because …'
- In the think bubble, have pre-written: 'But it could be even better if …'

Now let the group consider and record how they would reply.

Invitation 8: Park bench

The 'Park bench' is simply two young people sitting on a bench. It is a powerful activity because it can be used to open very sensitive issues. In the speech bubble on the left-hand side, write the problem you want to explore through the eyes of the first young person. For example, it could be a day-to-day issue:

- 'I am falling behind in my homework. I can't seem to concentrate. I don't know what to do!'

Or very sensitive issues:

- 'I have been going out with someone for a month and I really like them, but now they keep pushing me to go further than I want to!'
- 'I think I am/my girlfriend is pregnant.'
- 'I am being bullied.'

It is helpful to offer some unfinished sentences in the other bubbles, for example:

- 'If that happened to me, I would say …'
- 'I would do …'
- 'I might tell …'

In both think bubbles, simply put:

- 'I am thinking and feeling …'

Invite groups to fill in the empty bubbles and share their responses – how do people feel about the strategies that have been offered? What might be the good and not-so-good consequences of these strategies?

Invitation 9: Quiz sheet

This is a blank quiz sheet. It can be completed by you to help explore what is known and what isn't, or constructed by students using fact sheets in order to test their peers.

Invitation 10: Attitude continuum

We have included a blank attitude continuum. You can provide statements to explore, or offer students an opportunity to construct statements to test out what their peers think about particular issues, and why they think as they do. As with all the invitations, feedback is vital, and can be as much of a springboard to learning as the exercise itself.

Invitation 11: Cloud sheet

The clouds on this sheet are for thoughts (prompt: What do you think about …?) while the speech bubbles are for what is actually said (prompt: What do you say to others about …?)
This is a more reflective exercise, and the ground rules need to be clear. If students are to write in their private thoughts, then they need to know they will not be pressed to reveal them, and arrangements are needed to protect the completed sheets, too. To students, the activity may appear to be a more risky version of Invitation 2 (Bus stop people) or Invitation 8 (Park bench), as it can bring into sharp focus the difference in some instances between what is thought and what people are prepared to say.

If there is a difference, feedback and discussion could focus on why. If you judge (and the class agrees) that students are well able to manage personal disclosures in a mature way, you may want to forewarn them that the invitation to reveal their thoughts will be there for the courageous. However, this will not be appropriate with issues that generate highly sensitive or incriminating thoughts and, in any case, nobody should feel pressured to say anything they feel uncomfortable about. Any refusal should be accepted without challenge.

Invitation 12: Caught in the middle!

Caught in the middle can be used in a huge variety of situations. It could be a research tool to uncover your students' thinking about something; a classroom resource as part of a planned session; or a focusing activity to open a session. It is designed initially to be completed individually, then shared to see what others think. Another option is to put it on a whiteboard and give the students sticky notes to create a whole class 'thought shower'. It is an activity to prompt thought and discussion, rather than an 'end in itself'.

One interesting way of using the invitation, is to have it as a resource that you can use spontaneously if a dilemma arises in a discussion and you want to offer the group a way of quickly analysing how they might respond.

A choice could be worded from two different perspectives and put into the two 'They say …' bubbles. For example, complete opposites such as 'Go on, give it a try!' and 'No, don't try it!' or just two different viewpoints: 'You should never hurt another person' and 'Sometimes you have to hurt another person'.

The student then works through the sheet, starting with:

- I reckon they think (on each side)
- What I think or feel about what they think (on each side)
- I would reply … because … (to each side)
- What I think is …
- If someone asked my view, I would say … because …

In the real world, we may find ourselves being confronted by people giving us different or conflicting advice and we need to weigh up what they are telling us and make our choice. Remind students that they might agree with one or other voice or they might have a view of their own that is a mixture of both, or something completely different. Another layer of complexity is added when we may like one of our advisers, or even dislike them. Are we more likely to listen to dodgy advice if it comes from someone we like? Or reject good advice from someone we find unpleasant? And what if an advice-giver has a hidden (undeclared) agenda – one wanting to satisfy curiosity or get excitement, the other perhaps being overly frightened of being hurt or getting into trouble? Can we be strong enough to ignore attractive bad advice and to sense a hidden agenda? The invitation can help students identify more accurately some of these potential influences.

It is important also to remind students that all the thoughts and voices in this exercise are *actually their own*. They *must be* the thoughts of the person holding the pen. When we are faced with a choice or dilemma we may find our 'voices in our heads' giving us different or conflicting advice, and sometimes we may be able to identify the exact origin of these thoughts. We may sometimes even hear the recognisable voice of Mum, Uncle, friend. However, if the voice is inside our head, the thought is now ours, which means we can listen to it, follow it, ignore it, or change it. We need to be aware of our *own* 'hidden agendas'. Just as in the external world, we need to listen carefully and weigh things up, we may need to do this with our own 'voices' in our internal world.

Invitation 13: 'Parent', 'adult' and 'child' (1)

This invitation is designed to explore the 'voices' we may hear telling us what we should or shouldn't do, how we should or shouldn't feel and what we should or shouldn't say. They can also take the form of 'self-talk' telling us how stupid we are, how we can't do something, how we'll never manage this or that (negative self-talk), or how sensible we are, how we can do it or learn it if we try, that we should stand our ground, and reminding us that we are, basically, 'OK' (positive self-talk).

The thought bubbles on this sheet are for the thoughts that may arrive, unasked and insistent, from inside our heads. As the students become more familiar with the material and the approach in *Health for Life 15–16*, so they will become more familiar with the concept of the 'parent', the 'adult' and the 'child' within. The ability to refuse to be *dominated* by inner 'parent' or inner 'child' and, instead, to allow them their say while the inner 'adult' stays in charge is a skill that does not come quickly for everyone. Some people never adequately manage it, particularly those who are damaged and don't fully heal. The process of identifying the voices inside, and whose they are ('parent', 'adult' or 'child'), and learning to deal competently with them, can be a highly significant influence in helping students to become responsible, thoughtful, rational, balanced people.

This sheet provides the chance to explore the voices and the value of the messages they convey. It can be used as a private exercise, or may be the start of a discussion in pairs or groups to show the variety, or otherwise, of the many 'parent', 'adult' and 'child' voices in the class. It can be used whenever there seems a need. It may be worth having a supply of the sheets ready to hand out at any point where internal reflection and clarity seem useful.

If offered as a private, reflective exercise, then arrangements may be needed for secure storage or disposal of the sheets if the students don't want to keep them.

Invitation 14: 'Parent', 'adult' and 'child' (2)

This sheet is a similar one to Invitation 13 but involves a conversation or interaction between two people. One could be the student, but doesn't have to be and, in fact, they may feel safer when it isn't. The two people could be characters in a scenario illustrating a point you are making or dealing with an issue in question. A more risky-feeling option is for the two people to be chosen as real people, *though students need not declare if this is so.* The sheet can be used to illustrate what happens when two 'child' voices get the upper hand and interact, two 'parents', a 'parent' and a 'child', etc. If the students are imaginative, the results can be hilarious – but they may still make a point about how situations may be better dealt with.

General uses are similar to those for Invitation 13, and a ready supply of handouts may be helpful at any time. Again, the same ground rules and security care may be needed for any private use.

Invitation ① Looking back/Looking forward

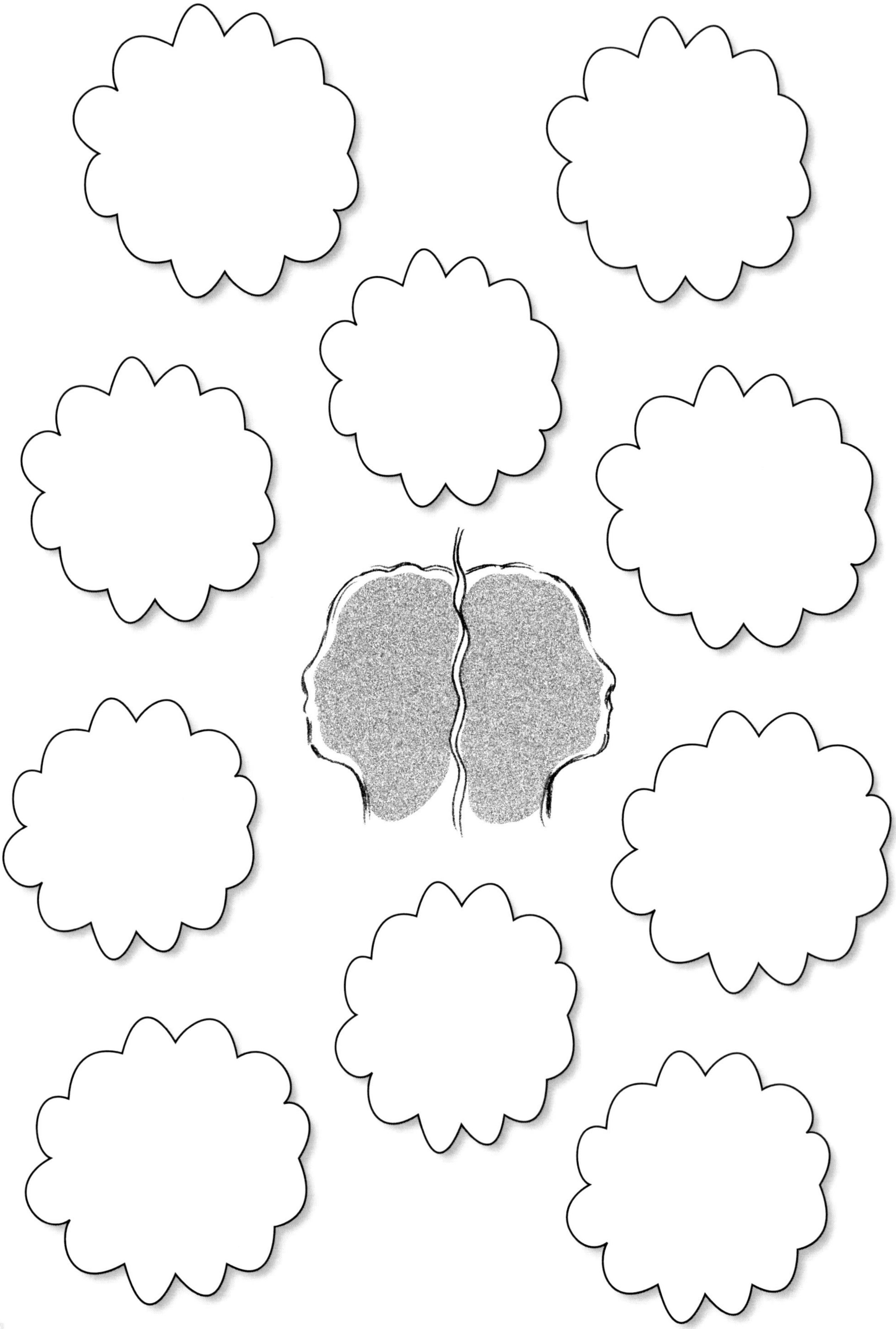

Invitation ② Bus stop people

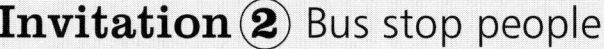

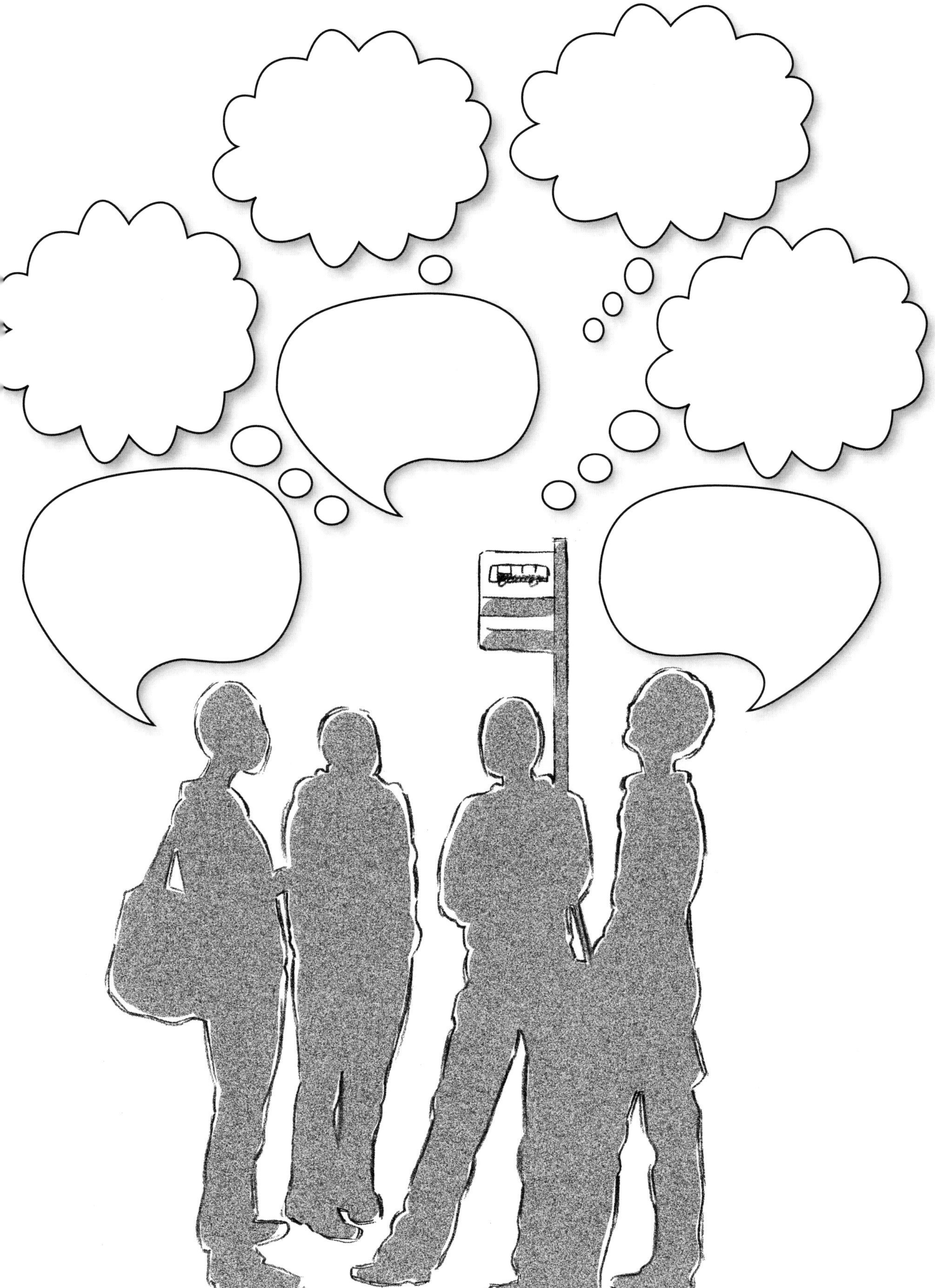

A group of people from our school have met at the bus stop on the way home. They are all talking and thinking about …

Invitation ③ Adults

Imagine a group of adults from _____ have met together.

They are talking and thinking about _____

_____

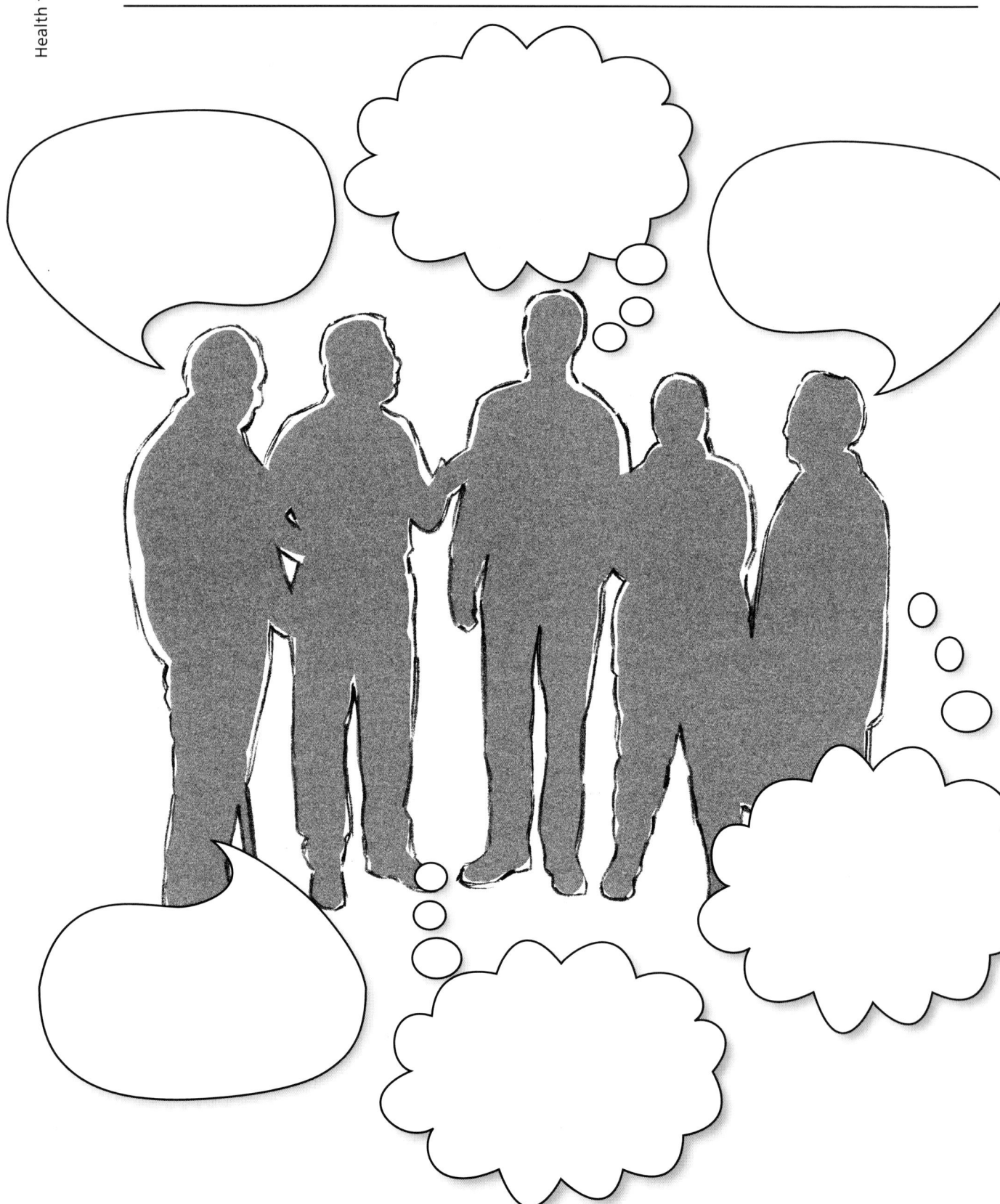

What do you think they are thinking and saying?

Invitation 4 Draw someone of your age
(or a little older than you) who …

Invitation ⑤ The storyboard

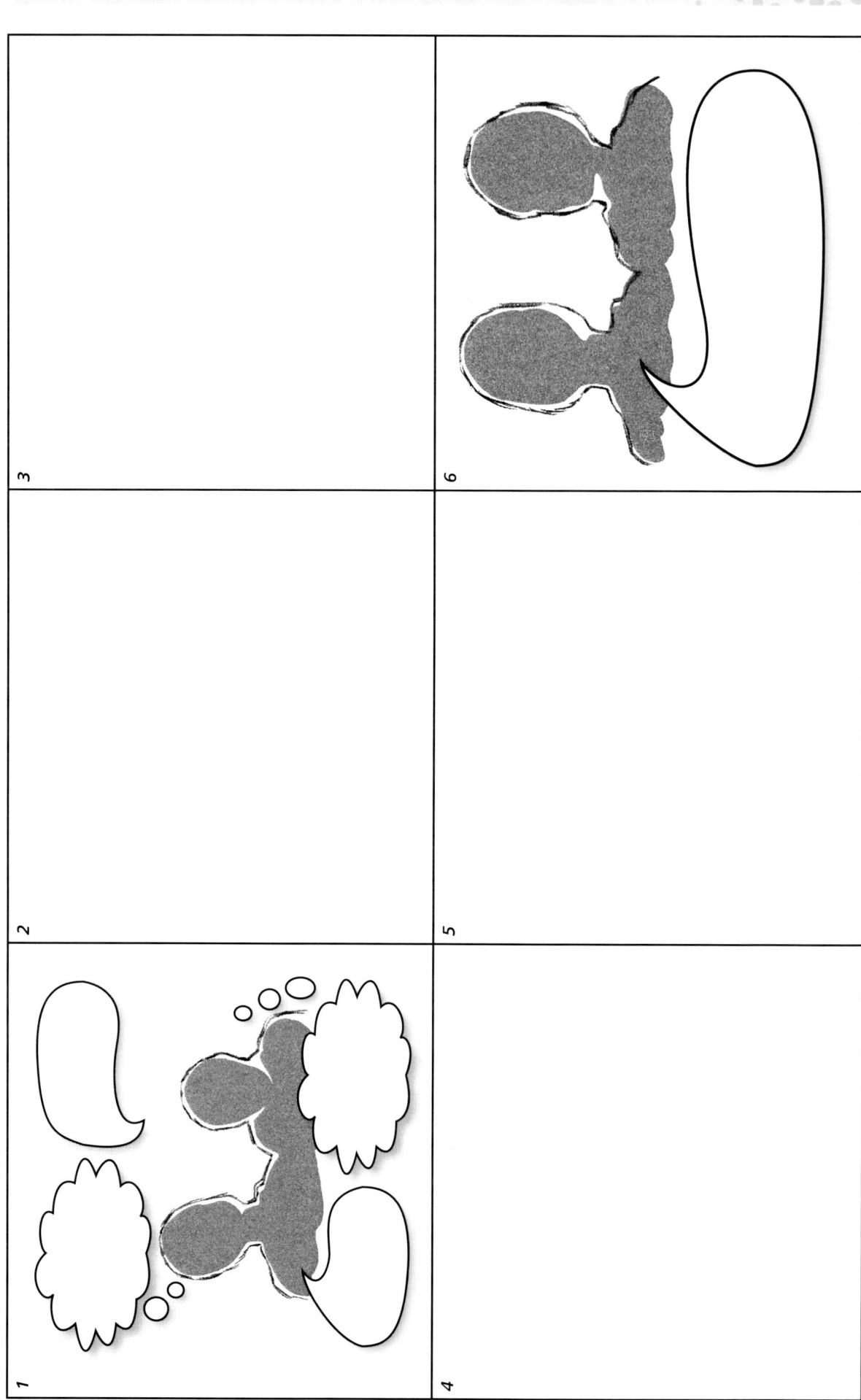

Invitation ⑥ I'm new here!

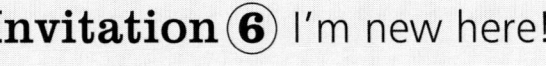

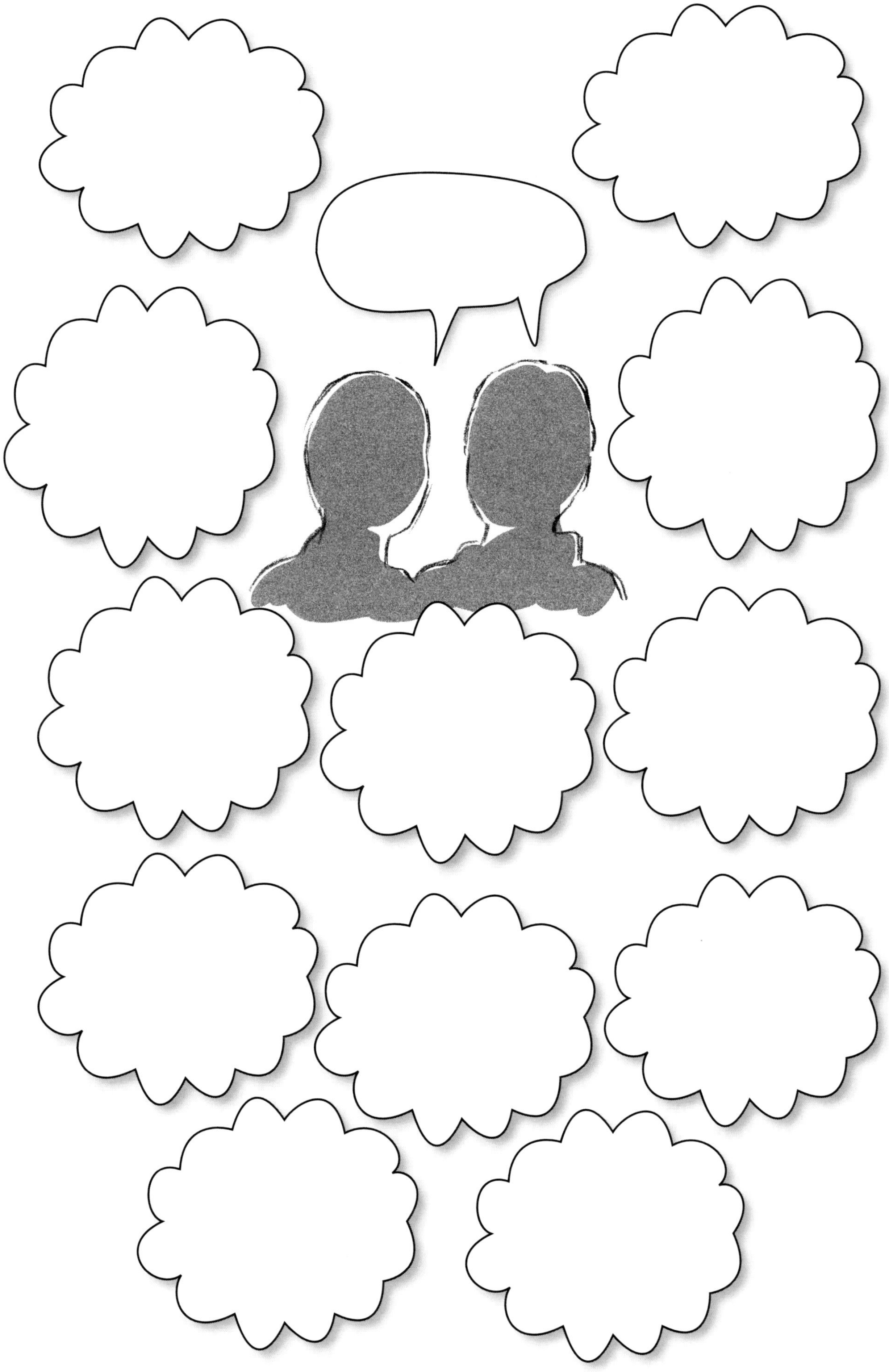

Invitation ⑦ Bubbles

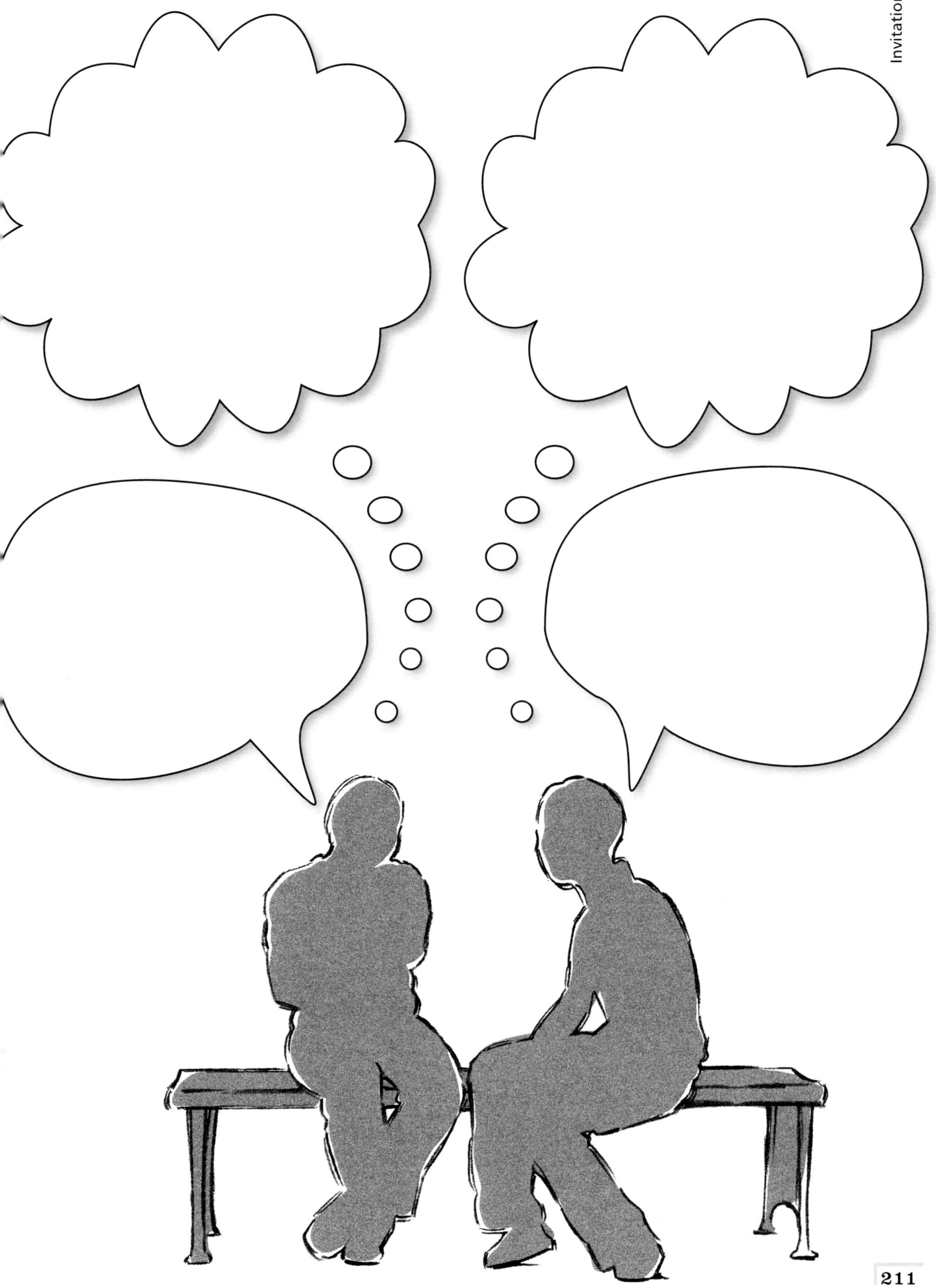

Invitation ⑨ Quiz sheet

	That's right	Not sure ...	That's wrong

Invitation ⑩ Attitude continuum

So how do I feel about ...?	Strongly agree	Agree	Not sure	Disagree	Strongly disagree

Invitation ⑪ Cloud sheet

What do you think about ...? What would you say to others?

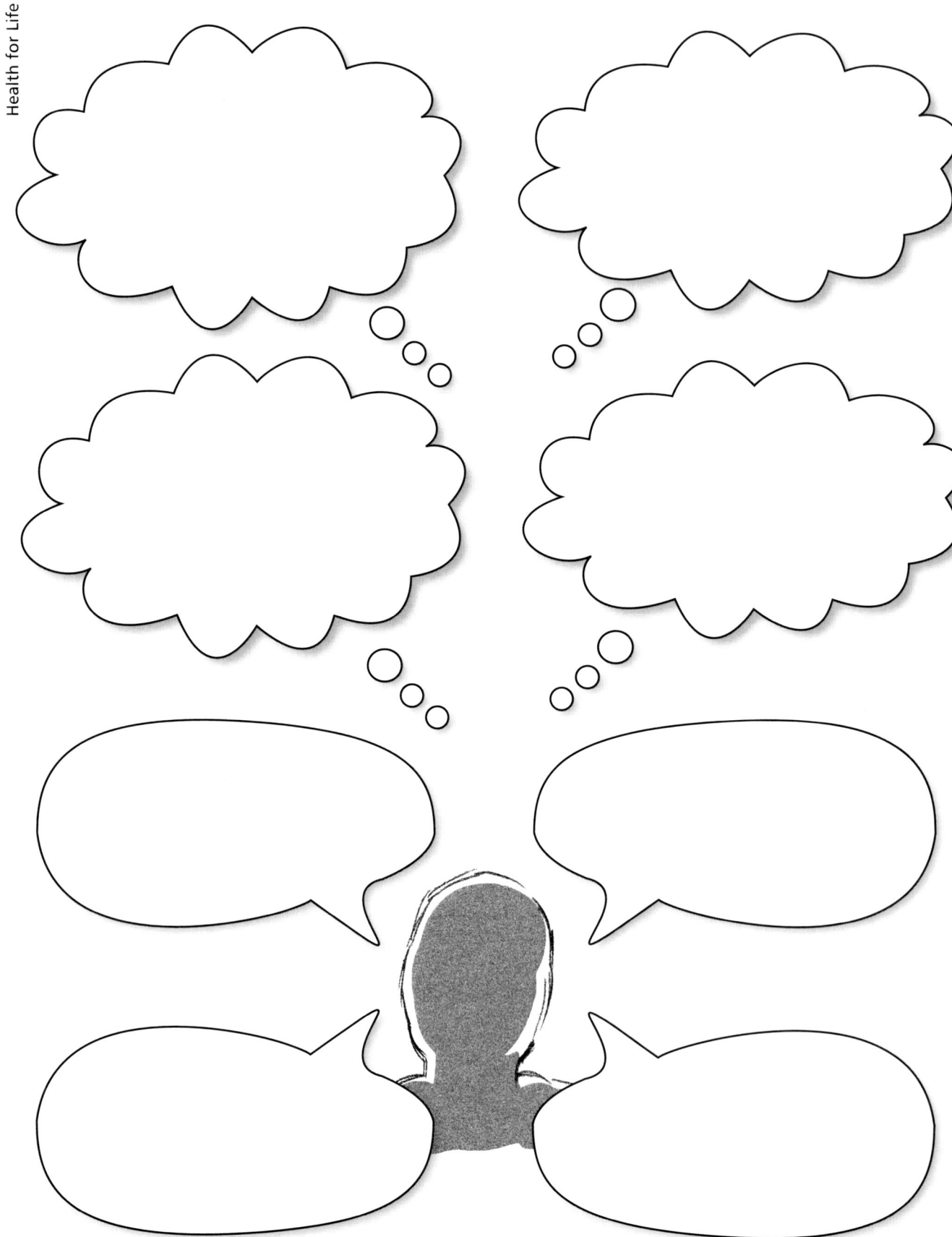

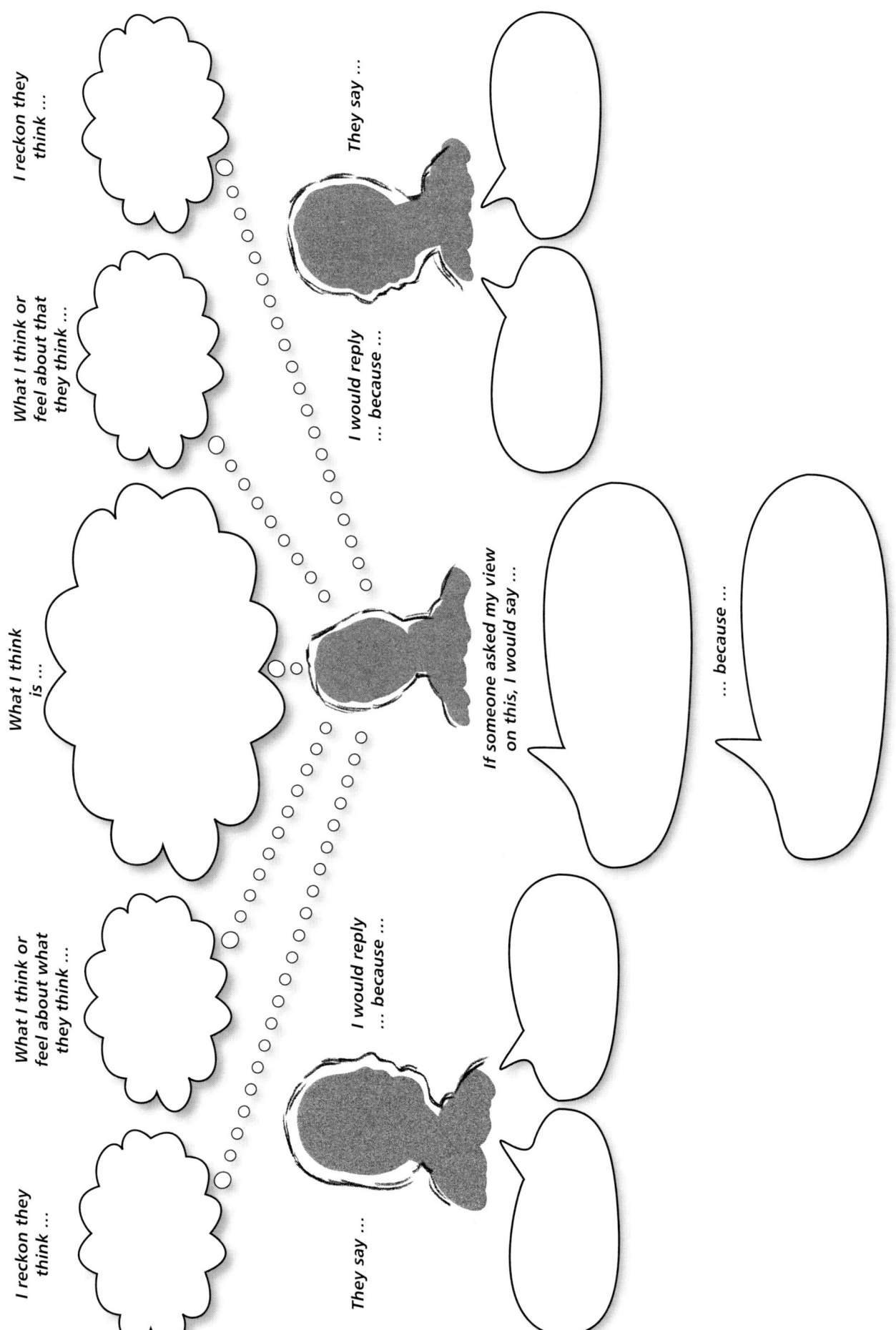

Invitation ⑬ 'Parent', 'adult' and 'child' (1)

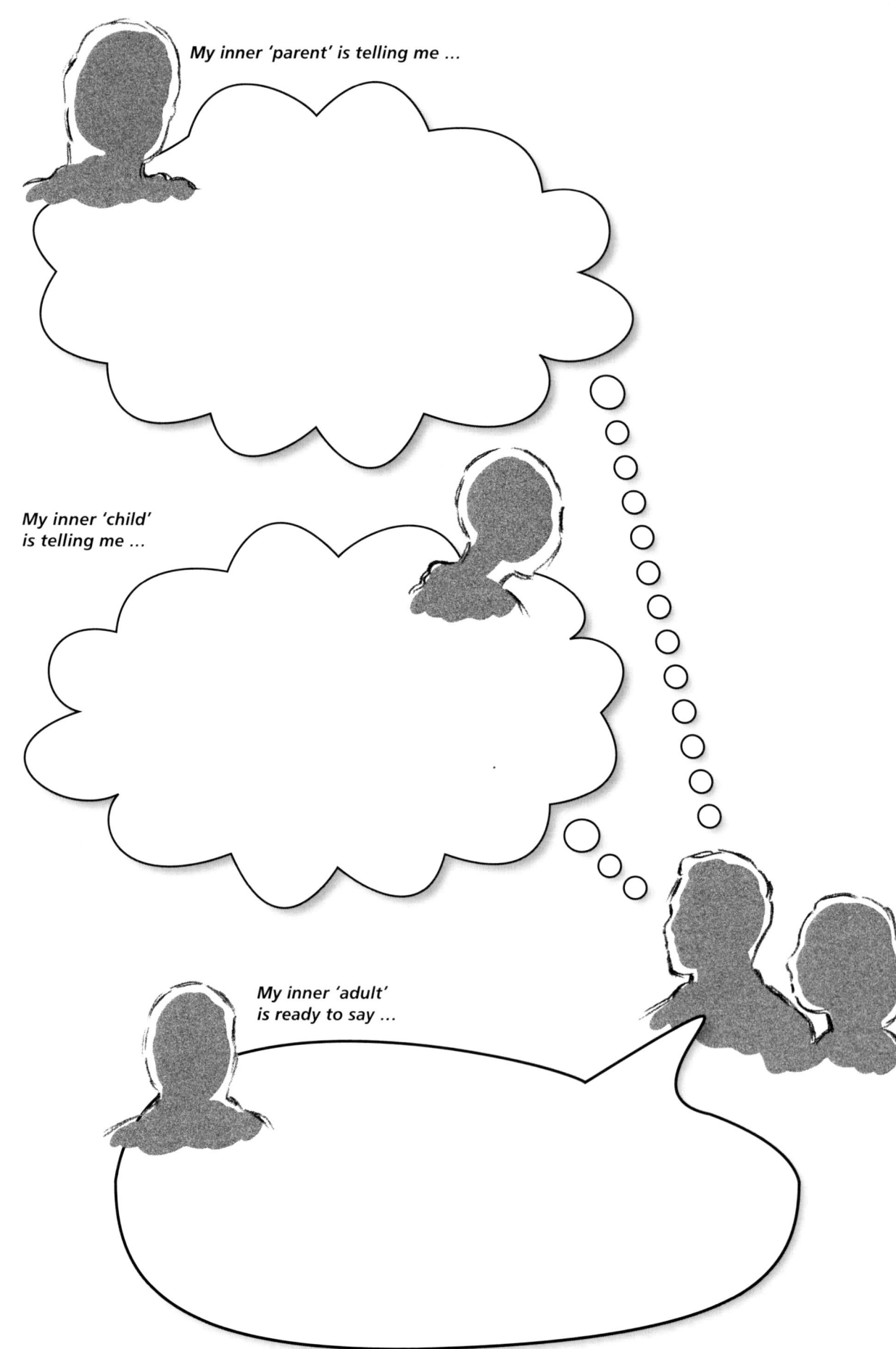

My inner 'parent' is telling me …

My inner 'child' is telling me …

My inner 'adult' is ready to say …

My inner 'child' is
telling me ...

My inner 'parent'
is telling me ...

My inner 'adult' is
ready to say ...

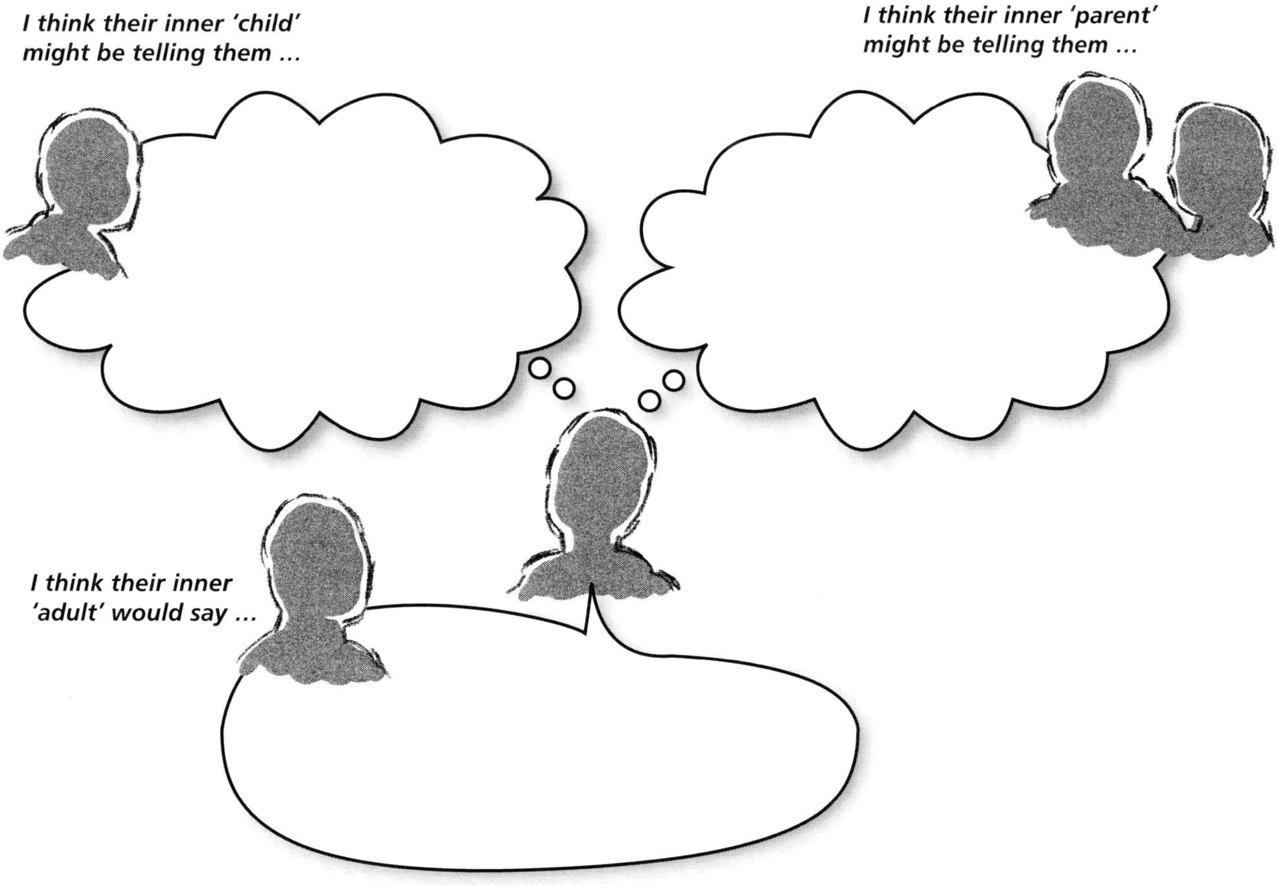

I think their inner 'child'
might be telling them ...

I think their inner 'parent'
might be telling them ...

I think their inner
'adult' would say ...

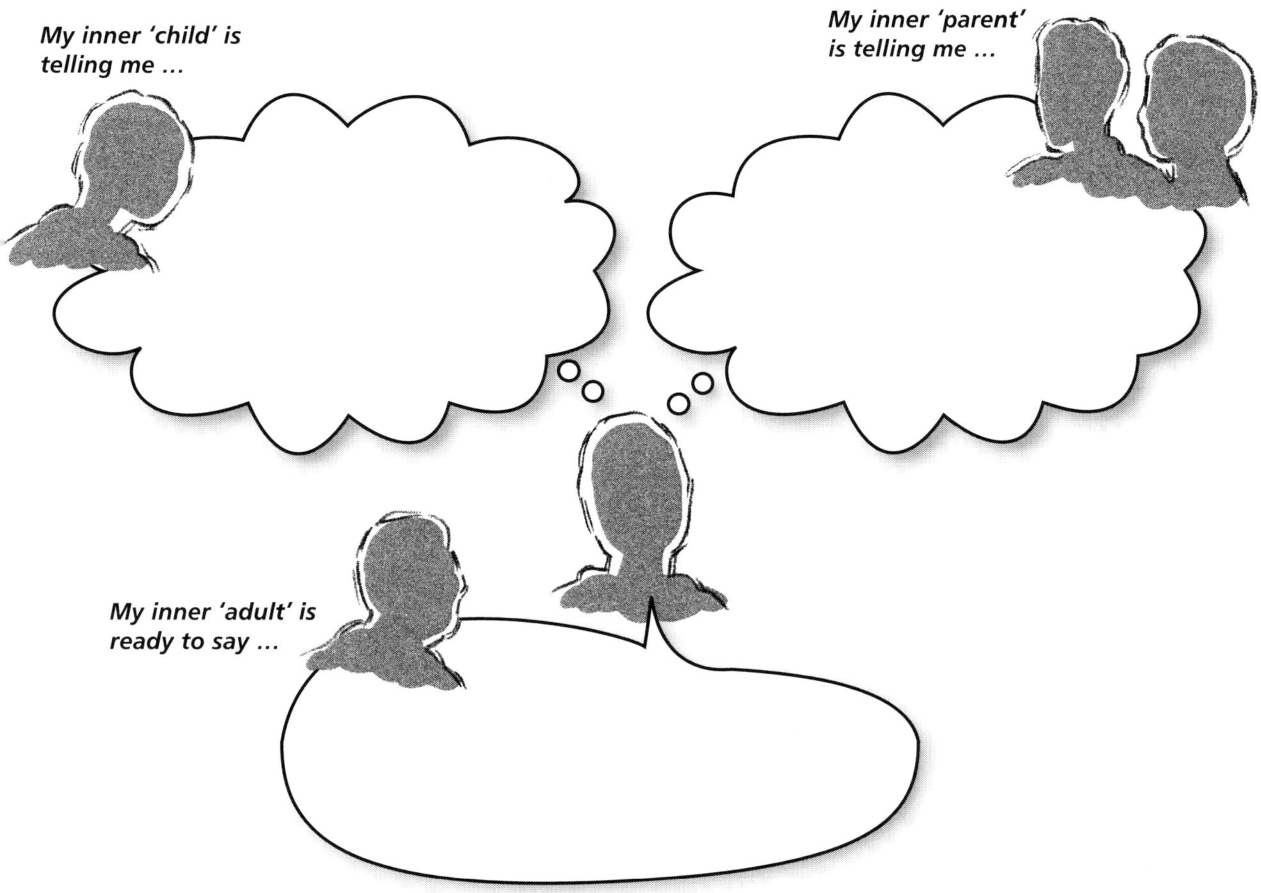

3.3 Knowledge frames

The following knowledge frames show the broad areas of knowledge that we believe students should have acquired by the time they reach 16 years of age. For reference, the knowledge frames from *Health for Life 11–14* are shown in normal type. The areas that may need revisiting and reinforcing are in *italics*, and additional knowledge that builds on this earlier work is in normal **bold**. The frames are very comprehensive and some of the knowledge in italics may not have been learned by the age of 14.

The lists are by no means definitive, and you may wish to add some of your own knowledge. You may well want to prioritise some over others, in order to fit your own local context. The age at which you will want to introduce information is also likely to depend on the needs of students. They will attach greater meaning to knowledge as it becomes relevant to them, and even when something has been taught earlier in the secondary phase it still may need revisiting.

It is important to build the imparting of this knowledge into a process that helps students reflect on it and make their own personal meanings from it. For example, use the knowledge:

- during group work to increase creative thinking: 'Look at this situation. If I give you this information, what are all the possible good and not-so-good things that could happen next?'

- during discussion or debate to increase critical thinking skills: 'If you now know this piece of information, does it change your point of view?'

- during an analysis of a case study to explore decision making: 'If the person knew this piece of information, do you think they would feel or react differently, and, if so, what could they say or do?'

- during risk assessment activities: 'If you now know that this is the case, do you rate the activity as a high, medium or low risk? If you still did this activity, what would be the risks now, in the short term, in the long term? If you decided not to do the activity, would there still be risks? So what risks do you find acceptable?'

- during research activities. Information can be gathered by students, providing suitable resource material is available: 'We have collected up what we already know; now I am going to give you a question and a series of fact sheets. Research your answer and convince the rest of us that you are right!'

Some cultures, families or individuals may have strong views about what is appropriate and inappropriate behaviour. It is crucial to recognise that students have a right to sound information. Providing information is not the same as obliging someone to make use of it. Ignorance is seldom protective, and good information enables students to better understand the consequences of their and others' decisions, though it cannot guarantee that decisions subsequently made will seem responsible or sensible from our perspective.

Knowledge frames are provided for:

- Drugs
  - Basic knowledge around drugs; the generic knowledge that applies to all drugs.
  - Specific knowledge around alcohol use.
  - Specific knowledge around tobacco use.
  - Specific knowledge around over-the-counter and prescribed use.
  - Specific knowledge around illegal and illicit drugs. (It is essential to check the relevance of these to your context.)
- Sexual health
- Healthy eating
- Emotional health
- Learning
- Aspects of personal safety.

Some thoughts on self-esteem are also offered. 'Building everyone's self-esteem' is demanded of schools, but what exactly does this mean? Self-esteem is complex, and the model and descriptions are only offered as a suggestion. It is intended that the approach taken by this resource supports the development of self-esteem.

Frameworks are also included for:

- the 'language of persuasion'. This is in response to the wide range of information and communication available to students and a growing sophistication in the way that the patterns of language can be crafted to influence beliefs, values and decisions.
- basic economic awareness
- internet safety.

Knives and first aid

Knives can and do cause injury. If young people are the first on the scene at an accident, they will be best able to help if they know first aid. The British Red Cross promotes simple but important first-aid techniques that it says can be learned in five minutes. This is what it says for bleeding:

> 'Make sure there's nothing embedded in the wound. Put pressure on the wound. Sit the person down and raise the limb above the level of the heart. Apply a bandage – a clean tea towel or pillowcase will do. Then call 999 if necessary.
>
> **Remember**: 'apply pressure and raise the limb, cover, and call 999.'

Contact The British Red Cross or St John Ambulance for more detailed support in this connection.

Drugs

It is vital to reinforce the earlier work around alcohol and tobacco. These remain the 'gateway drugs' and can obviously be problematic in both the short and long term. It is likely that a number of students at this key stage will be drinking alcohol and smoking tobacco regularly, and a smaller number will have tried illegal drugs. Research also suggests that the majority will be offered an illegal drug by the end of this key stage. Our programmes must reflect the needs and experiences of our students and the context within which we are working. This framework is offered only as a starting point.

While it can be inappropriate to single out a particular drug, some emphasis in this key stage on alcohol use is strongly suggested, especially issues surrounding binge drinking and its possible consequences. The substantial health risks may be seen as less relevant than other risks, especially poor judgement or over-confidence. These can lead to accidents, poor decisions and other problems, including the risk of becoming a victim (or even acting out of character and being the initiator) of serious crimes such as mugging and rape.

It can be helpful to set this work in a context such as a party or disco/club and to explore the risks and the connections between the risks. For example, alcohol leads to poor choices; which lead possibly to unintended relationships; which lead possibly to unprotected sex or violence.

Reinforce the need to treat over-the-counter medicines (especially painkillers such as paracetamol) with respect, and to use prescribed medicines only as instructed.

Re-emphasise the possibility of drug testing at job interviews or during the medical following a successful appointment. Re-emphasise the lasting nature of drugs, especially cannabis, in the body, as it is possible to test positive many weeks after even a single use.

Emphasise the dangers of any drug use on road safety, driving or being driven by someone who has recently used any drug. Reinforce the potentially lifelong implications of a drug conviction on future travel and career prospects. Emphasise that these restrictions are for life. Reinforce emergency procedures, reminding students to always get medical help if they think someone is having difficulties with their drug use and to always telephone for an ambulance if someone is unconscious.

By the end of Year 11, every student should be able to say:

Basic drug knowledge	Health issues	Social issues	Legal issues
I know ...	I know ...	I know ...	I know ...
All medicines are drugs but not all drugs are medicines.	Misusing drugs may result in immediate health problems (e.g. solvents).	Some industries and individuals will try to persuade me to try legal and illegal drugs.	The misuse of any drug, legal or illegal, is very risky. Just because a drug is legally available, it does not mean it is 'safe'.
There is no 'safe' way of using any drug; all drug use carries risk, from low risk to very high risk.	Misusing drugs may result in long-term health problems, including reduced fitness and increased risk of disease.	If I purchase an illegal substance, there is every chance I am being sold something else.	*Drugs are classified by the law into three levels: A is the highest, then B, then C. Penalties are variable, but drugs in the higher categories carry the higher penalties.*
Drugs are inert substances. It is my and others' behaviour that can make them dangerous, and we are responsible for our behaviour.		Many people try out different drugs. This is known as **experimental drug use** and is very risky.	*That once I am over the age of ten, I am deemed*

Basic drug knowledge	Health issues	Social issues	Legal issues
Drugs can come in the form of powders, pills, liquids, on small pieces of blotting paper, or as part of a plant. Drugs can get into my body by sniffing (through the blood vessels in the nose), inhaling (through the lungs), swallowing (stomach lining), or injecting (directly into the bloodstream). The drug is then carried to the brain and other organs of the body through the bloodstream. Some drugs are used under medical supervision – these are prescribed to us by a doctor, dentist or nurse practitioner. Some medicines we can choose to take ourselves – these are available from chemists, supermarkets and other stores. Some drugs are used for non-medical purposes because they change the way we feel. Some of these drugs can: • give us energy and reduce tiredness. These are called *stimulants* • slow us down and induce sleep. These are called *depressants* • change the way our brains make sense of the world around us. These are called *hallucinogens*. Some drugs are legal, some are illicit (legal but not considered acceptable by society, i.e. solvents) and some are illegal.	When I take any drug I am running a number of risks: • I do not know what the drug is. If this is a medicine, or purchased alcohol or tobacco, it is probably what it says it is. If it is an illegal drug, the supplier may not know what it really is, even if they are my friend. • If I do not know the strength/dose of the drug or if it has been mixed with something else. Most medicines and legally purchased drugs are produced carefully and are well tested. Illegally produced drugs are not carefully produced, not subject to hygiene or quality control, and have not been medically tested. • I do not know what effect it will have on me, only what it did to someone else. If I have used it before, I know there is no guarantee that I will have the same experience next time. • I know the way I take the drug into my body may cause problems. Drugs change the way we feel or change the way our bodies work. As my body gets used to some drugs, I need to take more for them to have an effect. This is called **tolerance**. This change can also make it very difficult to stop using the drug. This is called **dependence**. Some people call this **addiction**. It has similarities with a 'habit' that cannot be easily stopped.	Some people enjoy their drug or drugs and use occasionally or regularly. This is sometimes called **social/recreational** drug use. *Some drugs may change the way I and others feel and the way we behave. This means we can make poor choices when we are using drugs. We may regret these choices later or we may make a choice that gets us hurt.* *Many drugs, even in very low amounts, can affect our judgement. These include: alcohol and other depressants; stimulants; cannabis and other hallucinogens and some medicines.* *Others who use drugs may put me at risk through their behaviour. Some people who are intoxicated may hurt me.* *I cannot judge someone else's level of intoxication just by looking at them. To be safe on the roads requires all our concentration. Very low levels of intoxication can present very serious risks on the roads or anywhere where we have to make fine judgements.* Becoming 'dependent' on a drug can be very expensive. If it is an illegal drug, it can present serious difficulties since you have to engage in criminal activity either in using the drug or in getting the money to pay for the drug.	*in law to be capable of committing a criminal offence.* *Possession of an illegal drug is a serious offence. The drug does not have to be 'mine'. Holding a drug for a friend is still an offence. The drug doesn't have to be on my person, it could be in my bag or in my home.* *Drug trafficking includes supplying an illegal drug to another or possessing an illegal drug intending to pass it to someone else. No exchange of money or goods needs to be involved; it could simply be collecting a drug for someone else.* *Just agreeing to supply an illegal drug is an offence. The drug does not have to be real; even pretending to sell someone an illegal drug is an offence.* *Allowing 'my premises' to be used for making or supplying drugs or allowing cannabis to be smoked on 'my premises' is a very serious offence. The 'premises' includes any outbuildings or grounds attached to the premises. This even includes premises we may have rented for a party.* *Drug testing is becoming more common and may happen at a medical following an interview for a job. It is possible to test positive for some drugs such as cannabis many weeks after even one use.*

Basic drug knowledge	Health issues	Social issues	Legal issues
	Although some young people become dependent on drugs, many are seriously hurt just trying drugs out. I do not need to use drugs regularly to have problems with drugs, which may include: ● accidents ● allergic reactions ● accidental overdose ● accidental poisoning ● contracting diseases. Prescribed drugs should only be used by the person to whom they have been prescribed, in the dose prescribed. 'Over-the-counter medicines' can still be very dangerous if misused. I know they should only be taken in the doses recommended on the packaging and not with any other medication, prescribed or otherwise. If in doubt, I should ask a doctor or pharmacist. Injecting any drug without medical supervision or direction is very dangerous and sharing injecting equipment with anyone puts me at potential risk of a number of infections, including hepatitis and HIV. Where confidential help for drug problems is available locally and nationally.	*A conviction for a drug offence and the subsequent criminal record can result in:* ● *a possible fine or imprisonment* ● *a loss of future job opportunities* ● *a loss of travel to a number of countries including the USA* ● *a loss of life.* *To treat anyone who appears to be having a problem with drugs as a medical emergency. I know to lie them down in the recovery position and to get help by calling 999. I know how to put someone in the recovery position.*	

Specific alcohol knowledge

It is likely that most students will have tried alcohol by the end of Key Stage 2. Most will have experienced alcohol in their home, but a small minority will already be independent drinkers. From this age on, an increasing number will begin to become independent drinkers, many choosing very strong alcoholic drinks. It is also likely that, as students socialise with older peers, they become at risk from others' alcohol consumption.

By the end of Year 11, every student should be able to say:

Alcohol	Health issues	Social issues	Legal issues
I know …	**I know …**	**I know …**	**I know …**

Alcohol — I know …

Alcoholic drinks contain a drug called ethanol. It is one of the most toxic of the drugs we use in society.

This is a depressant drug; it slows down the working of my brain, starting with the parts that control my ability to make judgements. I know that this drug can make me feel confident that I can do things better than I really can.

Alcohol is absorbed through the lining of my stomach into my bloodstream and then directly to my brain. Eating before drinking will slow the process down; 'fizzy' drinks will speed this process up.

Alcoholic drinks are measured in 'units' (10mg of ethanol). The following drinks all contain 1 unit:

- *½ pint of ordinary beer or lager*
- *1 single measure of spirit, e.g. whisky, vodka*
- *1 small glass of wine.*

Alcoholic fruit drinks ('alcohol-pops') can contain high levels of ethanol and can be similar in strength to wine.

An adult liver can process 1 unit of alcohol per hour, but a young person's liver will process alcohol more slowly.

Alcohol is sold in bottles or cans with 'alcohol by volume' (abv) written on the label. This indicates the percentage of ethanol in the product. The higher the abv, the stronger the drink.

Adding a 'mixer' to an alcoholic drink does not

Health issues — I know …

As people use alcohol more regularly, their bodies get used to the drug; this is called **tolerance**.

The more I regularly drink alcohol, the less effect it will appear to have on me, as my brain and physical responses adapt to it.

Regularly drinking alcohol does not reduce the effect alcohol will have on my ability to make judgements.

Using alcohol regularly increases the long-term risks to my health.

Since alcohol is a drug, it can be misused. The risks include:

- *making poor judgements*
- *accidents*
- *choices I later regret.*

Consequences of overdosing range from being sick or ill through to coma and death.

Although there are advisory drinking limits for alcohol, these only apply to fully grown adults and not to young people. Adult bodies react differently to alcohol, and the adult liver is larger. The long-term effects on juveniles are at present unknown.

Small amounts of alcohol may improve the health only of men over 40 years and post-menopausal women.

Using very small amounts of alcohol, even 1 unit, can affect my judgement. There are no 'safe limits' for driving, swimming or any other complex task.

There is some evidence that even low levels of

Social issues — I know …

People have used alcohol in social settings for thousands of years.

Other people's alcohol use can cause me problems through accidents or aggressive behaviour.

I cannot judge by the way they look or by their speech whether a person who has been drinking alcohol is safe to drive. Drivers are recommended not to drink ANY alcohol beforehand.

Individuals and the alcohol industry will try to influence my decisions about alcohol.

In social situations, it can be difficult to control my alcohol intake. Drinks I am offered by friends may be stronger then I realise, especially 'punch' at a party.

I should treat anyone who has drunk so much alcohol that they are drowsy or unconscious as a medical emergency. I should lay them on their side, on a blanket, and keep them warm. If they lose consciousness, I should place them in the recovery position. I should quickly get medical help for them. I know someone should stay with them until help arrives.

Being intoxicated can inappropriately increase my levels of confidence, encouraging me to make poor choices that may lead to endangering myself and others, including leaving me vulnerable to being a victim of serious crime.

Legal issues — I know …

It is legal to drink alcohol over the age of five, but that legal and healthy are not the same thing.

It is an offence for anyone under 18 to purchase or to be sold alcohol.

Driving while under the influence of any drug is a very serious offence. It is virtually impossible to judge your own 'safe limits' for driving. It is safest not to consume any alcohol if you intend to drive a car or ride a bicycle on the roads.

If I, or someone else, consume large amounts of alcohol during an evening, I, or they, may still be affected by alcohol the next day and still be unsafe to do difficult tasks (e.g. work machinery or be within the legal limit to drive). This is because each unit of alcohol takes an hour to be processed by an (adult) liver. For young people, it may take longer.

Alcohol	Health issues	Social issues	Legal issues
change the amount of alcohol present. *Each type of alcoholic drink can come in a variety of strengths (e.g. a can of strong cider or export lager can be equal to four single whiskies in alcohol content).* *Coffee (no matter how strong) has* **no effect whatsoever** *on the alcohol I have consumed or on my ability to make judgements.*	*alcohol may harm my ability to learn and retain what I have learned.* *Alcohol, even in small amounts, should never be mixed with any other drug (the drugs can react together with potentially dangerous outcomes).* *If a pregnant woman drinks alcohol, it may seriously affect the development of her baby.*		

Specific drug knowledge – tobacco

Although every student should have acquired this knowledge by 13, many young people make their decision about tobacco use far earlier. Research suggests that this knowledge should be in place by nine years of age. Secondary schools should be reinforcing tobacco education carried out by the middle of Key Stage 2.

By the end of Year 11, every student should be able to say:

Tobacco	Health issues	Social issues	Legal issues
I know ... Tobacco comes from the dried leaves of the tobacco plant and is taken in many ways including: ● smoked in cigarettes ● smoked in pipes ● smoked in cigars ● chewed, sometimes in pouches ● sniffed as a snuff. All tobacco use is dangerous to my health. *The smoking of tobacco is directly responsible for 130,000 deaths per year in the UK and is our biggest cause of lowering of life expectancy and poor health.* Tobacco contains a drug called **nicotine**. People who smoke tobacco say it helps them to feel calmer and more relaxed.	**I know ...** Nicotine is a poison. Nicotine is highly addictive and *extremely* hard to give up once addiction has occurred. Help is available from my doctor if I start smoking and wish to stop. When tobacco burns, it produces many dangerous substances, which include: ● a gas called carbon monoxide, which the body attracts more readily than oxygen. ● a sticky brown/black material called tar which gathers in the lungs. Smoking causes or helps to cause: ● lung and chest diseases, e.g. a chronic cough, bronchitis ● heart diseases ● diseases in other parts of the body.	**I know ...** Other people's tobacco smoke can seriously harm me and others if we breathe it in. Smoking tobacco can stain my fingers and make my breath and clothing smell. Smoking of tobacco is not allowed in many social settings and public places. Other people and the tobacco industry may try to persuade me to smoke tobacco and that I may face strong pressures to try this drug. Addiction to tobacco can be very expensive.	**I know ...** It is illegal to buy or to be sold tobacco under the age of 18.

The drug is actually a stimulant which raises blood pressure and speeds up the heart.	including cancers of the lung and throat and thrombosis (or blood clots) that may cause brain or heart damage ● damage to the retina of the eye leading to a significant increase in the risk of blindness. If a woman smokes while pregnant, the nicotine can go into her blood and affect her baby. Chewing tobacco may increase the chances of mouth and throat cancer.		

Specific drug knowledge – over-the-counter and prescribed drugs

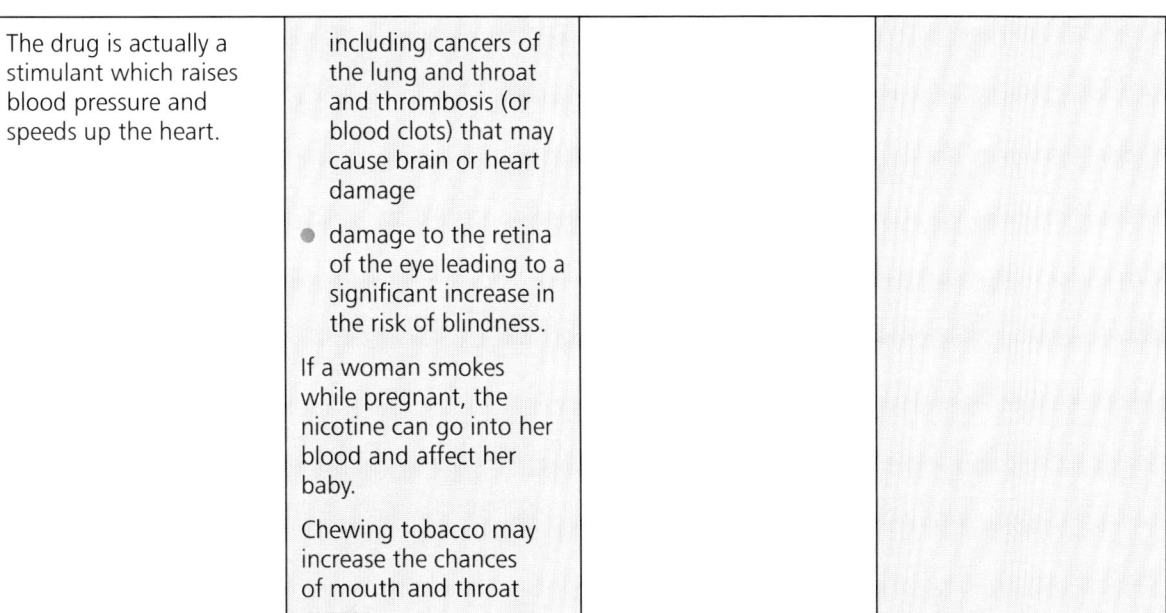

During Key Stage 3, some young people may be beginning to 'self-medicate' with over-the-counter drugs or be using prescribed drugs with greater independence. It is essential that they understand that these substances need great respect, especially paracetamol, which can be fatal if used incorrectly.

By the end of Year 11, every student should be able to say:

Over-the-counter and prescribed drugs	Health issues	Social issues	Legal issues
I know … Paracetamol is contained in many medications that I may purchase. Drugs such as paracetamol, ibuprofen, cough mixtures and aspirin are powerful drugs which must be used with great care. Prescribed drugs, especially sleeping tablets and tranquillisers, should only be taken as directed (and in the case of antibiotics, until I am told to stop). I have some say over whether to take medicines. My judgement and wishes should always be taken into account. I can always ask for a doctor, nurse or pharmacist's advice.	**I know …** To always check the dosage on any medication and never to exceed the recommended dose. If I intend to use two different medications, always to check with a pharmacist that I am not in danger of overdosing (especially if paracetamol is contained in each). An overdose of over-the-counter medications could be fatal, and to always contact a doctor **immediately** if I have any doubt about myself or someone else.	**I know …** *Some over-the-counter or prescribed drugs can affect people's ability to make judgements. This can lead to accidents. Advice will usually be on the jar or packet.*	**I know …** A prescribed drug is only to be used by the person to whom it is prescribed. *Giving a prescribed drug to someone else may be a serious offence.*

Specific drug knowledge – illegal and illicit drugs

The list of illegal or illicit substances a young person may encounter is vast. New drugs appear and some drugs lose their popularity, perhaps being surpassed by more effective ones. Very few illegal drugs are identifiable by anyone choosing to use them. A powder may be amphetamine or heroin but could just as easily be gravy powder; a tablet may be ecstasy but could just as easily be aspirin. By the end of Key Stage 3, the knowledge students need to have about the most commonly encountered illegal and illicit drugs is described below. It is desirable that students by the end of Key Stage 3 know at least the major issues surrounding **solvent**, **cannabis**, **LSD** and **amphetamine sulphate**. Teachers would need to work with students and local agencies to identify if more comprehensive knowledge around other drugs would be useful because of local needs or circumstances.

By the end of Year 11, every student should be able to say:

Solvents	Health issues	Social issues	Legal issues
I know ...	**I know ...**	**I know ...**	**I know ...**
Solvents are chemicals that are sold in many products, including some glues, paints and virtually all aerosols.	Solvent can cause me serious harm, even the first time I inhale it. It may cause:	Most people start to use solvents because their friends use them.	Selling solvent, if the shopkeeper believes it is going to be misused, is against the law. It is an offence to sell Butane (gas) in any form to anyone under the age of 18.
People inhale solvent because it makes them feel drowsy or light-headed.	● heart damage	Most solvent users stop when their friends stop.	
Some people hallucinate when they use solvents.	● a loss of my brain's ability to control my breathing and my heart.		
Although not illegal, sniffing solvent is extremely dangerous, even the first time it is used.	**Both of these can be fatal.**		
	Some people find using solvent hard to give up and may need to use increasing amounts (psychological dependency).		
	Serious accidents can happen when misusing solvents including:		
	● falls		
	● suffocation, either from a plastic bag if used or from vomit if the user becomes unconscious and is sick		
	● burns (most solvents are extremely flammable).		

Cannabis (puff, blow, grass, spliff, draw, weed and more)	Health issues	Social issues	Legal issues
I know … Cannabis comes from a plant. It comes in many forms, but the most popular is a small piece of brown substance similar to part of an 'Oxo' cube, called resin, or as part of a plant that looks similar to dried grass. Cannabis can be smoked, eaten or brewed as a tea. It comes in different strengths, some being so strong that they can cause hallucinations. It can also come as an oil, although this is rare, and is much stronger than the other forms.	**I know …** Smoking cannabis carries at least the same risks as tobacco and perhaps many more (see 'Tobacco', page 224). Some people become dependent on cannabis and this can cause serious health problems, especially to the throat and lungs. Persistent use can lead to a lack of motivation and lethargy, which can affect my ability to learn. Cannabis can affect short-term memory. *Getting intoxicated on cannabis can affect my judgement in a similar way to alcohol, but for longer. I therefore run increased risks of having accidents.* *I may become very distressed or anxious whilst using cannabis.* *Cannabis use may cause problems during pregnancy.* *For people with some mental instability, using strong cannabis can increase the likelihood of serious mental health problems.*	**I know …** Smoking cannabis can change my mood, perhaps for the better but equally for the worse. Some users become very sleepy; others get a strong desire to eat. *Some people who use cannabis feel everyone is out to get them (paranoia and anxiety attacks).* *Intoxicated (**stoned**) people can make poor choices. Getting a lift in a car from someone who has used cannabis (possibly within the last two days) may be risky.* *Cannabis stays in the fatty tissue in my body for a long time. I can therefore test positive for cannabis weeks after I have last used it (perhaps in a medical for a job).*	**I know …** *Having or passing cannabis to someone else or allowing 'my premises' to be used for smoking cannabis is a serious offence.* *Having or passing cannabis oil to someone else is a very serious offence.* *A criminal record for having, passing or allowing the use of cannabis on 'my premises' has the same implications for career or travel as any other drug conviction.*

LSD (Acid)	Health issues	Social issues	Legal issues
I know … Most LSD is sold in small paper squares of blotting paper, although it can come as tiny pills or coloured tablets. LSD is swallowed. LSD is a hallucinogenic drug, making me see and hear differently. This is called **a trip** and may be very pleasant but can be very frightening.	**I know …** *The main risk of LSD is having an accident because I can't make sense of the world whilst under its influence. These include:* ● *road accidents* ● *falls* ● *walking into obstacles.*	**I know …** LSD can be put into my drink without my knowledge. This can amplify the mental risks.	**I know …** LSD is an illegal drug. Having or passing LSD to someone else is a very serious offence.

LSD (Acid)	Health issues	Social issues	Legal issues
A trip can last for six hours or more, and once started cannot be interrupted or shortened.	*If I have a mental problem, even one I don't know about, LSD can make it worse.* LSD can affect my memory and the way my brain functions. Some people have 'flashbacks' or hallucinations many months, or even years, after using LSD.		

Amphetamine sulphate (speed, billy, whizz)	Health issues	Social issues	Legal issues
I know ... Amphetamine is a stimulant drug. It appears to give you energy. Amphetamine can be smoked or swallowed. Because it is usually a powder (it can be a pill), anything could be mixed with it and usually only 3–8% of the powder is amphetamine, the other 92–97% is any powder that is a similar colour.	**I know ...** Amphetamine raises my blood pressure and may lead to haemorrhage or strokes. It is possible that the powder used to bulk out the drug may be harmful to take. After the effects of amphetamine have worn off, I can feel very tired because it does not really give me energy, it only releases my natural energy. Although unusual, some people find it very hard to stop using amphetamine. Long-term use can lead to neural (nerve) damage.	**I know ...** Amphetamine can make some people aggressive. Amphetamine can make some people think others are 'out to get them' (or paranoid).	**I know ...** *Having or passing amphetamine to another is a very serious offence.*

Anabolic steroids	Health issues	Social issues	Legal issues
I know ... These are drugs that build up muscles, although research is still uncertain if these drugs do really improve performance. Some anabolic steroids are produced by the medical industry, some for humans and some for animals. Some anabolic steroids are produced illicitly.	**I know ...** Users can become very aggressive. The use of anabolic steroids may: ● damage my liver ● increase blood pressure ● affect my growth ● damage my reproductive organs ● be difficult to stop	**I know ...** Some users can become aggressive – even extremely violent.	**I know ...** Anabolic steroids are prescribed-only medicines. It is illegal to supply anabolic steroids to others if you are not a pharmacist who is providing them on presentation of a prescription from a doctor. Most are illegal to possess.

Anabolic steroids	Health issues	Social issues	Legal issues
	• put me at risk of HIV and other diseases if I inject with shared syringes.		

It is desirable that students also have background knowledge about the dangers of heroin, cocaine and especially 'crack' or freebase cocaine. These drugs are not normally associated with young people and their use by school-age students remains rare, but trends are liable to sudden changes.

MDMA or 'ecstasy', GHB and ketamine are usually associated with the dance scene. These are less commonly used by school-age students, although the age of experimentation may be dropping. The main risks of these drugs can be found in the generic drugs framework on page 220.

Other popular drugs include amyl and butyl nitrite. These are called 'poppers'. They come in small glass bottles and are inhaled or sniffed. Though not illegal, amyl nitrite is officially a medicine, and should only be dispensed by a pharmacist. The main risks are damage to the heart, especially if the young person has an undiagnosed heart condition or if the popper is drunk rather than inhaled or sniffed. **Drinking poppers is extremely dangerous.**

By the end of Year 11, every student should be able to say:

Heroin	Health issues	Social issues	Legal issues
I know …	I know …	I know …	I know …
Heroin comes from the opium poppy. Heroin is a powerful painkiller. Heroin is usually a brown powder sold in a small, folded paper square. Heroin is a physically addictive drug.	Heroin can be smoked or injected. It is easy to lose control of the use of this drug and become dependent, either by smoking or by injecting. Injecting is dangerous because of potential overdose, adulterants and, if I share the syringe or any other equipment, serious infections.	Dependence on this drug can • be very expensive • draw me into a very poor lifestyle • lead users further into theft, dealing or prostitution in order to raise money.	Possession of heroin, dealing in heroin, or allowing 'my premises' to be used for its use is a very serious offence.

MDMA (ecstasy)	Health issues	Social issues	Legal issues
I know …	I know …	I know …	I know …
MDMA usually comes in tablet form. The effects of MDMA are like a combination of a stimulant and a mild hallucinogen.	There is no safe way of using MDMA. The effects of this drug are still not fully understood, and the risks are unpredictable. There is no way of telling if the tablet I am offered has any MDMA in it, and	Many people are offered or sold other tablets (virtually anything) instead of MDMA. Analysis has shown that some tablets have proved an expensive way to buy a combination of ketamine and caffeine!	Having or passing MDMA to another is a very serious offence.

MDMA (ecstasy)	Health issues	Social issues	Legal issues
	(if it has) how much. Each use of MDMA is a unique event, and previous 'safe use' is no guarantee of future safe use. There is evidence of some young people suffering from depression and other mental illness following the use of MDMA. Although drinking water and staying cool may help prevent heat exhaustion, if I use MDMA in a disco or club, it is still very risky.	Some people feel 'closer to others' when they use MDMA. Some people find it hard to make judgements when using MDMA.	

Sexual health knowledge

Although only a small proportion of students are likely to be sexually active at this time, students will be moving at their own unique rate through and out of puberty, and both their bodies and feelings will continue to undergo significant changes. The media present confusing messages and images about the appropriateness of sexual behaviour among young people, ranging from moral outrage through to a virtual celebration of sexual prowess. As parents recognise their children are on the edge of becoming sexually active beings, many feel deskilled or uncomfortable in discussing sexual behaviour with them. Parents often say, 'This is a place we don't want to go' or, in conversation with their children, are heard to cry out, 'Too much information!'

Schools, therefore, remain a principal source of accurate information. The small numbers of students who do become sexually active in Years 10 and 11 may be at risk. Sexual behaviour may range from mutual masturbation through to, in a minority of cases, sexual intercourse, and the diversity of actual sexual experience within a group will be widening. Apart from issues of legality, bodies are still developing and are especially vulnerable to infection. Early sexual experiences may be fully planned and have been safely and comprehensively prepared, whilst others are opportunistic, *un*planned and *un*prepared with the risk of an unintended pregnancy or infection remaining high. Research suggests that girls remain more knowledgeable than boys at this age and may demonstrate greater maturity. It is essential that boys continue to receive comprehensive sexual health education. In Key Stage 4, an apparently comprehensive knowledge can still mask considerable ignorance. Fictitious sexual exploits and carrying condoms can help create status among boys, but this often masks innocence, confusion and even fear.

By the end of Year 11, every student should be able to say:

Basic issues	Health issues	Social issues	Legal issues
I know …	**I know …**	**I know …**	**I know …**
The physical and emotional changes that take place during adolescence, that these happen at different times for different people and that this is OK.	The menstrual cycle can be erratic and that following intercourse, sperm can live for many days in a woman's body. There is therefore no 'safe' time to have unprotected sexual intercourse; unprotected sexual intercourse may lead to an unintended pregnancy or infection.	*Feelings of attraction towards others of the same sex or opposite sex now or later may be confused; this is quite normal.*	*The law regarding sexual behaviour and how it protects me.*
How sexual intercourse takes place.		*Not everyone feels attraction towards the opposite sex; people are different and have a right to feel differently. All feelings of sexual attraction can change over our lifetimes.*	*Within certain legal boundaries we have a right to choose what we do with our bodies.*
In detail the human reproductive system, including the menstrual cycle and fertilisation.	Younger women and those with multiple sexual partners are among those at a higher risk for chlamydia infection. Early sexual intercourse may increase the chances of infection in both sexes, and later health problems for women, including cervical cancer and infection with chlamydia. (The signs and symptoms of chlamydia can remain hidden.) Chlamydia can lead to pelvic inflammatory disorder and can later lead to ectopic pregnancy or infertility.		*Where to get help if I feel threatened or upset by something that has happened to me, and the consequences of getting help.*
How the foetus develops in the uterus and the role of the placenta.		The potential strength of feelings or emotions at this time of life.	
That sexual intercourse may lead to an unintended pregnancy or sexually transmitted infection (STI).		What the term 'love' means to me and the difference between 'love' and 'lust'.	
How to acquire and put a condom on and have practised this on a model.		Some relationships involve sexual activity and others need not. I do not ever have to have sexual intercourse if I don't want to. Sexual activity that does not involve penetration may be just as satisfying.	
Condoms help lower the risk of infection (but never completely).	'Safer sexual practices' means activities that do not involve body fluids being passed from one body to another. Some activities are 'safer' but few are 'safe'.		
Oral contraceptives will not prevent in any way infection with an STI.		When relationships end it can really hurt.	
Oral contraceptives must be used as directed by a doctor, failure to use them properly may result in a pregnancy.	About cervical smear testing.	Different individuals, families or cultures have different views on what is appropriate or acceptable sexual behaviour.	
If I am worried about my sexual health, the sooner I seek help generally the greater are the choices that I have. I should always seek professional help urgently.	*Comprehensively about contraception and protection from disease, the availability, advantages and disadvantages of different methods.*	*Peers can influence us to become sexually active before we are ready, and many feel the need to pretend to be sexually active in order to gain respect or status. I do not need to pretend about myself or my relationships.*	
Where to get advice and support for issues concerning my sexual health (including gay/lesbian support) and the degree of confidentiality I can expect.	*Comprehensively about STIs, including those we can cure and those we can only treat, and the importance of seeking medical help if we are concerned, knowing that once infected they will not go away even if the*	There is no 'right age' to begin any sexual behaviour, it is up to me.	
If I wish to have sexual intercourse in the future, it is safest to use both		The social, financial, psychological, career and health costs of an unintended pregnancy on both the father and the mother.	

231

Basic issues	Health issues	Social issues	Legal issues
a contraceptive pill to avoid pregnancy and a condom to minimise infection (known as 'double-dutch').	*symptoms do.* *The availability of emergency contraception, where to get it and the limited time within which it is likely to be effective. (I know the failure rate can be as high as 10%.) The difference between emergency contraception and a termination of a pregnancy.*		

Sexually active by 15–16 years old?

By this age, an increasing number of students will be sexually active. We are preparing some for their future health behaviour, for others, we will be providing support for their current health behaviour. We need to help students know the location of support services but, more importantly, help them to access those services. We know that the first contact with any support service is always the most difficult. Ideally, we need to help students meet support services, either through an organised visit or inviting health workers to visit the classroom. Our guidance for all visitors is on page 257.

Know and understand:	Feel:	Say:	Do:
Reinforcement from previous key stages, especially contraception and disease control information. The consequences of pregnancy on lifestyle, finance and career to both father and mother. The responsibility of being a parent, including screening for hereditary and congenital conditions, nutrition during pregnancy and nutrition of newborn. Their own personal ethic with regard to sexual activity, the consequences of this ethic on themselves and others, how it compares with family, friends and the wider society. The contexts within which sexual activity may take place (parties and so on).	Clear about their own personal ethic and feel able to pursue it. Able to recognise and understand our feelings about being with someone or in a group situation where someone, or a member of the group, is considering doing something risky.	• No. • That's OK. • I won't. • Help! Being able to apply our vocabulary of feelings in order to share them with others and being able to tell others about our feelings and concerns.	Practise managing conflict and aggressive behaviour in a variety of situations. Practise being able to make informed decisions about drug use. Assess accurately potential risks from our own and others' sexual behaviour. Experience opportunities to take responsibility for our actions. Be able to access help, if necessary.

Healthy eating

By this age, students are taking greater responsibility for their diet and may soon take this on completely. Many report being dissatisfied with their body image and many report dieting. Food is tied closely to love and care and, for this reason, exploring issues of diet needs great sensitivity. It is vitally important that students understand how critical their diets are to their present and future health. This can be challenging since there is pressure from the media to make certain choices, and because others may decide much of their diet. It is important to be sensitive to students' culture and financial circumstance, and not to give the impression that a poor diet at home reflects a lack of love or care. This resource adopts the position that there are no 'good' and 'bad' foods, rather 'foods you should eat lots of', 'foods you should only have a little of' and 'foods you should eat only every now and again', which may be regarded as 'treats'. Healthy eating is about balance. Treats are, by their very nature, appreciated particularly for their 'occasional' character!

By the end of Key Stage 3, every student should be able to say:

Basic issues	Health issues	Social/cultural issues
I know ...	**I know ...**	**I know ...**
I am what I eat, and what I eat now will have an impact on my present and future health and wellbeing.	In order, the foods I eat most often should be:	There are laws controlling the quality of food and these are monitored by environmental health and trading standards.
Food is arranged in groups:	● bread, cereals, pasta and potatoes (approximately 30–50%)	Food is a massive industry and will aggressively promote its products.
● Milk and dairy foods.	● fruit and vegetables	Different cultures prepare foods in different ways.
● Fruit and vegetables.	● meats, fish and alternatives (proteins should make up about 12% of my diet)	Foods that are acceptable in some cultures are unacceptable in others, sometimes totally unacceptable.
● Bread, cereals, pasta and potatoes.	● milk, dairy foods and alternatives	
● Foods containing fat, foods and drinks containing sugar.	● small amounts of foods containing fat and sugars.	Sometimes farmers in other countries receive only a fraction of the money we pay for a product. 'Fairtrade' products seek to ensure farmers receive a fair price for their produce.
● Meats, fish and alternatives.		
I need a balance of these food groups in order to grow, develop and repair my body.	The main nutrients in:	
Food sold in shops has dates printed on the label that we should know about.	● bread, cereals, pasta and potatoes are carbohydrates (starch), some calcium and iron, vitamin B and fibre	It is possible to eat a healthy vegetarian or vegan diet, as long as I include all the basic nutrients in healthy proportions.
● 'Display until' means that a shop should only display the food for sale until that date.	● fruit and vegetables are carotene, vitamin C, folates and fibre	
● 'Use by' is the date after which it is unsafe to eat fresh food.	● meat, fish and alternatives are iron, protein, vitamin B12, zinc and magnesium	
● 'Best before' indicates that after that date, whilst the food may still be safe, it will not taste as good.	● milk and dairy foods are calcium, protein, vitamin B12 and vitamins A and D.	
These are important to ensure food is safe to eat.	There are different kinds of fats – 'unsaturated' fats (polyunsaturated and monounsaturated) are good for my health, 'saturated' fats (including hydrogenated or	
Many manufacturers have systems (often colour coded) to help us understand the nutritional make		

Basic issues	Health issues	Social/cultural issues
up of food. We need a regular intake of vitamins and minerals within our diet. We need to keep our bodies hydrated; ideally, we should drink between 1.5 and 2 litres of water a day. Many commercial soft drinks contain large amounts of sugar.	trans-fats) are not good for my health (saturated fats are normally solid at room temperature). Some unsaturated fat within my diet is essential to my health. (Omega-3 may be particularly beneficial and comes from oily fish, flaxseed, hemp seed and canola oil.)	

Emotional health

Emotional health could be considered to be enhanced by two types of skill or intelligences: interpersonal skills or having the language and skills to manage our relationships with others; and intrapersonal skills or the skills and understanding to manage our own emotional health. At this time in students' lives, they are likely to be impulsive, find it difficult to empathise with others and experience rapid changes in mood. These are natural, and reflect changes that are happening in their brains as significant reorganisation takes place, especially in the frontal lobes.

Key skills include knowing when we are in charge, when our feelings are trying to take over, and when they have taken over.

We also need to know that, just as we need to be careful what we take into our bodies, we need to be careful what we take into our feelings and our memories.

'Managing bullying' is included in this frame, the context of which could change to include the workplace. It is essential that students understand what is and isn't bullying, the school's policy towards this behaviour, and that they are taught strategies to know when and how to safely confront bullying, and when and how to get help. It is not enough to simply say help is always available. Students need to be given the strategies and language to attract the attention of the appropriate person at a time when they are feeling vulnerable, confused, hurt and perhaps angry or depressed. They also need to know that anyone can behave in a way that is perceived by the other as 'bullying'. We therefore have a responsibility to consider our behaviour, a responsibility to protect others from bullying and a right to live a life free from bullying behaviour.

By the end of Year 11, every student should be able to say:

Basic issues	Health issues	Social issues
I know ... ● *When I am in charge.* ● *When my feelings are trying to take over.* ● **When my feelings are pulling me in more than one direction.** ● *When my feelings have taken over.*	I know ... *If I get mood swings – times when for no reason I feel either really good or really bad – that this is natural.* *If I am worried about how I feel, who I can go to in order to get support.*	I know ... My words and actions can hurt others' feelings, and this can affect their subsequent behaviour towards me. Strategies for avoiding people and situations where my feelings might be hurt.

Basic issues	Health issues	Social issues
Strategies for re-establishing control. Just as I have to be careful what I take into my body, I have to be careful what I take into my feelings and into my memory. My feelings can be hurt as well as my body. An increasingly comprehensive vocabulary to help me express accurately my feelings to others. Being hurt on the inside can be really bad. People can have 'off days' when they feel 'down' or need some space. This doesn't mean they don't like me. The difference between being assertive, aggressive and submissive. *At times, I and others may react without really thinking things through. I need to practise stopping, thinking, thinking a bit more and making a decision before doing.* The difference between when: ● I really don't want to do something (and don't need to and shouldn't have to) ● I really do want to do something but I am frightened to 'give it a go' (including things it might be best for me to try). When I am beginning to feel stressed both in my body and in my feelings. Stress happens to everyone – it comes in at least four types: ● High and wanted – challenge ● High and unwanted – stress ● Low and wanted – relaxation ● Low and unwanted – boredom. Strategies include managing the **causes** of stress (confronting difficulties constructively, managing time, etc.) and managing the **symptoms** of stress (including diversion and relaxation techniques to help me manage my emotions, including stress, and especially to help me stay calm and in control).		Other people's feelings can be hurt badly. *How to give or get support for someone who is really hurting on the inside.* Other people can have mood swings the same as I do. When people really lose their tempers, different parts of their brains have taken over and it can be hard to reason with them. It can be better to wait until everyone calms down. *What the term 'bullying' means and how to manage it if it happens to me, or if I feel it is happening to others, including:* ● *how and when to assertively and safely confront bullying* ● *who to tell if this doesn't work or such a confrontation is (or seems) unsafe* ● *how to attract their attention* ● *what to say and how to persist until I get help* ● *what my school's policy is and what the consequences are (or should be) of me seeking help.*

Learning

The key knowledge about how we learn is likely to be taught throughout the whole curriculum. Being prepared for a future where constant change will demand lifelong learning will require students to be 'experts' in learning. Perhaps the most important skill students can acquire in school is that of 'learning', and then acquiring the motivation to develop and practise that skill.

Many students have no idea how their brains work and how to learn in 'brain-friendly ways'. If we want students to be partners in learning, this lack of knowledge is ridiculous. Although it is beyond the scope of this resource, many schools are building the concept of coaching throughout their entire schools, with all members sharing responsibility for everyone's learning.

If we are to demand that students take examinations, we also have a responsibility to provide them with the most sophisticated revision and examination techniques. A critical skill that is often missed is helping students to manage their emotions and achieve a 'performance state'. Just as no sports coach would ever allow a top-class athlete to compete without appropriate emotional preparation to get 'in the zone', no student should enter an examination without adequate emotional preparation.

It is extraordinary that many schools still consider that simply extensive academic revision is sufficient to control emotions during examinations and to ensure an optimal performance state. Since the areas of the brain that generate anxiety or fear (the limbic system) will impede (we get confused or forgetful) or override (our brain goes totally blank) the areas of the brain that support higher order thinking (the neo-cortex), helping students to stay calm and focused seems common sense. Sadly, many examinations are as much a measure of how we manage performance under artificial stress as they are a measure of our true ability.

By the end of Year 11, every student should be able to say:

Basic issues

I know ...

I learn with my brain, which requires food, fresh air, rest and sleep and fresh water.

I can learn how to use my brain.

When I learn my brain physically grows, I can never 'fill it up' and it can carry on learning all my life.

We all learn in different ways and I know which ways I learn best.

Why my teachers structure lessons in the way they do, and why the beginnings and endings of lessons are so important.

Learning often happens in 'bursts' and getting stuck is OK, it often means I am about to learn something new.

There is no 'failure' only 'success' or 'new learning' – when I 'fail', I have learnt that a strategy doesn't lead to success.

How to manage my self-esteem and motivation when success seems hard to find – how to stick at it!

How to organise my independent learning, both in terms of physical space and time management.

When I learn best on my own, with another person or in a group – how to give and receive 'coaching' to and from my peers.

How to access and assess the quality of different sources of information.

Basic issues

My brain learns by making connections, and a variety of techniques such as 'mind mapping'™ can help me organise these connections.

Regular review and practice strengthens these connections and increases my ability to recall and perform.

How to make accurate and concise notes.

How to revise effectively, including:

- constructing a revision timetable that structures in regular review loops (revise constructing notes or mind maps™, review notes one hour later, 24 hours later, seven days later and one month later to fix the information in my mind)

- how to construct revision notes (especially mind maps™)

- the importance of 'active revision' including setting myself my own questions or challenges and answering/meeting them

- how to construct and use mnemonics to help me remember.

Good examination techniques, including how to ensure a positive and resourceful state of mind when I enter an examination, to always read the instructions and how to use the available time to maximise my marks.

Aspects of personal safety

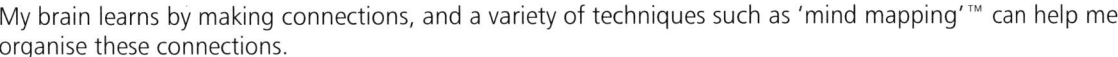

Most of us go through life without ever being physically attacked, but students are in one of the highest risk groups. Again, it is a balance. These are some key considerations to help keep students safe when out, perhaps on a date, and in the workplace, where young people are among the highest risk group for accidents.

It is important not to over-exaggerate issues of personal risk to avoid the risk of being ignored. Perhaps it is better approached by offering these suggestions and asking students what they think of them. Staying safe is not about stopping young people from having a great time, but the reverse: it is about ensuring that young people stay safe so that they can have great times.

This is also one of those issues where we might need to challenge 'hormones'. It can be difficult for a young person who perhaps is really attracted to someone they have just met to recognise that they are a 'stranger', and that it might be a bit early to offer them their trust. Most personal safety is common sense, but taking sensible precautions needs to become a habit and it is easy to get complacent.

Before I meet someone

If I arrange or agree to meet someone I have only recently met, I need to honestly ask myself:

- how well do I know this person?
- do I know them well enough to be meeting them at this location? Could I still have a great time but meet in a safer location?
- if our meeting/date doesn't seem to be working out, or if I feel uncomfortable, can I get home safely?

When I go out

I know, in my preparation, to think:

- about my style of dress – is it appropriate? Might it make me vulnerable? Can I change at my destination?

- about my journey – are there risks? Do I know exactly where I am going? If I am meeting someone, do I know exactly where and when? Can I travel with someone I trust? If I am travelling alone, can I put myself in places where there are other people – for example in a more crowded railway carriage?

- about how I will plan to get home, especially if it is going to be late at night. If someone is picking me up, do they know exactly where and when?

- about my personal belongings. If I am carrying an expensive mobile phone and I think it could make me a target, do I keep it hidden unless I am using it? Am I showing jewellery or a watch that might make me a target? If I am carrying money, do I keep it hidden rather than show it off? Am I carrying sufficient money to get home safely, especially if I need a taxi?

- about whether I choose to use alcohol or other drugs. Will they impair my ability to stay safe?

- about whether someone always knows where I have gone and what time I am expected to arrive or to get home. (This is not to control or limit you, it is to identify when something may be wrong and will enable someone to action help. Pilots call this 'filing a flight plan'.)

- about needing to carry a mobile phone, with credit and a fully charged battery, but not to 'flash it about', especially if it is an expensive one

- about whether I am intending to ring someone for a lift home. Do they know in advance that this is my plan?

- about carrying a small torch, for example on a key ring

- about carrying a small 'attack alarm'.

The issue of knives is also raised in the Year 10 action planner, box **K13**. A suggested session to expand this box is on page 107.

When in the street

I know:

- to stay 'threat aware'. (This just means being aware of your surroundings and not day-dreaming!)

- to avoid wearing headphones that might restrict my hearing, especially when crossing roads

- to walk confidently with my head raised

- without staring, to make quick eye contact to let other people know I am aware of them

- to occasionally look behind me

- that if I am asked by a stranger for the time, to say 'I don't have a watch' or 'My watch isn't working' and walk on. (This is a common prequel to a mugging, you look down at your watch, are distracted and they attack.)

- that if a car stops and the driver asks for directions, to step back, say I am not from around here and walk on, and never to lean into a car to look at a map.

When using minicabs or taxis

I know:

- to find out the numbers of my local licensed minicab and taxi services and store them on my mobile phone, so that they are always at hand

- to make sure a minicab is licensed, pre-book it, ensure the driver knows my name when he/she turns up and look for the official licence markings (these can be different in each region – check with the local police)

- that if I accept a lift from a minicab that I have not pre-booked, it is highly likely that I will not be insured in an accident

- when booking a minicab, to ask for the driver's name and colour/make of car so that when I get picked up, I will know that I am getting into the right licensed cab that I ordered
- to arrange with my friends to share a taxi home, as it's always safer to travel in a group and cheaper to split the cab fare between several people
- never to let my friends get into an illegal cab as the driver may pose a threat to their safety.

When in a club

I know:

- never to leave my drink unattended in case someone adds something to it
- never to accept a drink from a stranger, even if I really fancy them! (If someone offers to buy me a drink, I know to go to the bar with him or her.)
- not to leave with a stranger or accept a lift home from a stranger, no matter how fantastic they seem!

When in the workplace

I know:

- to recognise when using my initiative is a good idea, and when using my initiative might put me or others at risk
- to always follow all safety procedures I have been trained in, no matter how stupid or time consuming I may think they are
- to talk to my line manager if I think there is a risk to my own or others' safety
- to talk to my line manager or my personnel department if I am asked to do something that I feel uncomfortable about.

Self-esteem

Self-esteem is best thought of as a 'disposition' – a set of beliefs about ourselves (self-beliefs) that enable us to confidently utilise all of our other inner resources.

There are many models of self-esteem, but perhaps the most useful for teachers is to consider self-esteem as the gap between our image of ourselves (self-image) and our ideal image of what we feel we would like to be, or perhaps should be. Both of these images are likely to be constructed as a result of external messages from a variety of sources, including peers, teachers, family and media. These messages are accepted or rejected, depending on the existing self-esteem of the individual. Individuals with low self-esteem can feed off negative messages and reject positive messages as being incongruent with their self-belief. Individuals with high self-esteem can feed off positive messages and reject negative messages for the same reason. We are always working with an existing level of self-esteem; no one is empty of self-esteem, and so we must be sensitive to the learners' existing self-image and beliefs. Our level of self-esteem is likely to impact on our:

- self-efficacy, how capable we feel about carrying out tasks
- self-regulation, how willing we are to reflect on ourselves and our work
- locus of control, our beliefs about the degree of control we have over our lives
- ability to form productive relationships with others.

If we consider the above model, we might have three tasks.

1 To ensure that the student's ideal image is realistic, whilst still providing an aspiration. If the ideal image is potentially destructive, for example an aggressive bully, the image would need to be deconstructed to find out the attractive qualities ('They are popular and I want to be popular'), and then possibly reframed ('Are they really popular or are people really afraid of them? What makes people popular? How could I be like that?') If the ideal image is unattainable, once again it would need to be deconstructed, the positive qualities identified and some form of reframing take place. ('What is it about them that makes them attractive? How could you get the same thing in your life?')

2 To ensure that the student's self-image is as accurate as possible. We need to strike a balance, challenging limiting self-beliefs, promoting a belief in the student's ability to control their own destiny, helping to make that destiny aspirational, but not creating an over-confidence that might lead to inappropriate choices or risk taking.

Although we need to provide opportunities specifically to help students focus on their self-esteem, a metaphor for the building of self-esteem is 'filo pastry' – building layer upon layer. If we think in terms of building layers, another powerful metaphor for self-esteem is a 'laminate' that is very strong. We build or damage self-esteem layer by layer through messages received from the curriculum, the protocols and procedures the school adopts and the overall school culture.

3 To build students' self-esteem on the widest possible raft of 'pillars'. The notion of self-esteem resting on pillars is a useful metaphor. If our self-esteem is built on only one high pillar, should something happen to that pillar, our self-esteem quite literally crashes. (For example, redundancy if self-esteem is built solely on excellence in a particular career; or a debilitating sports injury if self-esteem is built solely on excellence in sports.) The more pillars our self-esteem is built upon, the greater the resilience if one pillar should fall. In schools we need to ensure that we celebrate as widely as possible our students' achievements.

Beliefs about ourselves are likely to lie in more 'primitive' parts of the brain and are therefore less susceptible to reason. A single word or cutting remark from a significant other can damage our self-esteem, even though our reason tells us it is unimportant. However, to separate the limbic system from the neo-cortex and the conscious mind from the unconscious mind is a mistake; they are all part of the same system. Therefore, although events that hurt us emotionally may continue to hurt us, having an understanding or mental models to help us rationalise why we are being hurt can also be protective. Understanding our self-esteem is therefore part of 'learnacy'.

If our self-esteem is built or damaged through the micro-interactions that take place in the school, then every single event in the life of the student could raise or damage self-esteem. If we truly want to enable students to develop a positive self-image and an empowering set of self-beliefs, we need to examine every single aspect of the life of the school from the macro (overall school aims and objectives) to the micro (the individual words heard by a student). We also need to recognise low self-esteem as a 'special need' and worthy of intervention.

The following framework is not 'developmental', although some parts would need a careful selection of language and pedagogy to be explored with younger students. It is a manifestation of high self-esteem. At different ages we could expect to see any of these being exhibited in different ways. The framework could be used either as a planning guide for teachers to consider how they could help a student attain this descriptor, or as a diagnostic framework to identify whether a student is showing evidence that they are 'struggling with', 'starting to work towards' or 'now attaining' the descriptor. These descriptors are not in a hierarchy nor do they read across the columns.

We know self-esteem is being built when every student can say:

I know and understand these things …	I believe and feel like this …	I am able to say these things …	I am able to do these things …	I have these experiences …
I know what makes me feel good about myself. I know I am as valuable as anyone else, no more, no less – my beliefs and opinions are of equal worth and I have a right to be heard. Because I know this to be true, I do not need to compete with others to have my voice heard over theirs. I have a comprehensive language of emotion. This allows me to differentiate between and precisely identify my feelings. I am then able to articulate these feelings to others. I understand cognitively, and have a mental model for, the concept of 'self-esteem'. I understand how my self-belief can be built or damaged. Although I may still be hurt by events or remarks, I understand what is happening inside me and can rationalise what is going on.	I like me and I can tell you why. I feel good about what I am good at; I feel OK about what I am not so good at yet. I feel good about getting better at these things. I believe there is no such thing as failure, only success and new learning that enables me to try different strategies. Because of this, my self-esteem is built on my successes rather than others' perceived failures. I value all of my life's successes within the school and outside school. I recognise that society needs success in a wide variety of fields and that the academic is only one. I feel OK to change my perception of myself – I recognise that change happens and that I can instigate and manage change.	I can tell you when I am feeling good and when I am feeling not so good. I can tell you what I am good at, what I am not so good at and why I feel this way. I can tell you the things I want to learn, the things I don't want to learn, and why.	I can openly accept appreciation and praise and store it so that I have the resilience to be undamaged by occasional adverse criticism or put-downs. I am able to differentiate between those people whose opinions of me I need to consider or accept and those I may (or even should) ignore. I am able to accept and grow from appropriate feedback and ignore or remain undamaged by inappropriate or hurtful opinions. Because I am good at lots of things, I am able to cope if I sometimes don't succeed in something or receive a setback. Because I can offset the occasional criticism from others against a wealth of positive experiences and praise, I can maintain a sense of perspective.	I attend a school that recognises that high self-esteem and its associate components are essential for creating 'lifelong learning' – it is therefore a planned, managed, monitored and evaluated part of the life of the school. I have a network of 'others' who show me that they value me and will support me when I am in need. I have teachers who enable me to develop my self-knowledge and my own value system. I attend a school that believes in offering me choices – I share control over how I learn. My teachers recognise that I am an individual and what builds my self-esteem may be unique to me. I attend a school that values all of my abilities, not just the academic.

I know and understand these things ...	I believe and feel like this ...	I am able to say these things ...	I am able to do these things ...	I have these experiences ...
I know what I am good at and what I am not so good at yet. I understand clearly what success looks, sounds or feels like, especially when I am working to someone else's criteria. I know and understand what criteria my teacher uses for 'good'. I know what I want to be like. I know where my ideals come from – I know which I chose, which were given to me (or demanded of me) by others, and which I might be 'catching' from other sources such as the media. If my ideal image is embodied in a role model, I understand that I may only know a little bit about them – they may be far more complex than I believe. If I have a role model, I recognise that I can admire some parts of them or parts of what they do but not necessarily all them or their behaviour. I can model the bits I like and leave the rest.	I feel able to change my ideal image – to let go of unhelpful images and replace them with more helpful or achievable images. When I am given a new responsibility, I believe I have the skills to carry it out or am confident I can learn them. I believe, as I grow up, that I will have increasing control over my own destiny. I will have choices in my life.		I am confident to take risks – but I am able to carefully assess these risks against my abilities. I am neither overly timid nor over confident. I can recognise what is a realistic aspiration – 'I can achieve this' and I recognise what may be an inspiring aspiration – 'I may not be able to achieve this but striving for it could be worthwhile.' I can see that in life 'big successes' may not be frequent and are often made up of lots of small successes. I can take pleasure from even the smallest of my successes or achievements, and I can 'aim high'. When I feel not so good, I have positive strategies for sharing my feelings with others and examining their cause.	I attend a school that recognises that I am not my behaviour – my behaviour depends on the social context I find myself in – but it is not 'me'. I attend a school that recognises that the very smallest exchange between two people can significantly boost or significantly damage my self-esteem when I feel vulnerable. I attend a school that identifies 'low self-esteem' as a 'special need' requiring suitable intervention. I attend a school that believes in success or feedback to inform new strategies. There is no 'failure' in my school. My school promotes this belief with parents and carers. Because of this, I feel able to take risks with my learning.

The language of persuasion

It is important not to be too cynical about language. Most people mean well and have our best interests at heart. However, with the internet and television allowing global communication into our homes or even bedrooms 24 hours a day, we need to encourage students to recognise language that may be attempting to manipulate them, their beliefs and their behaviour. Young people, many of whom are seeking meaning in life and shaping their adult identity, are especially vulnerable to this.

The use of persuasive language is the subject of rigorous study. Courses on persuasive language are offered to sales personnel, speech writers, the advertising industry and others. As with any technique, language can be used ethically – to support, empower people (therapists and coaches) and increase people's choices – or unethically, to influence, manipulate, limit people's choices and gain power over them. It is possible to be influenced by these patterns even when we read them. Most of us create a voice or voices in our heads when we read, and we know that the written word can significantly change serotonin levels in our brains and hence our moods. (If in doubt, try reading a really sad novel or, better still, a good comedy!)

What is said ...	What may be meant ...	Challenge with ...
'Everyone does ...'	'We do and we want you to as well.'	What? Everyone?
'Everyone knows ...'	'We believe something is true and we want you to believe it too!'	What? Everyone?
'By now I think it is generally agreed that ...' Variations include: 'There is wide acceptance of ...'; 'All "right thinking" people believe ...'; and 'Intelligent people such as yourself know ...'	'I think it and I am trying to convince you that if you don't agree with me, you are odd and wrong!' This is loved by politicians and is usually delivered in a very 'reasonable' and sincere voice.	Agreed by whom? Accepted by whom? How do you know? Who have you asked? Even if most people do agree (and they often don't), this statement tries to argue that 'agreement' = 'truth'. There was a time when most people believed the earth was flat. It isn't!
'They say ...'	Be wary of 'generalisations' or times when someone claims everyone in a group of people 'say', 'think' or 'do' the same.	Who precisely are 'they'? How do you know what 'they' think? All of them? Why should you accept what 'they' say?
'You want ... (a truth)' 'You want ... (a truth)' You want ... (a truth) 'You want ...'(What I want you to want.) Variations include: 'You know... (a truth)'	This is called a 'yes set' or 'agreement set' and is *very* powerful. It can be used unscrupulously in advertising, sales and politics for example. It begins with three statements that the speaker knows you will accept as truth. (These statements may be so general that people can interpret them in their own way, see 'fat language' below.) The fourth statement is then added and, if you're not careful, your brain will simply accept this as another truth. This technique is especially powerful in a group situation that is also caught up in the language pattern, and is even more powerful if there is fast pace to the language and quick reinforcers without offering any thinking time.	This is hard to challenge because others may be caught up in the pattern. You may find you are the only one who is saying to yourself, 'Hang on a minute, that doesn't follow'. You need to listen for them. When you catch them being used, be very, very wary. Someone is trying to manipulate you and what you think or believe.

What is said …	What may be meant …	Challenge with …
'You know… (a truth)' 'You know … (a truth)' 'You know…'(What I want you to believe is true.) If people react positively, it is often quickly reinforced with a positive comment: 'Great decision.' 'That's right!' 'We know, don't we?'	It can also be used ethically by coaches to encourage positive performance states: 'We have trained hard. We know our techniques. We are good at this. We are going to be great today!'	Ethical people will always show you respect, welcome questions and give you space and thinking time.
'You should …' 'You ought …' 'You must …'	'I think you should, ought or must do what I think is best for you.' Clearly, this can be helpful advice ('You really should look before crossing the road') or it can be manipulative ('You ought to give this a try.')	If in doubt, ask yourself: 'What if I didn't? What would be the consequences to me and to others? How do I feel about those consequences?'
'We all want to have fun!' 'We all want to enjoy ourselves!' 'We all want truth, justice, freedom, etc.' 'We all believe in education!' 'We all want to be healthy!' 'We all want to be rich!' 'We all want the best for our children!'	'I don't care how you interpret what I am saying; I just want you to believe that we think the same way, have the same values and want the same things so that you will support me.' This is sometimes called 'fat language'. They are words that are so open to interpretation that most of us can't help but agree, even if we later discover we all interpreted it in our own unique way. (Is one person's understanding of 'health' or 'education' the same as another person's? Actually it is fairly unlikely.) Manipulative people may target their language to appear to offer solutions to others' fears. (For example in a time of fear of redundancy, 'You want to be able to support the people you love!' etc.) This is even more powerful when combined with an agreement set above.	Any disagreement or challenge is often met with incredulity or even ridicule. 'You mean you *don't* want …' The last thing the speaker wants is to be detailed or specific and they may attempt to make you look stupid. You need to unpick 'fat language' and understand the details before you offer your agreement or support. Challenge the speaker by asking: 'What *precisely* do you mean by …?' 'How *exactly* do you propose we get …?' What *exactly* are the consequences to me and others of …?'

What is said ...	What may be meant ...	Challenge with ...
'We all think …'	'… and therefore so should you!' If you are with a group that believes something to be true, you can come under real pressure to agree (or 'conform'). Sometimes it is in a group's interests to recruit new members. The more people who agree with the group, the more its beliefs are strengthened. 'If so many people agree with us, we must be right.' (This is the difference between 'a popular belief' and 'something that is actually true'.) The power of conforming to 'group norms' should not be underestimated. It is possible to convince an individual to agree that $2+2=5$ or that red is green if 30 of their peers confidently state this is the correct answer. If just one other person disagrees, the 'spell' can be broken. (This should not be tried in the classroom – it will leave that individual in a very vulnerable position!) You should be very wary of groups that want you to keep things secret from other people you know or trust. Be very wary of groups who discourage or don't allow open discussion with others, or want to control or limit your behaviour. This is often about their own insecurity and need for power over you.	'Can we agree to be friends but differ on this issue?' If the answer is yes, great; if the answer is no, then ask 'Why not?' Assert: 'I don't want to be a friend of someone who makes conditions about what I think or believe!'
'So you don't find it easy to agree with what I am saying?'	'So you find it easy to agree with what I am saying.' This is a clever form of language used by people who understand that the brain tends to delete negatives. (Don't think of a pink elephant right now. I said *don't* think of a pink elephant!) Someone who is highly trained will 'analogue mark' the word 'don't', perhaps slightly softening it in the sentence and then slightly strengthen 'agree with what I am saying'.	'I find it easy to disagree with what you are saying!'
'I am right, aren't I?' 'This is true, isn't it?' 'You agree, don't you?' Variations include: 'You know this makes sense, don't you?' 'You know this is the right thing to do, don't you?' 'You know this is (… you are making …) the right choice, don't you?'	This is an advanced technique. This appears to be a question but with a clever trick; it becomes a command that transmits authority and implies agreement or compliance. The trick is how the question is finished. When we ask a genuine question in English we finish the question by raising the tone of our voice. When we give a command we lower the tone of our voice at the end of our sentence. If we use what is known as a 'command tone', a question becomes a command and more difficult to challenge.	'Are you really asking me for my opinion or are you telling me that you are right?'

Economic wellbeing and the world of work

In this new section, only the knowledge believed to be essential has been offered. It is likely that you will want to broaden and deepen this knowledge within your own programme. This section could be taught in earlier years.

Personal issues My finances	Social issues
I know ... How to set up my own bank (or similar) account and why I need one. Criteria for choosing a provider for a bank account. What a National Insurance number is, how I get one and what it is used for. What sources of funding are available for further education and how to access these. What sources of funding are available if I need to borrow money in the future, and what the implications are for me of borrowing such money.	**I know ...** How to calculate compound interest, so that I can see the true cost of borrowing money over a period of time. Who I can talk to or meet with if I have questions over my personal finances and want accurate impartial advice or guidance. The principles of taxation as they will affect me and who has responsibility for ensuring that my taxation is correct. What 'credit rating' means and the implications of having a poor 'credit rating'. How to purchase safely on the internet. The difference between credit and debit cards. To keep 'pin numbers' secret and to keep them, my debit and credit cards and cheque book separate at all times. How to use 'automated cash dispensers' safely. The advantages and disadvantages of using credit and debit cards in the future. What the terms 'retirement' and 'pension' mean, and why it is important for me to think about them while I am still young.

Me as a consumer	Social issues
I know ... My rights as a consumer. How to make a complaint if I feel I have been treated unfairly.	**I know ...** Who I can approach locally for support if I believe my rights as a consumer are being infringed.

Me as an applicant	Social issues
I know ... How to write a letter of application, complete an application form and produce a curriculum vitae. What I need to disclose to a future employer if I have a criminal conviction. When legally I can take up, and how to apply for, part-time employment if I wish to work at weekends of during holidays.	**I know ...** Where I can get accurate information, help, advice and guidance about future college places or future employment. Appropriate websites that offer accurate, impartial advice to help me broaden my choices. How to conduct myself in an interview in ways that will enable me to fully demonstrate my knowledge and skills. What a 'CRB check' is and when an employer is likely to ask for one.

Me at college or work	Social issues
	I know ...
	That organisations have 'health and safety' policies that I must respect for my own and my colleagues' safety, and that failing to do so could have very serious (including legal) consequences for me and others.
	That colleges and employers are required to address issues such as 'bullying in the workplace', 'discrimination' and 'equality of opportunity'.
	What to do, and what support is available to me inside and outside an organisation if I think an employer or college has treated me unfairly or inappropriately.
	The role of unions and professional associations and how they can support me.

Internet safety

To many students communication through ICT is a major part of their lifestyle, and telling them simply not to use it is not an option. However, many are quite naive when it comes to managing their own safety online. The internet offers instant communication between peers across the globe and is treated, quite rightly, by many students as a huge 'playground' for gathering information and social networking.

There are, however, serious risks to personal privacy and emotional and physical safety. There is a sense that, if we are accessing ICT from the privacy of our own home and possibly using a fictitious e-mail name, we are anonymous, the sites we visit and files we download are only known to us. In fact the reverse is true. Our own research revealed that there was considerable ignorance, even among our most able students, of the risks they were running with their use of ICT. Young people will often 'upload' personal information, details or images, not fully understanding how widespread the availability of this data becomes. Images that are amusing as a young person may seem less so in years to come, and the sharing of sexually explicit images, especially of a minor, even among minors, can be a very serious offence with lifelong consequences.

Bullying using ICT should not be treated as a separate issue from the school's general approach to bullying. The intention and behaviours are the same, it is just the medium and potential to be relentless that is different. As with any bullying, it is important to separate the initial bullying from 'revenging'. Cyber attacks can allow previously powerless individuals who have been bullied to strike back from a distance. Because mobile phones are constantly carried and many young people access computers in their bedrooms, it can be really hard to get away from hurtful, abusive or bullying communications. If we are experiencing bullying using ICT, we can be confronted with it virtually 24 hours a day and it can penetrate every location in our lives. It is important that schools have clear policies about the use of ICT and support for students who feel at risk through this medium.

Note: This is a new section and may also need to be taught in earlier years.

Using my mobile phone	Being tracked back	Sharing files with others
I know …	**I know …**	**I know …**
To share my mobile phone number only with people who I trust. Images or videos taken on a mobile phone and shared with others can be recorded and passed on to people I do not know, or put on the internet where they can stay forever. To keep a record of any annoying or hurtful texts or messages and who I can report these to.	Whenever I use the internet I leave tracks, like digital footprints. These can be used to pin down what I have been doing, which sites I look at, who I was chatting to and where I log on from. I know I am not anonymous when I am on the internet. Every website can keep a record of the computers that look at it. Every e-mail I send passes through other people's computers. There are special programs capable of monitoring what I am doing. Some computers have 'spy-ware' that can track everything I type. Every internet-connected computer is identified by a number, called an IP.	That some file sharing is illegal and when I am breaking national or international copyright laws. That file sharing might open private files on my computer for others to access. Passing images of other people could be a serious offence if the image is sexually explicit. If the image is of a 'minor', it is considered in law as passing child pornography, with the risk of a conviction and my name appearing on the sex offenders' register. (Images taken and shared 'for a laugh' can have very serious consequences.)

Protecting my privacy	Visiting chat rooms	If I need help or support
I know …	**I know …**	**I know …**
If registering with a website, never to give personal details such as my home address, telephone or mobile phone numbers, bank account details, images of myself or others or my e-mail address if I do not trust the site completely. To respect the privacy of others and not share their personal details or images online. Reputable internet sites should offer a privacy policy. However, even reputable sites can be faked. To always cover or switch off any webcam when I am not using it, and to be careful who is watching me and what I am doing when it is switched on. That images captured by others from my webcam can be shared with people I do not know and put on websites. That, in the future, others might carry out an 'internet search' using my name to produce a quick and cheap character reference on me. Unexpected e-mails *no matter who they claim to be from* asking me to provide my personal or financial details are always fake. I know not to reply to any such	That I should never give any personal information (such as personal address, postcode, school details, telephone or mobile phone numbers), share images of myself or others or agree to meet with anyone I meet in a chat room or through a messenger service. If I do decide to meet someone, I should only agree to meet them in a public place and take along someone I trust.	Who I can ask for help within school. Who I can ask for help outside of school. For example, The Child Exploitation & Online Protection Centre (CEOP) – a division of the Serious Crime Squad with international links.

Protecting my privacy	Visiting chat rooms	If I need help or support
requests but, instead, either delete them at once, or visit the company, bank or organisation's website to find their instructions for spoof e-mails and follow them. I know to telephone the company to check if I am in any doubt. I know financial institutions will not phone me and then ask for personal details. If I receive a call from someone claiming to be a bank or building society asking me for passwords or account details, I know to hang up and then phone the bank myself.		

3.4 Future pacing: imagining your future

Through PSHE, it is hoped that students are able to access their beliefs and to recall and confidently use their knowledge, language and social strategies at critical moments. This is a valuable asset for life. Adults, too, often know exactly what they should have said or done, or even always intended or wanted to do, after a situation is over.

The benefit of the technique known as 'future pacing' is that, at the end of any session, after the reflection, teachers can facilitate students to imagine a future time where they are using what has been covered in the session.

> **Future pacing**, a technique widely used in sports coaching, can be very powerful. Because PSHE explores sensitive issues, you need to use it with care, especially in a group situation. Do not use the technique if you have any reservations about the reaction of any member of the group. Instead, use role play or have a discussion about a character.

What is future pacing?

Future pacing is what happens when we use our imaginations to travel safely into our own future and rehearse a strategy. A 'future pace' might be thought of as similar to a short guided fantasy or visualisation. However, for some people, it might be a more auditory than visual, or even a more kinaesthetic, imagined experience.

It is suggested that this technique is used sparingly, when you have explored with students a specific situation, language or skill you want to strengthen. It can be very helpful in exploring situations that have an outcome people really want. For example:

- going to a party and being confident about walking in and socialising
- being able to approach someone you really like or need to talk to about something important
- going into an examination feeling calm and positive.

It is important that students see the situation in their imagination as if they are 'seeing it through their own eyes' or experiencing it in real time. This is known as being 'associated'. Being associated is different from imagining 'watching yourself' in a situation – known as being 'dissociated'. Here is a simple explanation of the difference:

'Supposing somebody stood by the door of this classroom and took a photograph of all of us. We could all look at the photograph and we would all be able to see ourselves in the picture. However, right now, I can see each of you and each of you can see me, but none of us can see ourselves. We're able to see bits of ourselves, say by looking at our hands or our feet, but because we're actually here, looking through our own eyes, of course none of us can see our whole self.

We're going to do an interesting exercise that involves imagining something as though we're actually there – rather than looking at a picture of ourselves in the situation.'

Because we are encouraging students to be 'fully associated' into a situation, it is important to be very sensitive to the use of this technique – because when people are fully associated, they will often feel the feelings involved in the situation.

Here is a carefully worded script that you can use. Of course, it is only one possible script. However, if you use something different, it is important to follow the same principles as in this script. **Most importantly, remember to avoid suggesting specific content for what the students are seeing, hearing or feeling in the situation they are future pacing to**. Notice how neutral language has been used in the script.

In this script, the words in **bold** type should be emphasised in order to help students quickly direct their thoughts.

You are going to **use your imagination** – for the next [5–10 minutes] you are going to be encouraged to daydream in a lesson! Some of you might find it easier to do this, and **do it really well**, if you **close your eyes now**, although some of you will find that you can **do it really well even if your eyes are open** – you might be curious as to which sort of person you are.

Imagine that you are going to make a film or a soap about the type of situation we've been looking at, talking about and exploring today. I'm going to ask you lots of questions to help you think about what's happening, but you can **do it without answering me out loud.**

You are on the set now. You are the scriptwriter, the director and the star! You are going to give it a happy ending for your character, an ending that's really good for you – one that you really want.

As you are there on the set, the action starts to happen for you as your character. What's happening? What can you see? What can you hear? What are people doing? Some directors and actors **notice things in the scene and see them very clearly**, some directors and actors **get more tuned into the dialogue** – others **just feel you know everything that's happening**. What's happening now? What is your character feeling right now? What are you feeling as that person? OK … pause the action on the set.

You can relax because with the action stopped you can decide how you are going to make it end the way you want to. You can **enjoy your ability to do that**. What are you going to say and do next? You are going to be able to use everything we thought about during the session to make it end well for you. Now start the action again and make it happen …

Notice what you are saying. What you are doing. Notice what other people say and do. Keep it going (or run the scene) till you get the ending that's good for you. Notice how you feel when that happens.

Now end the scene and **come back** from the set and **be yourself, in the classroom** with all of us. If your eyes have been closed, **open your eyes now**. Look around at everybody and listen to me.

Of course, **you know** right here, **right now** in the classroom, **that action on the set isn't really happening**. However, you can think about what you've brought back from when **you just imagined it** that you know would be useful in real life in the future – and in different situations from what **you just imagined**.

3.5 Using visitors in the PSHE classroom

The use of visitors in the classroom is an important part of many schools' PSHE programmes. Teachers cannot be expected to have a complete and current knowledge of every topic covered by a comprehensive programme, especially in the 15–16 age range.

As with any piece of learning, the questions to ask yourself when deciding whether to invite someone to visit your class are: 'What am I trying to achieve?' followed by 'Is inviting a visitor the best way to organise this learning?' and 'Can this visitor provide something worthwhile that I can't?'

It is important to think about a visitor as a classroom resource and not a substitute teacher. The term 'visitor' rather than 'speaker' is used because, while some professional organisations train their personnel who are expected to work with young people, many do not. Many of your visitors will therefore have had little or no training or experience.

Students will benefit not only from the expertise, experience and factual knowledge the visitor brings, but from interacting with someone they have not met before to gain insights or information that is relevant to them. For this reason, bringing a visitor into the classroom should be an active rather than passive experience. The skills of selecting and interacting with a visitor are transferable, whilst the actual information they impart may swiftly date.

What can a visitor bring to the classroom?

- They can bring knowledge and expertise that you as a teacher do not have, nor should be expected to have.
- They can act as an expert witness, recounting events in their lives from a personal or professional perspective.
- They have novelty value and we know the brain recalls novelty. If you try to remember visitors from your own classroom when you were a child, the chances are that you can recall them and have an impression of what type of person they were. The chances are also quite strong that you can't remember much of what they actually said.
- They can establish a 'first contact' to a helping agency. For example, it can be hard for a student to approach any source of support 'cold'. Establishing a relationship in a classroom session can help to overcome this.

Planning the session

As the session facilitator, regardless of who is working with your students, you are responsible for managing the learning.

Students are always learning at a variety of levels. For example, a visitor will not only be providing their input, they will be transmitting and modelling messages about who they are and also the values of whoever they represent officially or by association. When you invite a visitor to work with students you get the whole package, not just the content of their input.

What messages, spoken and unspoken, are being transmitted to students by an interesting, dynamic and charismatic recovered habitual drug user with a fascinating and exciting life story, and who is now invited to speak to large audiences?

Some essential considerations

- *Who are the people I am inviting into my session?*
- *What skills, needs, expectations, experiences or knowledge do they bring?*
- *How do I know?*

These are essential factors to consider. Never confuse a leaflet, a fantastic website or the written testimonials of other teachers or headteachers (unless you can contact them in person) with the expertise needed to work with your students.

If the visitor brings a body of knowledge, does it come with a personal message or set of attached values? Do you know what these are and are they in harmony with your school policies? It is important not to confuse 'passionate and well intentioned' with 'appropriate and skilled'.

Is a visitor happy to act as a 'resource' with you managing the learning, or do they expect to run the whole session? If they do run the session, are you confident that they have the teaching and classroom management skills to do this with this particular age group, in your community, with students they have never met before?

If the visitor has been endorsed by another organisation, ask yourself what confidence you can have in that organisation to assess the visitor's ability to work with your students. Does that organisation have the expertise to really make a valid assessment?

In an ideal world, you should try to watch any visitor work in a similar learning environment before confirming their visit to your session, but more realistically ask what other local schools or settings they have worked in and talk to professional colleagues in that school or setting.

Negotiation

If you think there might be any professional role conflict, this needs sorting out before the session takes place and ground rules renegotiated if necessary with the students attending the session.

- *Does this visit fit into and build on my scheme of work?*
- *Is the input relevant?*
- *Does it build on, extend or enrich previous work?*
- *Does it offer a stimulus for future work and, if so, do I or my team have the skills and knowledge to capitalise on it?*

Visitors can make a considerable contribution to any programme, but a steady stream of visitors is no more a comprehensive PSHE programme than inviting a stream of bank managers, accountants and perhaps even bookmakers would constitute a comprehensive mathematics programme.

Any visit should be part of a spiral PSHE programme with continuity and progression, and never a 'one off'.

The only exception might be in response to a local, sudden and unexpected incident. Pragmatically, you might realise that an immediate local danger will not be covered in your programme for some time and that students need to quickly have their attention drawn to a particular issue or threat. Any 'one off' however can only raise awareness and perhaps offer some strategies. If they need to action these, they will be still drawing on the entire decision-making, problem-solving and communication skills they have developed through their previous PSHE programme. A 'one off' can't possibly teach these, but can connect them to an immediate threat or issue. It is highly likely that a 'one off' such as this will still need follow-up work.

What do you plan to do after the visit? For example, if a visitor has raised an issue, what:

- communication skills
- strategies
- research opportunities

might students need to manage this issue for themselves?

Do students have these skills already and require you to connect these to this new issue through rehearsing and applying them in this new context, or do you need to teach new skills?

If students raise questions or express anxieties after the visit, perhaps days or even weeks later, do you have a means to answer their questions or address their concerns?

Confidentiality and school policies

- Might any student be upset by a visitor's input?
- What if a student becomes upset or reveals something disturbing about their own or another's personal experience?

PSHE, perhaps more than any other area of the curriculum, works in the student's immediate reality and helps them explore how they feel about it. For this reason, it is important to be sensitive to students' prior experiences and be ready for them to share their present experiences and feelings. It is wise to have a protocol in place to support any student who becomes distressed.

No matter what policies the visitor (or any organisation they might represent) has with regard to confidentiality, your school's or local authority's policies should always take priority. It is essential that 'safeguarding' policies be adhered to.

Involving students

For a visitor experience to be really valuable, ideally students need to be fully involved in every step. Consider the following:

- How has this visitor been selected? Who selected them? What were the criteria:
  - for deciding a visitor was needed
  - for deciding who should visit?
- What do or will the students know about the visitor prior to their session? Who do they work for? What do they do? What is their role?
- How big will the audience be? What opportunity will there be to ask questions or break into smaller discussion groups?
- Were students involved in the choice of visitor? Practically, this might only be realistic if the visitor has been before, but offering a range of possibilities, considering the pros and cons of each is often possible if the actual visit is some time ahead.
- If you have selected the visitor, have you explained to the students the criteria behind your selection? Why do you feel you can trust this visitor as a source of information or advice? What gives you the confidence that they are a reliable source of support?
- Do students already have a relationship with, knowledge of or experience with this visitor?

Practical matters

- How will the visitor be invited? By letter, e-mail or telephone?
- Who will make the arrangements? Will they need a map? Where will you arrange for the visitor to be met and by whom?
- How will the visitor be briefed and by whom?
- Will the visitor be provided with questions in advance? How will you balance the input of their information with students' questions?
- If questions are to be provided, how will they be generated?
- If there are lots of questions, how will students prioritise them?
- Who will meet and greet the visitor?
- Who will chair the session?
- Who will escort the visitor off the premises? Who will thank the visitor and how?
- Will the visitor receive any feedback? Will they be informed about what students feel they learnt?
- Will you ask the visitor for their feedback? What did they find interesting or surprising? What has the visit made them think about for the first time, think more about or think differently about? What did they enjoy?
- Will there be an opportunity to ask the visitor follow-up questions? Will students be able to forward recordings of their subsequent work, for example e-mailing photographs of displays?

The best 'visitor sessions' are always a collaboration between you, the visitor and the students and this requires time to set up. A visitor to your classroom or setting should never be left unattended by you. This is no reflection on them, simply for mutual professional safety.

There is a world of difference between:

- having 200 students in a hall arranged in groups of six involved in a combination of expert input and question and answer sessions, with a previously selected panel of visitors with differing viewpoints that builds on previous PSHE work and can be extended through subsequent small group work that is part of a planned PSHE programme with an emphasis on skill development

and:

- getting 200 students of mixed abilities and life experience in a hall to be addressed by yet another 'one off' experience for an hour by a single speaker talking about the dangers of a particular health behaviour. This may be better than nothing – but only marginally.

Ideally visitors need to work interactively with small audiences where students can not only receive the benefit of their input, but practise the skills of gathering information from someone they haven't met before and begin to form a relationship with them and, if appropriate, their organisation.

You can photocopy the information for visitors on the opposite page and use it as a handout when briefing someone who is coming to visit your classroom.

3.6 Information for classroom visitors

In our complex and rapidly changing world, teachers don't always have all the information students need if they are to live knowledgably, safely, confidently and competently in their world. For this reason, they need the help of 'visitors' such as you. You might be an individual with an important story or valuable experience to share. Even if you have little or no experience of working with students, you can bring to the classroom a variety of valuable qualities. Perhaps you have:

- expert knowledge that students can receive, question and perhaps challenge
- personal experience that can act as a stimulus to get students thinking in new ways
- witnessed events or situations that will offer students a different perspective on an issue.

You will certainly offer students a chance to meet and work with a new person, and research shows that students remember visitors to their classroom for a long time. The impression you leave will often last longer than the detailed knowledge you provide. (Think back to a visitor you may remember from your own school days. Do you remember the detail of what they said? Or do you recall more clearly the type of person they were, and how strongly or passionately they felt about the topic they spoke about?)

If you represent an organisation, you also offer the beginnings of a relationship between the students and your organisation, a sort of 'ice-breaker'. Students will not only make an assessment of you, but will also extend that assessment to the organisation or group you represent.

Students will benefit in two ways from a classroom visitor. Not only will they take away the knowledge or story you bring, but, often more importantly, they will practise working with someone new, perhaps trying out their questioning skills or evaluating what you are telling them.

Questions to ask before your visit

It is essential to talk to the teacher beforehand about the purpose of the visit and what is expected from it. Your organisation may have given you training in working with young people, but the teacher won't assume this and, in any case, the teacher is always responsible for the students' learning.

Make sure that you have the answers to the following questions:

- What does the teacher hope their students will get from my visit?
- What do the students already know about me?
- What do students hope to get from my visit?
- Are these achievements possible? Can I offer all this? Do I need to renegotiate this?

- What do I hope the students will get from my visit?
- What exactly am I being asked to do? Am I comfortable with this?
- Who will I be working with?
  - A large audience, a class, a small group?
  - How old are they?
  - How able are they?
  - Will I be the only visitor or will I be joined by others, for example a panel?
- What have students already learnt?
- Is there anything I need to know about the students I am working with? For example, might any student be upset by my visit, perhaps because my input reminds them of an experience? In which case, how will they be supported?
- Will the students have a chance to give me their questions or interests in advance?
- Do the students need anything from me before my visit? For example, can I give them some information about me? Can I give them some questions, a case study or some information in advance for them to be thinking about?
- What will students be doing after I have gone?
- What is the school's policy if a student tells me something that makes me concerned for their safety?
- Am I able to leave any material or information behind after I have left?
- Do I have any questions or ideas that I could suggest they think about or work on after I have left?

Planning your session

If you are not used to working in a classroom, it can be helpful to think about these points:

- Lessons may be shorter than you expect. A 45-minute lesson can be less than 40 minutes by the time students arrive. This is especially true in secondary schools.
- Lessons tend to be in four parts:

1 An **opening activity** to engage the students' attention.
2 An introduction where the **overview of the lesson** is described with the key issues the lesson will cover. (This is a good opportunity to introduce yourself and ask the students what they hope to get from your visit.)
3 The actual **teaching**, which should be as active as possible.
4 The **plenary** when the lesson is reviewed and learning summarised. (This is the time to recap on the key points you hope students will take away from your visit.)

- It is better to **do less** and get over a few key points and then leave plenty of time for discussion and questions than to try to do too much. While interesting stories can hold our attention for a considerable time, even the most able of adults will often lose concentration after about 15 minutes of listening to a factual information-based talk. Our minds simply 'wander off' into daydreams, so try to break up your session. Try to mix any factual input with opportunities to talk in pairs about what you have said, take quick questions then back to the next part of your input.

- If you feel it is appropriate and you are willing, **share** what you feel (or felt) about whatever it is you are providing for the students. It is also appropriate to offer them an opportunity to share their feelings with you. Don't underestimate the value of this. Many of our choices or decisions are based on what we think we, and others, feel about a situation or issue.
- The more interaction between you and the students the better. A common technique used by teachers is called, **think, pair and share**. Instead of simply asking for questions, invite students to think for a few seconds, talk to the person beside them, then invite questions from pairs.
- The plenary is really important. It is a quick opportunity to **recap and reinforce** the learning of your session. To ensure that the students have learnt the key points, restate them. If in doubt, simply return to the original objectives and ask the students if you have collectively achieved them.

Confidentiality

There is always a chance that one of the young people with whom you are working will share something with you that may concern you. If you are giving a talk on a sensitive issue, it is possible that a young person will ask to speak to you in confidence after your session.

All schools are required to have a 'safeguarding' policy and you should have discussed this with the class teacher beforehand (see above). You need to be clear about what you can and cannot keep confidential before you begin the session, and whether the young people need to be briefed on this and by whom. The golden rule is, if in doubt about a young person's wellbeing, tell their teacher as quickly as possible and definitely before leaving the school.

Thank you for helping us learn!

Part 4

4.1 Focus on pedagogy

You can choose from literally thousands of techniques that enable individuals and groups to learn actively. Below are some of the best.

Learning techniques

First thoughts activities

Traditionally called 'brainstorming' or sometimes called a 'thought shower', this is simply collecting on to a board everyone's first thoughts. It is important not to process anything until the thoughts have all been collected and recorded.

Facilitated discussion

Most of the sessions require 'facilitating discussions'. Where possible, try to ensure that the students are engaged in thinking or talking, either in groups or through whole-class discussion 80 per cent of the time.

Where possible, avoid telling any student that their ideas, thoughts or opinions are 'wrong'. We need to have a high level of trust and respect in someone to let go of a belief after simply being told by that person that we are wrong.

Where possible, challenge misunderstandings or inappropriate strategies by asking: 'What would things be like if that were true?' or 'If we did that, what are all the things that might happen next, soon, in the future?'

We are more likely to influence new thinking if we help students explore the consequences of their strategies or misunderstandings through challenge rather than confrontation. We also want students to develop the skills and habit of using the thinking skill of exploring the consequences of beliefs or actions, and so modelling this skill is important.

Marketplace

'Marketplace' is an alternative to groups feeding back individually to the whole class. A marketplace requires two students from each group to stay with their work, and for the rest of the group to circulate and look at others' work. Steer this by asking those 'shopping' to look for ideas they agree with, want clarified, want to challenge, or new ideas they can borrow to take back to their group. After a few minutes, invite the groups to swap roles so the 'shopkeepers' can walk around. Bring the groups back together to allow them to talk through any ideas they have borrowed from other groups.

Home and away groups

If students always work with their friends, there is a danger that values of that group can be mutually supportive. While this can be positive, it can also be destructive. A key problem in health education arises when students overestimate the behaviours of their peers. For example, many students overestimate the drug use, alcohol use or sexual experience of their peers.

Home groups are the students' friends within the class; away groups are new groups where students have an opportunity to interact with other members of the class. It is important to consider which group or mix of groups is most appropriate for different activities.

Role play

Role play is a powerful opportunity for students to 'try on' new personalities, language or strategies in order to test out what this feels like or how useful any offered strategies are when actually put into practice. There is, however, a very real danger in role play; because of its power, it should never be used without extremely careful planning and management.

Role play is a powerful technique for practising positive strategies, however, if it is part of group activity, others in role may be practising very negative behaviours, language and strategies, some of which may be very emotionally enjoyable. Unless you are experienced in teaching drama, it is recommended that you restrict role play to pair and small group activity. 'Theatre', or asking groups to demonstrate their 'role play' to a wider group, is a different experience and also needs very careful, sensitive management.

It is vital to 'de-role' everybody who plays a character, in order to reduce the possibility of the student subsequently being confused with that character, or the character's feelings, limitations, views, negative behaviour, etc. which may be poles apart from the student's. One good way to achieve this is to get the student to state his/her name, making eye contact with the class, and state one thing about themselves which *is* true and draw one (or more) distinctions between him/her and the character they just played. For example, 'I'm Dave, I can't stand violence, and I don't easily lose my temper like [character's name] did.'

Class debates

As with role play, this technique needs to be treated sensitively. Debates can encourage flexible thinking and empathy. They can also develop research skills and structured arguments. With students who might be exposed to, or have already chosen, a risky lifestyle, researching and arguing the benefits of the positive health choice might positively influence their future choices or be the first stage in change.

Inviting students who already hold positive opinions or have made healthy choices to prepare and strongly argue in favour of a potentially risky behaviour may be cognitively demanding, may open up previously unconsidered points of view and increase empathy. However, it might also instal doubts in a previously strongly held 'positive' position; lower a previously strong resistance to that behaviour; and result in a loss of confidence in applying previously useful strategies. It may be better to debate the strengths of two possible potentially healthy options or positions, rather than two extreme positions.

Carousel

This technique helps students to share ideas, explore issues and try out brief conversations in a structured way. Ask the students to help you generate a list of questions or statements about an issue or idea worthy of exploration. Arrange the class in two concentric circles, those in the inner circle facing a partner in the outer circle. You will need enough slips of paper for each chair in the outer circle. Write one question/statement/comment on each slip (repeating some if necessary) and place one on each outer chair (where it stays when students move). Each pair has a brief conversation. After a short time, ask students to stop, and ask those in the *inner* circle to stand up and move one place to their left. After another brief conversation in their new pairs, ask the students in the *outer* circle to move one place to their right, and on to a new question or statement. Repeat, until the issue has been reasonably aired, or until a reasonable number of pairings have occurred. Invite class feedback on the issue.

Forum theatre

In this version of role play, the characters in role are 'directed' by the class. The characters only follow the script and strategies offered by the group. A simple way to manage this is to allow different groups to control different characters, with the characters indicating a 'time out' when they need to consult with their group for advice. The groups can also call for a 'time out' when they want to test a new strategy with their character.

A useful strategy is to 'freeze frame' the action at an important point. Anyone in the 'audience' may stop the action using an agreed signal, for example a single clap. This still image of characters, where position, expression and body language may be all-important, can be shown to the rest of the class, who comment on it. Once the obvious elements have been established (who is involved and what they are doing), individuals in the freeze frame can be asked to say, in character, what they are thinking and direct the action or suggest how the scene could be replayed differently. Either at this point, or immediately after the action has stopped, it can also be helpful to allow the person who clapped, or another volunteer, to enter the action in place of one of the characters. This will enable students to try out a different strategy or approach within the scene, to develop it along more desirable lines, or simply to explore other options.

Conscience alley

This is a way of exploring a significant choice that a character must make between two options. Divide the class into two equal groups. Ask the students to discuss the issues in a scene with their group. The task is for one group to generate statements to encourage the character to take one option (for example, 'Ask her out'). There should be one statement for each member of the group. The other group is to generate statements in favour of the other option ('Don't ask her out – she's already spoken for'). The two groups line up opposite each other and you, or a brave pupil, walk down the alley in role as the character in question and listen to alternate statements. The character may respond to any or all of the statements and, on reaching the end of the alley, the character decides what to do and explains why.

Goldfish bowl

This invites one group to either complete a task or process how they went about a task while others observe, often with a checklist of things to watch and listen for. It helps to uncover other people's thinking when faced with a problem. After a while, stop the discussion and ask the observers to feed back their comments to those 'in the bowl'.

Ranking

This simply provides students with a series of options and asks them to rank them in importance or using similar criteria. For example, most/least urgent, high/low risk, cost, acceptability, etc. The final ranking is less important than the discussion, and different groups can compare and justify their rankings. The exercise can feel more relevant if the students themselves generate the options or topics to be ranked.

Concept mapping

Mind mapping™ is only one of many excellent ways of helping students express their thinking visually. Other methods include flow diagrams, timelines, Venn diagrams, etc. These can help capture and structure thinking. *Mapwise – accelerated learning through visible thinking* (Oliver Caviglioli and Ian Harris, Network Educational Press Ltd, UK) contains a wealth of ideas for helping students to make their thinking and processing visible.

Micro-debates

Rather than whole-class debates, micro-debates are simply carried out in groups of four. Two students present their opposing cases to the other two who listen and decide who has the more convincing argument. The second pair then presents their debate to the first two. This smaller audience retains the intellectual exercise, involves everyone in presenting a viewpoint whilst minimising the potential nerves of presenting in front of a large and often passive audience. As with any debate, it is also important to 'de-role' afterwards, to make sure that no positive feelings created towards a previously negatively held position remain. It is recommended that you avoid asking a student to argue for a positive position on a high-risk situation. It is safer to debate two less extreme positions.

4.2 Focus on stress

Many people think of stress as purely a 'modern' phenomenon, suggesting that we are just applying a new label to something we all once 'just got on with' and that it is perhaps something people 'imagine' they experience. Nothing could be further from the truth. Stress is the body's response to the demands made upon it. Those demands can be experienced as stimulating and motivating, or they can provoke feelings of anxiety and/or tension. When feelings of anxiety and tension occur, your performance is impaired, even though you may not be aware of it.

Stress may be described as a physiological response to a physical or psychological stimulus. Following activation by the central nervous system in response to the stimulus, a twofold reaction takes place in the autonomic nervous system, which is responsible for regulation of smooth muscle, heart muscle and the endocrine system. There is a *neural* response via the sympathetic autonomic nervous system and a *hormonal* response via the endocrine system. The section 'The fight or flight response' on the next page looks at this more closely.

Stress affects everyone to varying degrees because we all react differently to situations according to our characteristics, past experiences and our environment. Experiences that provoke a stress response, called stressors, come from *wanted* and *unwanted* events. However, exactly the same experience (such as riding in a tiny cable car 30 m above the ground) could induce feelings of elation in one person and immobilising panic in someone else. The extent to which stress is a welcome challenge to be overcome and the 'buzz' that overcoming creates will be unique to each individual.

A model of stress

We are faced with demands on a day-to-day basis. They can vary from meeting deadlines at work, to getting jobs done at home and from moving house to preparing a meal. For a young person, we can think of things like homework, interacting with family and friends, playing in a team, sitting exams, etc. One way of understanding the stress is to show it as a model with four sections:

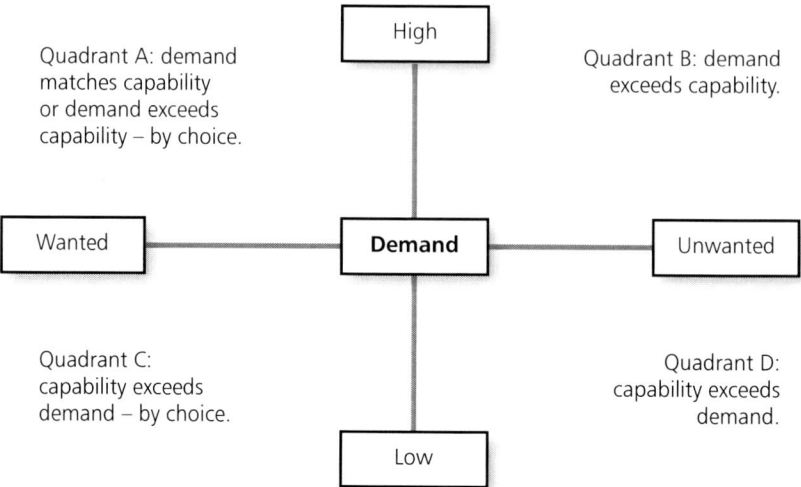

Quadrant A: demand matches capability or demand exceeds capability – by choice.

Quadrant B: demand exceeds capability.

High

Wanted — **Demand** — Unwanted

Low

Quadrant C: capability exceeds demand – by choice.

Quadrant D: capability exceeds demand.

For each demand placed upon us, there are four potential outcomes:

1   High stress that we *seek*. For some people, this might be off-piste skiing, solo rock climbing, or even a white-knuckle ride at a theme park.

2   High stress that we *don't want*. For some people, this might include a long, unavoidable drive at night in the rain, being made redundant from a job, losing someone close, exams, too much to do in a short time, tasks needing skills we don't have.

3   Low stress that we *seek*. For some people, this might be sunbathing, reading, watching soaps on TV.

4   Low stress that we *don't want*. For some people, this might be doing a boring repetitive job in a factory, having to wash the car, clean the room, do the cooking, etc.

The factors that influence these possible outcomes are:

- our perception of the demand
- our perception or beliefs about our ability to cope (which may or may not fit with reality).

If our perception of the demand is 'high', and we believe we can cope well, the result is that we feel *good* about the challenge – these good feelings are sometimes called *eustress*. This includes challenges we see as worthwhile and tasks we consider both achievable and stimulating. They may also be seen as a positive experience, leading to improved confidence and raised self-esteem. A training course, even a driving test we feel fully ready for, may be something we take in our stride. An exam in our best subject, when we've revised well, may be a breeze for some of us!

If our perception of the demand is 'low', but it's what we have chosen (and we can cope well), then we usually enjoy the experience. Eustress again. Leisure and recreation often come into this category. However, if low demands become the 'norm', this may turn to the stress we feel when we are bored through a lack of stimulation, particularly if our skills are high and are not being practised or valued.

Worse still, if our perception of demand is 'high' and we believe our coping skills are not adequate, this is the classic formula for unwanted stress or *distress*. The demand doesn't even have to be a major life event for us to perceive it as a high demand, particularly if coping mechanisms are already stretched. 'Too much to do, in too little time' can cause us *distress* even when we could manage fine with the demands if only time was on our side. An exam in a subject we find difficult, and haven't revised for (but don't want to fail), may be very stressful. Waiting for the results may not be much better either.

The fight or flight response

At the top of page 266, stress was described as '… a physiological response to a physical or psychological stimulus …' Faced with a stimulus or threat (perceived or real), the central nervous system activates a two-fold reaction. There is a *neural* response via the sympathetic autonomic nervous system and a *hormonal* response via the endocrine system. This is often referred to as the 'The fight or flight response' response.

So what happens? The first thing that happens when we react to a stressor is usually (often unnoticed) a sharp intake of breath ... This sends a message to a part of the brain called the hypothalamus and, in turn, the anterior pituitary and adrenal cortex ... which triggers the release of glucocorticoids, in particular cortisol, which affects the way glucose is stored in the body ... so more glucose goes to the muscles and the body's 'escape systems' are given the energy they need to escape from the stressor.

While this is going on in the endocrine system, the sympathetic autonomic nervous system has also kicked into action, stimulating the adrenal medulla which increases the release of adrenaline and noradrenaline. Adrenaline increases the heart rate, blood flow and raises energy, heightening muscle activity. Noradrenaline increases arousal and attention (psychological effects). Thus, the individual is ready for 'fight or flight' – to face what is causing unwanted stress (*distress*) or escape from it by running away.

The symptoms

But what actually happens to us? Why can stress be 'destructive'? To varying degrees, any of the following may happen:

- Pupils dilate.
- Mouth goes dry.
- Neck and shoulder muscles tense.
- Sweating begins.
- Heart pumps faster.
- Breathing is faster and gasping.
- Muscles tense for action.
- Brain activity increases.
- Blood pressure rises.
- The liver releases glycogen and blood glucose levels increase to provide energy for muscles.
- Digestion slows down or ceases.
- Sphincter action increases.

This response was, of course, designed as an adaptive one – to ensure our survival. In the days when our ancestors lived in caves and clubbing was not just a fun night out, we stepped out of our caves in the morning unsure if we would *get* breakfast or *be* breakfast. So our ancestors would have experienced the stress response, would have been able to take appropriate action (for example run from a large hungry animal or fight it) and then recover. However, in our modern society we have set ourselves up with lots of stressors where we can't really respond by 'fighting' or 'running away'. It is not possible, for example, to escape from areas of responsibility that we have to face in daily lives, or as part of education. Therefore, instead of the 'fight or flight' response being used appropriately and then subsiding, we literally 'stew in our own juice' and health problems can and frequently do ensue, *unless unwanted stress is effectively managed.*

All manner of health problems have been linked to unwanted stress – it increases blood pressure, alters glucose levels and lowers immunity (immune system cells have receptors for glucocorticoids and noradrenaline). So, quite apart from the tension headaches, aching muscles and anxiety reactions that occur, stress increases risks of infections, skin problems, cardiovascular problems, diabetes and even cancer. Inappropriate avoidance behaviours, such as smoking or use of alcohol or other drugs, can also exacerbate the unhealthy effects of stress.

In the long term, we *may* become so used to chronic stress that we develop a *false* belief that we can cope. The initial feeling of alarm at being unable to cope leads to resistance and a feeling that we're learning to cope but overcompensating so that we *perceive* little stress, which is nevertheless still having an impact. Unless the stressor is removed or lessened, it can lead to exhaustion, in addition to symptoms described above.

How to recognise stress

Most people, when asked, actually identify signs and symptoms of stress in others or themselves quite easily.

Psychological symptoms can include: general anxiety; apprehension; fears; phobias; gloom; despondency; being unable to enjoy life; depression and anxiety; 'short fuse' and mood swings; apathy and withdrawal; loss of self-esteem and confidence; loss of interest in sex; feeling guilt and inadequacy; and excessive worry about physical health.

Physical symptoms can include: physical tiredness; disturbed sleep patterns; aches and pains; headache; migraine; neck and back tension and pain; joint ache; clenched fist and/or jaw; chest pain; palpitations; and a 'lump in the throat' feeling.

Behavioural symptoms can include: irritability; being critical; touchy and uncooperative; impulsive actions; uncharacteristic mistakes; procrastinating over routine tasks; delaying decisions; longer and less productive hours at work; increased use of smoking/alcohol/drugs; overeating or loss of appetite; frequent and prolonged absence from work/school for minor illness.

Preventing stress

Unwanted stress is a very real phenomenon that can have adverse effects on health. The good news is that there are things that can be done about stress.

Stress *prevention* strategies include:

- removing or reducing demands
- refusing (appropriately!) tasks that are too demanding or too numerous
- changing perception of demands
- changing belief about coping ability
- developing a good support system
- practising assertiveness
- developing better time-management skills
- reviewing diet and sleep patterns
- increasing exercise.

Managing stress

It's important to teach students about stress early on. If they are to stay healthy and achieve their potential, they need to develop their stress awareness, prevention and management strategies. Stress management strategies include:

- positive self-talk
- treats/rewards as part of work-leisure balance
- learning new skills (training) to prepare for meeting demands
- flight, when necessary, even if it's just to think
- seeking support from that support system.

Just imagine, for a moment, how results could improve if students could overcome 'exam nerves'. What might that sort of coping ability mean for them in the long term?

4.3 Focus on risk

One of the most important concepts in this book is 'risk'. This four letter word is sometimes explicit (see, for example, action planner content boxes K1, K5, K14, K15 or D2, D6 and D15) and sometimes implicit (see, for example, action planner content boxes G1, G9 and G12). This section aims to help you think about risk, what it means in your life and your teaching, before planning any teaching that is about risk, or that relies on a shared understanding of risk.

There are several agreed definitions of risk, but most of them, whether technical or everyday definitions, are negative. These definitions focus on the harm that might happen, and all too often lead us to think about the worst possible consequences. These worst-case scenarios are often also the least likely consequences. As a result, this kind of thinking can cause us a great deal of anxiety. There are few of us who have not lain awake at night worrying about the worst thing that could happen in a given situation, only to wake up in the morning to find the actual outcome was much more trivial.

The approach to risk in this resource is more balanced, recognising both its positive and negative aspects, and providing questions that challenge students to reflect on their developing knowledge and understanding, and importantly on their feelings about risk.

Understanding risk

Research shows that children and young people develop their understanding of risk gradually. We also know that there are important differences between the way boys and girls develop that understanding and how boys and girls experience risk. It's important to begin to share responsibility for risk taking with young people as their abilities and understanding develop. They need practical experience, knowledge and adult support to learn how to identify challenges, hazards and consequences, and who can help them gain the maximum benefit with the minimum of harm to themselves and others.

At 15–16 years, some students may have a very mature understanding of risk, be able to see a range of consequences of their actions for themselves and others, and take wise decisions based on that understanding. Of course, the choices they make may be based on different knowledge and understanding of the circumstances than that of a parent or a teacher – so it is important to encourage students to talk with their friends, families and, where relevant, to seek advice and support from a wide range of agencies. Too often, students may see adult advice as coded disapproval, especially when some of the longer-term consequences of their choices may involve poor health or social outcomes.

The three-step risk model

It may help to use neutral language to begin a dialogue about risk, and this is where one of the most common models of risk can be helpful. Take care not to imply that all risky situations carry danger, or that the likelihood of enjoyment, thrill or achievement may not be great.

Teachers of this age group are aware that students will be entering the workplace – either for work experience, for Saturday or other casual jobs, or as part of vocational training. The workplace can be a very hazardous environment and, over the years, legislation has been introduced to try to ensure the rights of a worker to be safe at work, but also to underline the responsibilities all workers have for their own safety and that of others. As part of this, the health and safety executive has promoted a three-step model of risk: hazard recognition; risk assessment; and risk management.

1 **Hazard recognition** is being aware of what can cause harm in any given situation, and to whom.
2 **Risk assessment** is deciding if a risk is trivial, tolerable or intolerable. Judgements about this can be based on previous experience of the hazard, the needs of a particular worker, and changing circumstances, if any.
3 **Risk management** is considering whether tolerable, or even intolerable, risks can be managed so that they present less of a threat.

The model can be applied in a wide range of settings: change workplace for leisure centre, beach, club, home or street, and the same steps may apply. Sharing this model and working through examples can have a positive practical outcome for students, as their employers will increasingly expect them to take responsibility for their own safety and that of others in the workplace.

An alternative risk model

In contrast to this well-known model of risk is one promoted by leaders in outdoor and adventurous activities, and in business and enterprise. In their models the word 'risk' is often replaced by 'challenge', and the focus is very much on the positive outcomes of risk taking, whether that is in personal development or tangible achievement such as medal winning or financial gain.

Their model of risk can be summarised as four steps:

1 Identify the challenge.
2 Recognise the hazards.
3 Assess the risk (positive and negative).
4 Control or manage any risk of harm.

Those using this model also emphasise the importance of dynamic risk assessment. It is not enough to use a long-range, regional weather forecast before deciding to go canoeing in a gorge. Local weather conditions can change rapidly, so there may be circumstances where a fun, positive activity has to be curtailed because the risk (probability of harm) has changed.

Once again, this model can have wider application. For some students the biggest challenges are social: fitting in with a group of peers; having a strong, loving relationship with someone special. For others, the challenges may be academic: choosing subjects that stretch their abilities in order to get on a particular course; or be accepted for training in a chosen trade. Students identify a wide range of challenges they face when asked about risk, so it makes sense to ask them for their ideas first.

Questions about risk

One of the best approaches to this subject with students may be to offer these alternative models and ask them to devise their own. Is 'risk' the same as 'danger'? Is it the same as 'challenge'? Can all consequences be forseen? Are all consequences equally likely? Can the students devise a scale that combines the magnitude of the consequences (positive and negative) with the probability of harm or benefit, to help decide how to measure the risk? Would they ever choose not to do something because the harmful consequences for others outweigh the benefits to themselves, or because the longer-term harmful consequences outweigh the short-term benefits? This questioning approach is at the heart of this resource and at the heart of effective practice in PSHE.

Finally, it's worth considering the model of risk adopted in this resource. The column headings in the action planners give a useful clue:

Becoming everything that I can be can be summarised as: 'What are my choices?'

Enriching a healthy and safe lifestyle (Year 10) or *Taking charge of my healthy and safe lifestyle* (Year 11) can be summarised as: 'What are the possible consequences (positive and negative) for me and others?'

Managing my changing relationships includes: 'Who can help me?'

By focusing on choice rather than hazard, and by emphasising the role of others in helping to manage risks and achieve the possible benefits, this *Health for Life* model of risk can help you to help your students make choices that will enable them to become everything they can be.

4.4 Focus on the brain

Our brains are the most complex structures we know, and we have still barely scratched the surface of our understanding of how they work. *Health for Life 11–14* included a section on the brain and how it influences our social behaviour, and at ages 15–16 it is important to recap on this in our programmes.

Educational neuroscience is in its infancy, and evolutionary psychology is still theoretical. It is inevitable that any set of 'brain facts' like those given below will be huge simplifications and sweeping generalisations. What is important is that students recognise that their feelings and the behaviours they may be encouraging, while natural in origin, may not be appropriate in the world in which we now live. Students need to be able to challenge them, take control of them, make different decisions and behave accordingly. We are no more responsible for our feelings than we are for our dreams, but we *are* responsible for how we respond to them in our behaviours.

Broadly, evolutionary psychology argues that our brains have evolved over millions of years (the 'reptilian brain' about 400 million years ago, the limbic system about 150 million years ago and the neo-cortex much more recently, about 4 million years ago), but that our society has developed in recent years far more quickly. We therefore possess a brain that has evolved for a very different world from the one in which we find ourselves. Our feelings and subsequent behaviours can be 'out of sync' with our world. While we can control some parts of our brain, others such as the amygdala can suddenly shut down our conscious thinking and take over because this part of our brain still responds to threats as if we were a small animal, living 150 million years ago and faced with a very big and hungry tiger. Both those who try to support us and those who would like to exploit us study how brains work and use this information.

Over 400 million years in the designing, and with 150 billion cells, sharing part of its structure with reptiles, part with other mammals and with a part that is uniquely ours, each one individual and developed by responding to its own unique experiences, it is hardly surprising that when two or more brains get together fantastic things happen.

- **Our brains pay attention to novelty.** We seem pre-programmed to notice new or unusual things. This could be to keep us safe, since the familiar is less likely to hurt us than the unfamiliar. As teachers, we can turn this to our advantage by building novelty into critical pieces of learning. The chances are that you will remember a school field trip perhaps from many years ago but would find it impossible to remember the school day immediately before or after.

- **Like many other creatures who were originally prey for other creatures, we tend to be neo-phobic.** This extends the point above: for our survival many of us feel uneasy around the unfamiliar or new. As a result, we can feel uneasy when we are with new people, especially if we perceive them as different. We store our experiences as 'templates' and when we meet people from different cultures we may feel a little odd, because our 'templates' or experiences are different from theirs. Many people feel uneasy around people

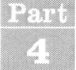

with disabilities or from different cultures or races. We have the power to recognise this in ourselves for what is. It is the way our brains work and, if we recognise this, we can take control, become 'open minded' and rise above it. Failing to do this has led in the past to terrible acts against people perceived as different, and our vulnerability has been exploited by some leaders to their advantage.

- **We seem programmed to seek patterns and connections between things.** Without this many of our greatest inventions would not have happened. The downside is that we may be imposing patterns where none exist. We all know that if we stare at clouds, we may start to see shapes, the 'castles in the air'. We are imposing our pattern over a random event. The downside of this is that we often 'read things into' events that are from our own imagination. Because this is so strong, other people can accept our interpretation, build on it and before we know it we have a 'conspiracy'. Because people feel so strongly once a 'conspiracy' is believed, it is really difficult to challenge, even if the actual evidence that there is none is overwhelming.

- **We are only programmed to fear two things, heights and loud noises.** All the rest are learnt from experience (either directly or indirectly) or by observing fear in others. It is great that we can learn to fear things that may hurt us from others; this stops us having to experience the pain or injury before we learn to avoid it. If this were not the case, we wouldn't be around for very long. However, we need to be careful whom we learn from. Fear can be 'caught' from others without us being aware that it is happening. Are we certain that we should be afraid of what they fear? There is a world of difference between learning to be afraid of being knocked down by a car, and learning to be afraid of another ethnicity or culture.

- **Fear can be more powerful than pleasure.** We are basically programmed to avoid things we don't like and do more of the things we do like. We once needed to make these judgements very quickly and having been made they can be very strong. This means our first impressions can be powerful, leading us to fear something that (or someone who) on further reflection could help us and to feel attracted to something or someone who could actually harm us. This is why first impressions are important, sometimes known as the 'horns and halos' effect, although actually it is a bit of a myth that we cannot re-evaluate these early judgements. It is also the reason why it can take a lot of work to rebuild a relationship with someone we have emotionally hurt. It isn't simply a case of one hurt being put right by one kindness, or one criticism being put right by one praise (it may be nearer one to ten!)

- **Living things are programmed to reproduce.** In human beings sexual relationships are very complex, but as a broad principle our drive to reproduce is strong. The early stages of new relationships can be very intense, probably to encourage reproduction. It originates in primitive or 'old' parts of the brain and at certain times can temporarily dominate our higher-level thinking ('I can't believe we just did that … We got carried away and before we knew it we had …'). This is why thinking about what decisions we want to make in advance is important, so that we have previously planned to 'lose control'! This is probably why we are rewarded for sexual behaviour with pleasure (an otherwise somewhat bizarre behaviour), but childbirth can be very painful. Unusually, we have sexual relations all year round, probably because women have no obvious sign of ovulation, therefore no 'mating period'. What makes us unique is that we can control our ability to conceive, separating sexual intercourse from having a child and allowing us to have sexual relations principally for bonding with another human being, as portrayed by sexual activity in the media. We share the ability to have 'sex for fun' with a small number of other species, including dolphins.

- **Our brain draws our attention to things we are interested in or evidence of things we believe strongly in, and deletes most of the rest.** At any given moment we are being bombarded by our senses with information, most of it being processed unconsciously and deleted. Our brains filter much out, and draw to our attention things we are interested in or evidence that supports our beliefs. (Perhaps when you buy an item of clothing you suddenly notice how many other people are wearing something similar.) Our brain is trying to be helpful and this is great if we are seeking berries or need to be wary of a particularly dangerous snake or spider. The problem is that this process, while useful, may distort what is really around us. Someone who believes that young people, or all people of a particular ethnicity, are a nuisance may disproportionately notice newspaper stories that support that view and unconsciously delete those that don't. This further confirms their conviction that the evidence supports their viewpoint. We need to be wary of this as our own world view can in this way become very distorted.

- **Parts of our brains are very primitive.** Reptile brains can only do about 27 things. One of them is to bow down before a larger reptile to avoid a fight. Watch people when they meet the royal family and you are actually seeing 400 million-year-old reptile behaviour as people bow – it's still wired into our systems. These older parts of our brains still respond to threat by taking over with the intention of keeping us safe. The problem is that the 'threat' used to be lions and tigers and bears but now can simply be a challenging look from someone we dislike. Sometimes this response is good, for example when we jump out of the way of a speeding car, but sometimes it can get us into trouble and we 'lose it', perhaps suddenly losing our temper and screaming things we later can't believe we said and now regret. Confronting someone who has 'lost it' with equal anger simply risks two mindless people screaming at one another as two sets of amygdala (now aided by another very old part of their brains, the reticular activating system releasing noradrenaline and adrenaline) fight it out. It is usually best either to try to calm them down or walk away until they have calmed down.

4.5 Focus on personal safety

Personal safety is a huge subject. In addition to keeping physically safe, we also need to keep our feelings safe. This section only offers some first thoughts on physical safety and safety in the street. Helping students to stay safe, one of the 'Every Child Matters' outcomes, could be thought of in two parts:

1 What we do as professionals and as a school community to keep children safe.
2 How we provide the learning that enables them to acquire the language, skills and strategies to keep themselves (and others in their present and future care) safe.

Although there are people and systems, such as safety at work regulations that are there to protect us, in the real world the police can often do little more than offer support once an incident has happened and try to make sure it doesn't happen again. For their success, safety regulations depend on people following them.

As we get older, the degree to which we have to take responsibility for our own safety steadily increases. There will be times when we have to hand this responsibility over to someone else, for example the pilot who flies the plane that takes us on holiday or even the person who cuts our hair, but in these cases we usually assume that they have the qualifications to look after us. (How many of us, when offered a lift, assume the driver has a valid licence, appropriate insurance and their car has a valid MOT?) There is a need to judge how to balance what we don't know against what we can assume.

In assessing our personal safety we need to ask ourselves if we, through the choices we make or the behaviours we choose, are making ourselves vulnerable. Some situations such as the workplace will probably place restrictions on how we behave, while others such as some sports or activities will have safety procedures that we should follow.

Just going out for a social event is a balance between our right to go where we please, carry what we wish and dress how we like against the possibility of making ourselves more vulnerable. Since the consequences of an assault are potentially so appalling, common sense says we need to consider how to protect our safety in different situations.

The world is actually a remarkably safe place and we should all have the right to be and stay safe regardless of who we are, where we are or where we go. In the real world, however, there is a small minority who may threaten our personal safety. These may be:

- predators – people who deliberately set out to cause us harm – who might be known to us and even trusted by us, or be complete strangers who attack with no warning
- people who we know and who might care for us, but whose behaviours or choices put us at risk (for example being with a friend who is getting drunk)

- people we know little about but whose carelessness, perhaps in the workplace, may put us at risk.

We need to consider some terms:

Self-protection is about what we do to minimise our vulnerability and keep ourselves safe. It is about:

- (in our planning) anticipating potential threats and safeguarding ourselves against them
- (at any moment) being aware of a potential or growing threat in the present, assessing it and taking action to avoid it.

Self-defence is about the actions we take when faced with an immediate threat. It is a subset of self-protection and is:

- escaping as quickly and/or as aggressively as we need to in order to protect ourselves.

Staying safe is a combination of what we know and how we feel about what we know. Safety is not only about knowing our rights and responsibilities; it is as much about feeling able to *access* our rights and *action* our responsibilities. For example, we can have comprehensive safety regulations in a workplace, but they are useless if we lack the skills to execute them or the confidence to challenge behaviour we believe contravenes them.

Advice on street safety

In the street many people walk in what is known as 'white light' – this is also known as 'downtime' when we are thinking about what is for dinner, what is on the television tonight and virtually anything except what is going on around us. (This is the state some muggers watch for, and can be tested by what is known as a 'by'. They walk past you twice, and if you look puzzled leave you alone. If you don't notice, you are in 'white light'!)

In the street we need to be in 'yellow light', simply aware of our surroundings and possible threats. This is not particularly dramatic, including things like not tripping over the kerb! It is simply sending the signal that you are switched on to what is happening around you and that you are going to be difficult to catch by surprise.

If we identify a threat, we move to 'orange light' – we evaluate the threat and decide if we need to take action. Common sense says the earlier we can do this the better.

We finally move to 'red light' – threat avoidance. We take action to get away from the emerging threat. Only if this proves impossible do we move to self-defence, and if we have to defend ourselves we need to be willing to hit first, hit hard and move away quickly.

(Source: Adapted from work by Peter Consterdine)

The vast majority of self-protection is avoiding the need for self-defence, which should always be considered a last resort. In the real world, an assault is usually very fast and will be very aggressive. Being hit unexpectedly brings considerable shock, and an assault is often over before the victim is even aware of the threat.

When travelling, some of the most risky times are known as 'transitions'. These are times when we are moving *between* safer locations, for example moving from

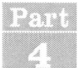

a crowded bus to the entrance to a busy nightclub, or moving from your place of work to your car. Although night-time brings obvious risks, many people underestimate the possibility of an attack in daylight.

Some people like to carry a personal alarm. These may drive away an attacker, but there is little evidence that they summon any help from bystanders. Carrying an offensive weapon, even for self-protection, is an offence (see page 107).

Traditional martial arts training is virtually useless in these situations, and 'self-defence' classes that claim to teach you how to protect yourself in a physical assault after a single or small number of lessons should be avoided. Even Special Forces personnel are frightened of knife attacks, so you certainly can't defend yourself against a knife attack after a handful of lessons!

It takes many years to learn a martial art to a level of proficiency where it can be useful for self-defence and, even then, the element of surprise can leave a highly trained martial artist hurt or injured. Most human beings, even those trained in martial arts, find it difficult even in a defensive situation to hurt another person. Sessions such as these can give a false sense of confidence.

A mobile phone can obviously be helpful, but showing off an attractive mobile phone may put us at risk. It is also important to remember that texts may take time to arrive. A text sent to someone to ask for an urgent lift may not always arrive quickly, and this is especially true at 'high traffic' times including weekends and public holidays.

4.6 Focus on transsexualism

There are people who, with the help of surgery, alter their gender. While most of these people were born as either men or women, in extremely rare cases a person's gender is not entirely clear as they have some features of both male and female bodies. As a whole, all these people are sometimes called 'transgendered'. Some transgendered people might describe themselves as transsexual, perhaps convinced that they are women or men in 'the wrong body', but not all transsexuals accord with this view of themselves. For some, it is a question of silencing feelings of extreme discomfort in their current gender.

This is *not* about sexual orientation but about gender identity.* There is scientific evidence for a neurobiological basis for this, and research into 'sexually dimorphic' brain structures supports transsexuals' assertion that some are in fact women or men in 'the wrong body'. The brain of the developing foetus has been 'sexed' as female or male and the body has developed at full or partial variance with this. Trans-women or trans-men can also be heterosexual, homosexual or bisexual, independent of their transgendered status, just like any other women or men.

In 2004, Parliament passed the Gender Recognition Act, which means that trans-women and trans-men now have full legal recognition as women and men. A person who has 'transitioned' to their true gender may, after two years and with medical evidence, apply for a Gender Recognition Certificate and then a new birth certificate.

---

* Many people think that transsexualism is the same as transvestism. It isn't. Transvestism, or cross-dressing, is dressing in the clothing of the opposite sex. People might do this for a variety of reasons, including sexual gratification. However, many transsexuals, particularly trans-women in the early stages of their transition (achieved through hormone treatment and surgery), are wrongly perceived to be simply cross-dressing.